DISASTER NURSING

A Handbook for Practice

Deborah S. Adelman, PhD, RN, NE-BC, CNS
Associate Professor
SUNY Delhi
Delhi, New York

Timothy J. Legg, PhD, RN-BC, GNP-BC, CHES
Assistant Professor of Health Sciences
TUI University
Cypress, California

JONES AND BARTLETT PUBLISHERS
Sudbury, Massachusetts
BOSTON TORONTO LONDON SINGAPORE

World Headquarters
Jones and Bartlett Publishers
40 Tall Pine Drive
Sudbury, MA 01776
978-443-5000
info@jbpub.com
www.jbpub.com

Jones and Bartlett Publishers Canada
6339 Ormindale Way
Mississauga, Ontario L5V 1J2
Canada

Jones and Bartlett Publishers International
Barb House, Barb Mews
London W6 7PA
United Kingdom

Jones and Bartlett's books and products are available through most bookstores and online booksellers. To contact Jones and Bartlett Publishers directly, call 800-832-0034, fax 978-443-8000, or visit our website www.jbpub.com.

Substantial discounts on bulk quantities of Jones and Bartlett's publications are available to corporations, professional associations, and other qualified organizations. For details and specific discount information, contact the special sales department at Jones and Bartlett via the above contact information or send an email to specialsales@jbpub.com.

The authors, editor, and publisher have made every effort to provide accurate information. However, they are not responsible for errors, omissions, or for any outcomes related to the use of the contents of this book and take no responsibility for the use of the products and procedures described. Treatments and side effects described in this book may not be applicable to all people; likewise, some people may require a dose or experience a side effect that is not described herein. Drugs and medical devices are discussed that may have limited availability controlled by the Food and Drug Administration (FDA) for use only in a research study or clinical trial. Research, clinical practice, and government regulations often change the accepted standard in this field. When consideration is being given to use of any drug in the clinical setting, the health care provider or reader is responsible for determining FDA status of the drug, reading the package insert, and reviewing prescribing information for the most up-to-date recommendations on dose, precautions, and contraindications, and determining the appropriate usage for the product. This is especially important in the case of drugs that are new or seldom used.

Production Credits
Publisher: Kevin Sullivan
Acquisitions Editor: Emily Ekle
Acquisitions Editor: Amy Sibley
Associate Editor: Patricia Donnelly
Editorial Assistant: Rachel Shuster
Supervising Production Editor: Carolyn F. Rogers
Associate Marketing Manager: Rebecca Wasley
V.P., Manufacturing and Inventory Control: Therese Connell
Composition: Circle Graphics
Cover Design: Kristin E. Ohlin
Cover Image: © Sharon D/ShutterStock, Inc.
Printing and Binding: Malloy, Inc.
Cover Printing: Malloy, Inc.

Library of Congress Cataloging-in-Publication Data

Adelman, Deborah S.
Disaster nursing : a handbook for practice / Deborah S. Adelman, Timothy J. Legg.
p. ; cm.
Includes bibliographical references and index.
ISBN 978-0-7637-5844-8 (pbk.)
1. Disaster nursing—Handbooks, manuals, etc. I. Legg, Timothy J. II. Title.
[DNLM: 1. Disasters—Handbooks. 2. Emergency Nursing—Handbooks. 3. Bioterrorism—Handbooks. 4. Burns—nursing—Handbooks. 5. Disaster Planning—Handbooks. 6. Mass Casualty Incidents—Handbooks. WY 49 A229d 2009]
RT108.A34 2009
610.73'49—dc22

2008028606

6048

Printed in the United States of America
12 11 10 09 08 10 9 8 7 6 5 4 3 2 1

Dedication

This disaster text is dedicated to all those who have had the misfortune of living through disasters of any magnitude and those everyday heroes who willingly risk their lives to help them. For as we all know, there but for the grace of God . . .

Contents

Introduction

The terrorist attacks that occurred on September 11, 2001, changed the mindset of all Americans. We experienced, many of us for the first time, the confusion, chaos, and fear associated with a terrorist threat. America is no longer naïve to terrorist threat. Although many of us can recall the 1993 attack on the World Trade Centers, the attack of 9/11 was something vastly different and left scars that for many, will never disappear.

Although a significant event, terrorism is not the only disaster that can befall humankind. Confidence in our dominion over the planet was shaken in 2005 when Hurricane Katrina devastated Louisiana. Considerable death and destruction accompanied the tsunami of Indonesia in that same year, adding even more horror over what the forces of nature could do to us. The invisible world of microorganisms also plays a central role in the culmination of events that can be considered a disaster. Most of us have probably heard of *E. coli* infections transmitted by hamburgers and tacos from two famous contemporary chain restaurants, resulting in a few deaths and leaving dozens of others significantly ill. Incidents of food supply tainting, both accidentally and purposefully, will always remain a concern in the collective consciousness of Americans. What about the fear of avian influenza or "bird flu" as it was dubbed by the television stations? What about pandemic flu—will we be ready for it when or if it should ever strike?

In the face of these realities, logical questions of our preparedness as a nation in general and as a profession in particular come to the forefront. The question is not one of *will* there be another major disaster; instead, it should be *when* will the next major disaster occur and how will we deal with its aftermath? While the American public, government, and public health system debate these issues, the reality is that most hospitals, long-term care facilities, residential care facilities, home healthcare agencies, RNs, and other healthcare professionals are not adequately prepared to respond to the myriad challenges that a disaster will pose. Many people are content in living life with the baseless idea that nothing like Hurricane Katrina or the events of 9/11 could happen near them. Many believe that they live in unimportant hamlets where no terrorist would be caught dead, let alone strike. But the truth is that none of us are immune, and all of us live some place important enough to face man-made and natural disasters.

As healthcare professionals, we may be called upon to respond in a disaster. Even for those who do not wish to do volunteer or professional disaster nursing, the possibility is all too real that each of us may find ourselves the only healthcare provider available in the midst of a disaster. This text is designed to educate nurses and graduate-level nursing students in how to respond to disasters as professional nurses. It will look at the role of the RN as first responder, either through membership in a first response team such as a regional medical response team; as an "innocent" bystander, happening upon some sort of disaster; as a home health nurse, such as those in the New York Visiting Nurses Association, trying to respond to their clients' home health needs in a disaster; or as a staff nurse, wondering if he should go in to work in a disaster or if she should stay at work, not knowing where family and friends are. The text will not cover specifics of nursing care, because no matter what the need, nursing care is nursing care. The evidence is that the provision of nursing care during a disaster should be situated among the core competencies of the professional nurse. Those competencies do not change, just the situation surrounding them. That is the goal of this text.

What's Inside

Chapter 1, "The Nature of Disasters," discusses the different types of disasters (e.g., natural and man-made, bioterrorism, and public health emergencies) and how local, state, and national responses work. It includes a discussion of various types of agencies that respond in disasters, from the federal level to local emergency response agencies, as well as volunteer organizations.

Chapter 2, "Volunteerism," looks at the various roles nurses play in disaster nursing. The chapter covers the role of the nurse as volunteer, first responder, as being preparedness focused, and before, during, and postdisaster. Also included is a discussion of all facets of volunteerism including preparation to respond to the call, issues that arise during the response, and recovery after the response.

In Chapter 3, "The Varying Faces of Disaster," disaster response in the field and in the healthcare organization is the focus. Attention is focused on how a hospital prepares for and responds to a disaster. Establishing hospital incident command and how to prepare staff and administration on all shifts for disasters is explained.

The role of the nurse administrator at all levels will be addressed in Chapter 4, "Leadership and Management in a Disaster." Covering not only the nurse administrator in the hospital, disaster nursing leadership and management is one of the topics in this chapter. The chapter includes an excellent discussion of real-life leadership lessons that have resulted from a wide variety of disaster situations.

As we found out in 2005 in the aftermath of Katrina, there are people with special needs who have been, and still are, left out of disaster planning and awareness. A national incentive is on now to plan for these special populations, which include the elderly, children, pregnant women, and disabled individuals. Chapter 5 provides us with an exceptional discussion of the role of nurse in caring for children and the pregnant woman during times of disaster. In Chapter 6, we examine care of the elderly and disabled and the unique challenges that nurses may face when working with members of these special populations.

America is known as a melting pot, but some authors liken America to a salad bowl in which the differences taken as a whole result in something spectacular. Instead of conformity, nurses are increasingly being taught to celebrate and appreciate the richness of our differences. However, this richness in difference does have some drawbacks in a disaster: How does one care for the disaster victim who speaks another language or does not eat certain foods for religious reasons? Dealing with the effects a disaster has on those of other cultures is the theme of Chapter 7, "Culture and Disasters."

Chapter 8, "The Psychology of Disasters," takes a look at the psychological implications of a disaster, for both the victim and the disaster worker. What does one say to the victim who is despondent and tells one he or she can not go on? How do you deal with people staying in temporary shelters who pierce the few rare moments of calm in the dead of the night with the screams from a nightmare? The outlook on how we respond to psychological needs, for both victim and disaster worker, has changed in the last several years, and this chapter offers insight into these changes.

The language of disaster work is not the language of everyday nursing in any specialty. Chapter 9 addresses the language of disasters. The chapter will discuss the terminology used among differing agencies, how to communicate between agencies, dealing with the press, and how to deal with disaster victims and friends and family not involved in a disaster.

What happens to the law when disaster strikes? What about ethical concepts? If 10 people need CPR, how do you decide which one will get it? How can you mark a person as dead and walk on to the next victim? Are you covered by your state's Good Samaritan laws? Can a veterinarian prescribe medications for a human? Can a nurse dispense medications? The answers to these questions, found in Chapter 10, "Law and Ethics in Disasters," may surprise you. Legal issues and ethical considerations that licensed personnel have to be aware of such as licensing in a disaster, practicing outside the scope of one's license, local to federal laws governing health care in a disaster, and nursing responsibilities in a disaster are presented.

Chapter 11 explores the field of HAZMAT (hazardous materials) disasters including types of HAZMAT disasters that can occur, professional responders that may be involved in the HAZMAT scene and how to handle a HAZMAT disaster. The chapter further explores the "ABCs" of responding to a HAZMAT disaster.

Chapters 12 through 15 are related, but remarkably different. As we mentioned earlier in this introduction, nursing care is nursing care. However, most nurses have had limited exposure to and limited experience with the patient suffering from burns. In Chapter 12 an overview of the multiple etiologies and pathophysiology of burns is reviewed. Assessment of resuscitation levels and determination of the need for referral is presented. Chapter 13 examines the management of the trauma patient who is burned, from prehospital assessment through rehabilitation. Chapter 14 builds on the concepts reviewed in Chapters 12 and 13, but explores the response to the disaster environment in terms of responding to mass burn injuries. Chapter 15 concludes the discussion on burns with an overview of the types of specialized burns including blast, radiation, and chemical burns.

Chapter 16, "Bioterrorism: The Use of Biological Agents," presents general information on biological agents used in bioterrorism. Most of these agents are also naturally occurring in the world and can produce epidemics on their own. An example of this would be smallpox before it was eradicated. The chapter also covers the three categories of biological agents and provides information on modes of transmission, signs and symptoms, and medical treatments for the major agents in each category.

The text concludes with Chapter 17 which explores the important role of education for nurses about emergency preparedness and disaster response. The authors then consider the role of best practices and their relevance to disaster nursing. The chapter closes with a consideration of the future of disaster nursing.

The appendices provide information for further consideration and other sources that the reader may wish to consult. The appendices include links to important Web sites and the handling of hazardous materials, treatment considerations, and protection in handling hazardous materials, radiation, and burn situations.

How to Use This Text

This text is designed to be of use to many different levels of nursing professional. The nurse educator in academia may find this text useful as a primary text for a course in disaster nursing, providing the basics in nursing care in a disaster and offering a series of integrated tabletop exercises that can be used for testing and improving critical thinking skills. These exercises, and other instructor materials, can be found online at *nursing.jbpub.com.* It can be used as a supplemental text for every nursing course, from medical/surgical nursing to mental health and home health nursing. The text may also be useful for other healthcare professionals.

For the hospital, administrative, and staff development nurse, this text can be used to help prepare nursing departments for dealing with external disasters. In the emergency department, issues such as how to handle patients brought in with exposure to dangerous chemicals and surge capacity planning are covered. Checklists are presented that can help identify areas of strength and weakness. The issues presented herein can also help healthcare organizations with development and/or revisions to existing disaster plans.

The home and public health nurse will find the chapters that discuss care of vulnerable populations of particular interest since nurses in these settings tend to provide nursing care and coordinate services for those individuals who are vulnerable. The role of reporting agencies and how they relate to the home health and public health department is addressed.

This text is also of value to nurses who wish to volunteer their services in a time of disaster. How to prepare oneself and where to go to offer one's services is presented. The text will also help the nurse caught in a disaster or the nurse who, through the "luck" of being in the wrong place at the wrong time, finds him- or herself the first one on-site in a disaster.

Each chapter begins with a statement of goals and objectives. We start the chapters with goals, because goals are broad statements regarding what the chapter intends the reader to "walk away with" as a result of reading the chapter. Objectives are more tangible and concrete; they are statements that list actual abilities that the reader should acquire as a result of reading the chapter on the way to reaching the chapter's goals. These goals and objectives can be used by educators to plan courses based on the text. Each chapter also has a list of key terms that can help the reader focus on the key concepts addressed.

What This Text Is Not

This text should not, by any means, be considered as the sole source of information on the subject of disasters. The generation of such a volume would be a task beyond capability because of the tentative nature of disaster, medical, and nursing sciences and the emergence of research on various fronts including government and private-sector endeavors. Laws and incident command standards are constantly changing, as well. Other authors have done a commendable job on generating texts on this subject, though no one text can be said to be *the* definitive work on the topic. This book should stimulate thinking, introduce the reader to a broad range of concepts, and, it is hoped, serve as the springboard from which the reader can delve into a larger body of knowledge on the subject.

The Realities We Face

Preparedness and safety are the first fundamentals taught in all disaster training, from disaster classes taught through the American Red Cross to special first response disaster teams. We live in a world where the question is no longer *if* we will have to deal with a disaster, but *when* we will have to deal with one. Nurses are continuously seen as one of the most trustworthy of professionals, and the public turns to us for answers. This text is designed to offer the nurse the basics needed to be there for self and others when disaster strikes.

Acknowledgments

It may sound cliché to say that no work of this magnitude is ever the undertaking of a single individual or group. The multiplicity of individuals involved in a work this large can never adequately be listed on a single page; however, we will try. Both Drs. Adelman and Legg would like to thank the talented group of contributors that appear in this text, without whom this work would not have been possible. They would also like to thank the editorial staff at Jones & Bartlett, particularly Emily Ekle and Patricia Donnelly. Dr. Adelman would like to acknowledge Dr. Mary Pat Lewis and the State University of New York at Delhi for allowing her the time to complete this work. Dr. Legg would like to acknowledge Dr. Edith Neumann and Dr. Frank Gomez of TUI University, California, for their support and guidance over a number of years. We would also like to acknowledge family and friends who stood by us as we tore our hair out in frustration and who kept telling us that we could do it!

Contributors

Deborah S. Adelman, PhD, RN, NE-BC, CNS
Associate Professor
SUNY Delhi
Delhi, NY

Rebecca F. Cady, RNC, BSN, JD
Children's National Medical Center
Washington, DC

Deborah A. DeLuca, MS, JD
Assistant Professor of Health Law, Biomedical Ethics, and Medical Sciences
Seton Hall University School of Health and Medical Sciences
South Orange, NJ

Josephine DeVito, PhD, RN
Assistant Professor
Seton Hall University College of Nursing
South Orange, NJ

Sharon Druce, MS, RN, CCRN
Nurse Manager, Progressive Care and Stroke Unit
Mission Hospital
Mission Viejo, CA

Maryann Godshall, MSN, RN, CPN, CCRN
Assistant Professor, DeSales University
Staff RN, Lehigh Valley Hospital
Doctoral Candidate, Duquesne University
Center Valley, PA

William Gray
Captain Paramedic Squad 8 (Retired)
Springfield, Illinois Fire Department
Springfield, IL

Carol S. Kleinman, PhD, RN, CNAA
Professor and Chair
Nursing Department
New Jersey City University
New Jersey City, NJ

Timothy J. Legg, PhD, RN-BC, GNP-BC, CHES
Assistant Professor of Health Sciences
TUI University
Cypress, CA

Sharon A. Nazarchuk, PhD, MHA, RN
Chair and Professor, Department of Social Science
Lackawanna College
Scranton, PA
Adjunct Faculty, Marywood University
Scranton, PA

Matthew Roberts, MPH
Illinois Department of Public Health
Springfield, IL

Jean Rubino, EdD, APRN, BC
New Jersey City University
New Jersey City, NJ

Dale Simpson
Fire Marshal, City of Springfield, Illinois
Illinois Certified HAZMAT Tech A & B
Former Decontamination Unity Leader
Springfield, Illinois Fire Department
Springfield, IL

Susan Sonnier, MS, RN
Patient Education Coordinator
Clear Lake Regional Medical Center
Webster, TX

The Nature of Disasters

Deborah S. Adelman and William Gray

GOAL

The goal of this chapter is to introduce the reader to the concepts behind disasters, what they are, and how disaster response is organized in the United States.

OBJECTIVES

At the completion of this chapter, the reader will:

1. Understand the concepts of emergency and disaster.
2. Describe the differences between a natural and man-made disaster.
3. Compare and contrast the different levels of disaster response, from local to national.

Key Terms

- Emergency
- Disaster
- Disaster response
- Natural disasters
- Man-made disasters
- Levels of disaster response

Introduction

The terms *disaster* and *emergency* are often used interchangeably. Before one can even begin to discuss disaster planning or preparedness, understanding the difference between a disaster and an emergency is important. According to the World Health Organization (WHO, 2005), an emergency is a situation where a sudden incident or event has occurred and normally used, local responses will suffice to care for the situation without calling in outside help. An emergency can be natural or man-made. Examples of emergencies would be a car accident or a water main breaking.

A disaster is any event that leads to a response beyond which the affected community can deal with locally. Disasters, like emergencies, can be man-made or natural. Disasters are a subset of emergencies and tax responding agencies beyond their capacity. Disasters for one community may not be more than emergencies for another community and degree of response can be like a spreading ring of concentric circles, influencing the outer rings less and less (WHO, 2005). Examples of disasters would include such things as the expected pandemic flu outbreak, earthquakes, technology destruction so great as to interrupt the economics of a country, or a war.

An example of how disaster response and declaration may be made can be seen in a train accident, where a train transporting dangerous chemicals derails in a small Midwestern town at 0224 on a Wednesday morning. The first to respond to this incident would be the town's local police and fire departments. As the seriousness of the situation grows and the town's mayor realizes that she does not have the manpower or equipment to deal with a chemical spill of this magnitude, the mayor decides to call in the county sheriff's department to help deal with the crowds forming as people are evicted from their homes and the local Red Cross is overwhelmed. While waiting for the railroad company to send help, the incident commander, mayor, and other local disaster response agencies discuss the situation and realize they have much more than an emergency on their hands; they have a disaster.

Because of the growing spill and dangers to her town, the mayor contacts the governor of her state. At this level, the local disaster is an emergency that the state government begins to assess and deploy help to the area. State departments of homeland security and public health, the state police, and other disaster response agencies in the state are activated. Not sure if this is an accident yet or a possible terrorist attack, the governor is advised that contact with the FBI, federal Department of Homeland Security (DHS), Federal Emergency Management Agency (FEMA), and other federal disaster agencies should be made and the governor okays the state's head of their homeland security to do so.

What once was a local emergency has now become a local disaster, as local responding agencies are overwhelmed, hospitals are filled with citizens exposed to dangerous and unknown chemicals or just afraid they were exposed and in a panic, and the chemical spill seeps into the ground, contaminating the local aquifer. As support comes in from state agencies, the governor declares the whole region of the state a disaster area and makes a request of the president of the United States to send federal assistance. The governor tells the president that the state does not have the supplies to deal with such a major chemical spill or the displaced populations and that healthcare and emergency responders are overwhelmed. In the space of a few hours, an event that was an emergency is now a local and state disaster, but still not a federal emergency (Figure 1-1).

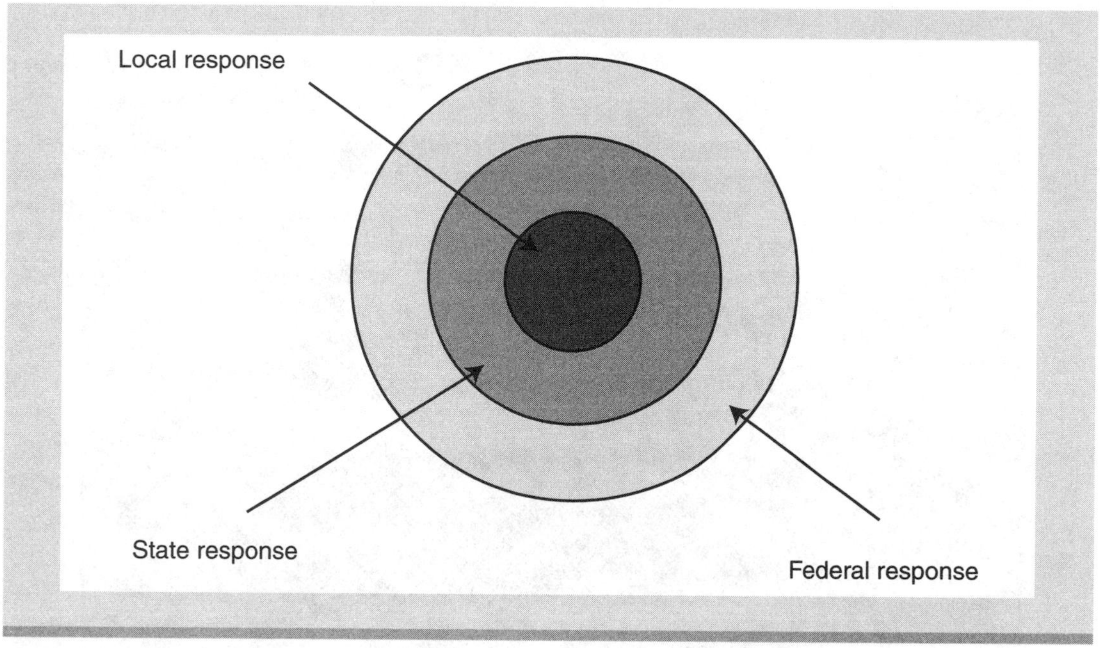

Local response

State response

Federal response

Figure 1-1 As each level of response spreads out from an incident, the degree of severity decreases, going from a local disaster to a federal emergency.

In this chapter, the nature of a disaster and who responds to it will be covered. Different types of disasters will be addressed in a general overview and gone into more depth in future chapters. As each level of response spreads out from an incident, the degree of severity decreases, going from a local disaster to a possible federal emergency or disaster.

Types of Disasters

There are basically two different types of disasters: natural and man-made. Natural disasters are such things as earthquakes, tsunamis, pandemic flu outbreaks, and tornados (see Figure 1-2). Man-made disasters include anything that a human being has done to cause a disaster, such as acts of bioterrorism, hijackings, and war. The type of response does vary in specifics, but, generally, it is the same for all disasters: assess, contain, respond, and recover.

Natural Disasters

Natural disasters often strike without warning, though most areas know what is "normal" for their areas and prepare for such occurrences. Assessing is done by reviewing the history of the region, looking at what weather and other disasters have occurred in the past. For example, at the southern tip of Illinois through

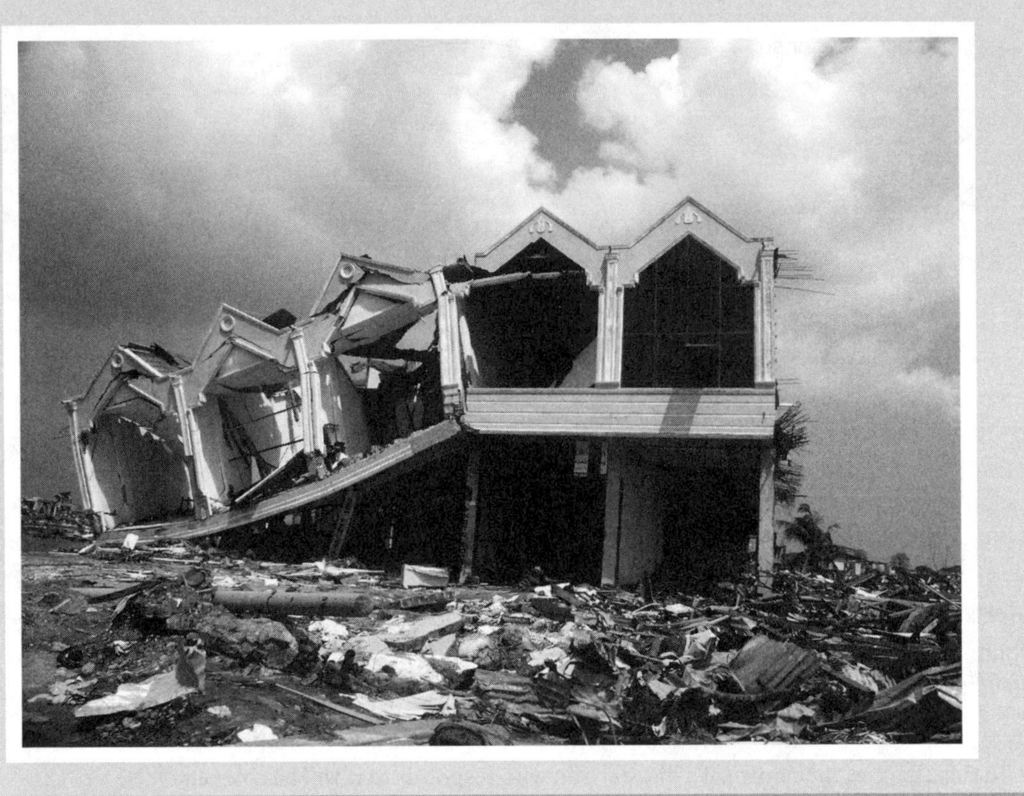

Figure 1-2 Ruins of houses in Acch, Indonesia after the Boxing Day Tsunami caused by the 2004 Indian Ocean Earthquake. *Source:* © A. S. Zain/ShutterStock, Inc.

Missouri and Arkansas is a fault line called the New Madrid Fault. The last time this fault moved and produced a major earthquake was in 1811–1812. The disaster covered more than 50,000 square miles, almost 10 times the size of the San Francisco earthquake in 1906. Because the potential for another major earthquake exists and the fault is due for one, almost all towns along the fault and through much of Illinois and Missouri are prepared to deal with such a natural disaster.

Some natural disasters occur with more warning than an earthquake or tornadoes. As the United States saw in 2005 with Hurricane Katrina, there is often enough warning to prepare for the disaster and to evacuate citizens when necessary. Wildfires are another example of natural disasters, though some are man-made, that provide time for people to evacuate or establish firefighting responses to the disaster.

Man-made Disasters

There are some man-made disasters that occur or can occur with some warning, such as knowing that a dam is weak and, without proper mitigation, it will break, releasing a flood. However, most of the serious man-made disasters are the result of unexpected accidents (e.g., an oil tanker running aground or a power plant blowing up) or deliberate acts of terrorism. There are also epidemics and pandemics that occur with some regularity and, while one may not consider these man-made, many are the result of people living with livestock, as in influenza, or living in crowded conditions, which helps spread tuberculosis.

In assessing the potential for these disasters, first responders, public health officials, and other healthcare agencies survey their communities for the potential for man-made disasters. Many people believe that their area of a country is unimportant and a terrorist attack would occur somewhere more "important." They believe that a city such as Atlanta would be more likely to be attacked than a city such as Ocilla, Georgia. This is not the case, though, for most major security agencies in the United States know that terrorists are looking at the psychological response from an attack as much as from destroying major landmarks or large numbers of people. Ocilla, being an average small town, would be a perfect choice to shock and numb people reading about such a "senseless" attack.

Levels of Disaster Response

It is important for every locale to prepare for potential disasters, natural or man-made. Part of preparing is understanding who responds when and how. There was much criticism leveled at responders to Hurricane Katrina, and many people wondered why FEMA was not in Louisiana and Mississippi *before* the hurricane struck. The reason is that there are different levels of response for a disaster, and no level responds before requested to do so by the lower level below it.

In the scenario presented above, a small town was overwhelmed by a train accident with a resulting chemical spill. The mayor utilized her local resources, which included the police and fire departments, hospitals, ambulance services, and the local American Red Cross. The town also had a Community Emergency Response Team (CERT), a group of local citizens who volunteer in times of need. After a short period of time, the mayor realized that she did not have the means to respond effectively, and she contacted the county sheriff's department. When the county sheriff found his agency overwhelmed, the governor was called and state response was requested.

Because the incident outgrew the state's ability to handle the incident, the governor called the president of the United States and asked for a federal response. What started as a local emergency eventually became a state disaster, and a chain of first responders was activated.

This chain of response can even go to a level beyond the ability of a nation to handle, and international disaster relief can be requested. At this level, such agencies as the International Red Cross and the United Nations will respond. In Table 1-1, the various levels of response and who has the power to call for help from that agency is outlined.

TABLE 1-1 LEVELS OF RESPONSE

Level of Response	Agencies Responding	How Requested
Local	Police	Called by local citizens
	Fire	Called by local citizens
	Hospitals	Notified by local EMS
	Ambulance/emergency medical service (EMS)	Called by local citizens or local EMS
	Local public health department (PHD)	Called by local citizens, mayor, or local EMS
	Community Emergency Response Team (CERT)	Called by mayor or mayor's representative
	Medical Reserve Corps (MRC)	Called by mayor or mayor's representative
	Volunteers in Police Service (VIPS)	Called by mayor or mayor's representative
	Red Cross	Called by local EMS or citizens
County	County law enforcement	Called by local citizens, county officials, or mayor
	County EMS	Called by local citizens, county officials, or mayor
	County emergency management agency (EMA)	Called by county officials
	County PHD	Called by local citizens, mayor, or local EMS
State	State EMA	Called by governor
	State EMS	Called by governor
	State Red Cross	Called by local Red Cross
	State PHD	Called by local or county PHD

(continued)

TABLE 1-1 LEVELS OF RESPONSE (Continued)

Level of Response	Agencies Responding	How Requested
	State law enforcement	Called by governor
	State homeland security	Called by governor
	State disaster volunteers	Called by governor
	National Guard	Called by governor
Federal	Department of Homeland Security	Called by president
	FBI	Called by local citizen, mayor, governor, or president
	CIA	Called by local citizen, mayor, governor, or president
	American Red Cross	Called by state Red Cross
	FEMA	Called by local EMA, governor, or president
	United States Public Health Service	Called by state PHD
International	United Nations	Called by leader of requesting country
	World Health Organization	Called by leader of requesting country
	International Red Cross	Called by leader of requesting country or American Red Cross

Timing is also a factor in responding to a disaster. Most agencies do not wait to be called to a disaster, but call and ask if help is needed or respond when they hear about the disaster. An excellent example of this occurred when the World Trade Centers, the Pentagon, and the plane crash in Pennsylvania took place on September 11, 2001. Many leaders of foreign countries called our president to ask if they could help us respond to the disasters. We were able to deal with the disasters without international help, but it was comforting to know that, should our resources be overwhelmed, we did have help available from other countries.

In the case of federal agencies, FEMA is an agency that does not automatically respond to a disaster. The same is true of Homeland Security and even the Strategic National Stockpile, which is a cache of medications and other disaster medical equipment kept in hidden and secure areas that can be called upon if local resources are overwhelmed. These agencies and resources on the federal level are generally only available after the first 48 hours of a disaster and take 12 hours to be mobilized.

Conclusion

In this chapter, a broad overview of what a disaster is and what agencies respond was provided. We learned that every emergency is not a disaster, but every disaster is an emergency. First responders are called out in levels, from the local to the county, state, federal, and international levels. In Chapter 2, a closer look at volunteerism in a disaster offers a first look at how people respond to disaster, because it is often local volunteers who are on the scene of a disaster along with the first responders from the local community.

Reference

World Health Organization. (2005). *List of definitions.* Retrieved July 6, 2007, from http://www.who.int/hac/techguidance/training/induction/definitions%20list.pdf

chapter 2

Volunteerism

Matthew Roberts

GOAL

The goal of this chapter is to define the role of the volunteer in disaster nursing.

OBJECTIVES

At the completion of this chapter, the reader will:

1. List the competencies needed to be a volunteer disaster nurse.
2. Apply these competencies to volunteer disaster nursing.
3. Analyze the various types of volunteer disaster response at the local, state, and national levels.
4. Understand what is involved in preparing for and responding to a disaster.
5. Define the recovery phase of volunteer disaster response.

Key Terms

- Disaster competencies
- Volunteerism
- Types of disaster responses
- Local disaster responses
- State disaster responses
- Federal disaster responses
- Preparing to respond
- Recovery

Introduction

In Chapter 1, a broad look at the nature, definition, and level of response helped us to understand what disaster nursing encompasses. In Chapter 2, we will look at volunteerism in disaster response, focusing on the role of a nurse volunteer in a disaster.

Disaster nursing fulfills a critical component of the health and medical emergency response, much as in common day-to-day health operations. This disaster nursing component applies directly to both the healthcare employee and the healthcare volunteer. The following chapter will address some of the competencies related to disaster nursing, especially in the context of the volunteer, throughout multiple phases of disaster response, including the preresponse or preparedness phase, during the response, and the postdisaster and response phase. These competencies will be woven throughout and will describe those functions that need to be considered both by the organization that recruits, as well as by the individual who hopes to assist in the response. A brief introduction to these competencies follows through works of the Medical Reserve Corps program and other sources (Center for Health Policy, 2004; Nursing Emergency Preparedness Education Coalition, 2003; Hospital Core Competency Subcommittee, 2004).

The Medical Reserve Corps (MRC) program was developed through the Surgeon General's office following the 9/11 terrorism attacks and will be explained in detail later. Reacting to the need to coordinate function of the program across the country, the program developed a core competencies matrix that illustrates general emergency response roles (Office of the Surgeon General, 2007a). This matrix is to be used by MRC units to further develop their teams and shape the individual volunteer experience so that a degree of cohesiveness can be inserted into the national model. Its tenets include considerations for personal safety, health, and preparedness; roles and responsibilities for volunteers; and overviews of public health activities and incident management principles.

Competencies and Volunteering in a Disaster

A more generic set of basic disaster competencies that any health responder, whether volunteer or paid, should appreciate include having a thorough understanding of the command structures to which one would report; knowledge of general roles and responsibilities, as well as policies and procedures; recognition of an emergency situation and its precipitators; familiarity with backup communication systems and constructs that would be employed; an understanding of the utilization of personal protective equipment (PPE) and other health and safety precautions; and a basic understanding of weapons of mass destruction (WMD) and chemical, biological, radiological, nuclear, and explosive (CBRNE) terrorism. All responders should have an understanding of the different types of terrorism and how to respond adequately to the differing types. Medical personnel should have a basic understanding of what various treatments are required for each type of terrorism, how casualties may present, and what plans are in place for dealing with these casualties, including decontamination procedures and mass medical triage plans.

Any disaster involving a health or medical response element will tax the normal function of the medical community, as discussed in Chapter 1. This has been evidenced in recent responses to Hurricane Katrina, the attacks of September 11, 2001, the sarin gas attacks in Tokyo, the first World Trade Center attack in 1993, the Oklahoma City bombing, and so on. Indeed, even small-scale responses will produce a significant surge and stress on local and regional responses.

Neither governmental public health nor private-sector healthcare agencies have much surge capacity inherently built into the system. Mutual aid agreements among these institutions and increased regional collaboration are two ways that these groups have added some depth to their response structure, but true surge capacity can only be reached by having additional local personnel to augment the response. This is most clearly the case in scenarios wherein regional sharing might not work well (i.e., events that drain resources at a similar rate throughout multiple jurisdictions, such as pandemic influenza scenarios or large-scale regional responses such as those found with Hurricane Katrina or the 1993 flooding of the Mississippi River). This additional response can and often does come from local citizens with special talents and skills who volunteer their services in a disaster.

The willingness of volunteers to respond, especially in times of crisis, can be overwhelming at times. For example, over 30,000 volunteers flooded into the New York City area after the 9/11 attacks to assist, far beyond any governmental agency's ability to handle, especially when these volunteers are not trained in disaster response. People want to help and will most definitely present themselves to lend assistance during a crisis. Fortunately, the emergency response volunteering process is improving over time, consistently resulting in a more seamless process.

Types of Response: Who Might Respond

Several volunteer organizations have arisen since the September 11th attacks, mostly due to federal preparedness grant monies that have been issued to state and local governments across the country. One such volunteer organization developed after the 9/11 attacks is the MRC Program (Office of the Surgeon General, 2007b), which is housed under the newly crafted Citizen Corps (Federal Emergency Management Agency, n.d.) and U.S.A. Freedom Corps (n.d.) programs. MRC units are developing all across the country to meet the expected surge needs, as well as bolster the day-to-day activities of public health by strengthening the overall public health infrastructure of local communities. Education, training, response gear, and other resources are available to these teams through the federal funding. Composition of MRC units varies widely, by design, to reflect local community needs, although similar preparedness goals run pervasively throughout the groups. For example, at the time of this printing, Illinois had 38 MRC units, with many local health departments (LHDs) in Illinois exploring this option as a way to bolster their response plans.

All MRCs seek nursing and other medically trained personnel, and most recruit clerical staff to assist with paperwork and logistics. One of the biggest missions that LHDs enlist nurses for is the Strategic National Stockpile (SNS) implementation.

Through this response, federally stockpiled vaccines, drugs, and other medical supplies can be sent to local governments for dispensing to the public in a response to a mass epidemic such as an influenza pandemic or an act of bioterrorism such as anthrax. Nurses have many roles in assisting at local dispensing operations, whether through physically dispensing medicines or vaccines (under orders of the local physician or pharmacist or under suspension of licensing rules and regulations in a disaster and when a physician is not available), providing patient education to the affected public at the dispensing site, screening individuals before entering the clinic, helping discern the appropriate medication for an individual to use (based on the patient's possible contraindications and potential drug interactions), or by providing a clinical consult for the patient. These potential roles will vary from area to area, based upon planning models and the degree of training that personnel will receive, in addition to the direness of the scenario.

In addition to the local disaster health missions listed above, nursing personnel are also needed to support mass care operations, including sheltering of impacted individuals or mass treatment of the injured from a mass casualty incident. MRC volunteers from areas impacted by the 2004 and 2005 hurricane seasons helped their communities by filling in at local hospitals, assisting their neighbors at local shelters, and providing first aid to those injured by the storms. American Red Cross nurses and responders may also be deployed to assist with a response (ARC, 2007a, b). Congress chartered this quasi-governmental organization in 1905 to assist in disaster relief efforts domestically and internationally, and nurses have played a major role since its inception.

The SNS also contains federal medical stations (FMS) or field hospitals that are for use by local and state governments when resources have been overwhelmed and additional noncritical hospital care is necessary. It is likely that local and state responders would be used to assist in staffing an FMS, including local ARC and MRC volunteers or other statewide volunteer teams.

Local and State Response

As presented in Chapter 1, when a disaster occurs at the local or state level, different types of responders are called out. Some of these may be volunteers. Regional volunteer groups were discussed in the previous section and include MRC, Community Emergency Response Teams, and local ARC volunteers. Many states have statewide volunteer responders as well. The ARC has a state-level response, when a local chapter is overwhelmed. Other types of healthcare professionals volunteer with statewide agencies, as well. This section will explore one state's volunteer response groups to show you how such a statewide volunteer response might be organized.

The Illinois Medical Emergency Response Team (IMERT, n.d.) and Illinois Nurse Volunteer Emergency Needs Team (INVENT, n.d.) are two Illinois-specific state volunteer response teams, coordinated at the state level, that assist local response as well as deploy across state borders via Emergency Management Assistance Compact

(EMAC) responses. IMERT is a statewide volunteer response team that can provide support for some of the acute medical functions associated with mass casualty incidents and other large-scale medical issues, like those from Hurricane Katrina.

INVENT is similar to IMERT, although it is generally deployed to augment the first responder capability of IMERT by providing a secondary follow-up supportive response. INVENT is a volunteer group of RNs from a variety of backgrounds trained to respond and provide nursing care during state disasters, emergency situations, and prolonged recovery efforts. INVENT, being a secondary response contingent, largely serves to assist IMERT or other first response teams in field response efforts, thereby creating a tiered response capability. Similarly, INVENT would be able to enhance local health department capacity for mass immunizations or medication dispensing and assist with localized hospital surges and/or staffing at alternate care sites, such as locations established by hospitals when a particular facility is overwhelmed or compromised.

Both IMERT and INVENT teams have been deployed to confront large-scale disasters and emergencies that overwhelm local personnel resources. For example, IMERT and INVENT assisted with a special needs shelter to meet the medical need that surpassed the capabilities of the local American Red Cross shelters and local health providers during ice storms that affected central and southern Illinois in 2006. Together, IMERT and INVENT have about 500 nurses and are always recruiting more.

In the event of an outbreak scenario or disaster, there is always a high demand by the public for information about the disaster and response. The Illinois Poison Control Center has phone banks designed to field questions from the public and from clinical providers to serve as a hotline for information sharing in the event of a pandemic or other emergency. INVENT nurses are currently being trained to staff these phone banks, and a recent drill tested the state's capabilities to execute an information hotline function. Over a 4-hour time span, the capability of the system to handle a surge in calls from the public was explored. Most of the calls (85%) were handled immediately by an INVENT nurse. Lessons from the drill are being used to adjust automated messages, build capabilities to field inquiries from the public and healthcare providers, and direct callers to useful information. Other potential uses for INVENT include staffing megashelters (when regional resources have been exhausted and state facilities need to be established), that would likely be state-operated facilities, designed to execute a well-defined scope of care and manage noncritically injured or ill patients.

Federal Response

One of the first FMS deployments was to Louisiana for the Hurricane Katrina response. This response was partially staffed by IMERT volunteers who actually assumed command of the FMS in New Orleans because the first responders in that state were overwhelmed and unable to respond themselves. The FMS contains all the necessary components for a very basic field hospital, but does not deploy with sufficient personnel to staff it; thus, volunteer staff must be brought in to support the complement of medical supplies. This solution works well when a hospital becomes overwhelmed with patients or becomes environmentally or structurally compromised by the effects of a disaster. It is likely that the FMS would constitute much of the physical composition of the alternate care sites or mega-centers that could be staffed by volunteer response teams such as IMERT and INVENT or local responders.

Federal medical and nursing teams are also available and are assembled through the National Disaster Medical System (NDMS) (U.S. Department of Health and Human Services, 2007). Nurses have many opportunities to join different teams within the NDMS and have their licensure and certification recognized by any state to which they respond, in addition to federal protection in malpractice suits. The two main NDMS teams that utilize nursing professionals are the Disaster Medical Assistance Teams (DMATs) and the National Nurse Response Team (NNRT).

Volunteer groups will need, in conjunction with local, state, and federal authorities, to determine the roles they will have in local Hospital and Health Emergency Response Plans and work to coordinate the plan development, while familiarizing themselves with the incident management procedures and techniques of the volunteer organization and other responding agencies (Toner et al., 2006). Hospitals are required to test their surge capacity plan annually via either a surge in volunteers or a surge in victims from an emergency, and a partnership with the leadership of a volunteer disaster team should be forged with the hospital management to utilize these surging volunteers in a response (American Medical Association & American Public Health Association, 2007). Clinical personnel, namely nurses, will have an important role in assisting in this plan development, as well as bringing the plans to life by being part of the actual response.

Preparing to Respond

In 1995, Rebecca Anderson, an LPN, was killed while responding to the Oklahoma City, Murrah Federal Building bombing. She heroically worked to save lives immediately after the blast, but was struck by falling debris and ultimately died days later (Oklahoma City National Memorial and Museum, 2006). Her courageous yet tragic death serves to remind any responder of the importance of protecting oneself and ensuring his or her health and safety, as well of that of fellow responders. Personal and family plans are as important for the responder and the volunteer as for those of the responding institution: With no capable responders, an agency's response plan is nothing. Ensuring the safety of the responder ensures there will be one less victim and more help for those in need.

All levels of government are working to provide simple plans so the average citizen can respond better to an emergency. The Red Cross has developed these plans for some time (ARC, 2007a). Illinois recently activated its emergency response Web site for the public, complete with a link that can be added during a response to provide important updates to the public (State of Illinois, 2007). The federal government developed a comprehensive website that covers various levels of preparedness for individuals and businesses (U.S. Department of Homeland Security, n.d.) as well as a look at WMD and CBRNE considerations, and also utilizes a specific website for pandemic influenza activities that shares information to the public (U.S. Department of Health and Human Services, n.d.).

It is very much in the best interest of the volunteer responder to pre-affiliate with a response organization before a disaster for a number of reasons. Joining a team that is a good fit will align the responder with the right type of response that fits his or her scope and skills. Additionally, an affiliated responder will be more capable of responding in an appropriate fashion and more likely to be included in the response element because he or she will have had credentials verified, received proper training, and will be more familiar with fellow volunteer responders as well as the governmental or healthcare-sector employees working alongside the volunteer through exercises and orientation meetings. Therefore, it behooves the potential volunteer responder to examine the different types of teams that are available and the proper team for him or her to join. Joining a volunteer team is an important and sought after decision, but it should be an informed decision. Some considerations one should ask are included in Table 2-1. Answering these questions will assist the potential volunteer in deciding which program to join and whether or not volunteering is a good idea.

During the Response

Medical personnel in general and nursing professionals specifically have a huge role in a disaster medical response, whether they are employed by a responding agency or

TABLE 2-1 QUESTIONS TO CONSIDER BEFORE VOLUNTEERING

Lots	Some	Little	Questions to Consider
☐	☐	☐	How involved do I want to become?
☐	☐	☐	Do I want to be deployed frequently and receive lots of training?
☐	☐	☐	Do I want to respond outside of my immediate area? Outside of my county? State?
☐	☐	☐	Would a deployment hurt my family life?
☐	☐	☐	Do I need to be paid during any deployment?
☐	☐	☐	Does the volunteer team I like cover liability issues?
☐	☐	☐	How could this affect my current employment?

Source: Adapted from Peterson, 2006.

are responding in a volunteer capacity. For instance, if a human influenza pandemic occurs, as patients begin to present to their doctors and to medical facilities for treatment, it will be up to the clinicians to report cases to public health authorities in order to direct the management of the response. The same conditions apply for food-borne outbreaks and generally any other large infectious disease or disaster response involving health issues or injuries. As mentioned earlier, a surge in caseload and a complimentary drain on resources is to be expected both in the outbreak scenario as well as a mass casualty incidence.

Beyond surveillance, during a major outbreak, practitioners may be forced to implement isolation of infected patients, conduct infection control procedures, and develop PPE policies. Nurses and other clinicians in medical settings will be relied upon to execute these interventions. As frontline personnel directly engaging the ill, nurses will also need to protect themselves and then extend stringent infection control standards when caring for each other and for their patients. This was clearly evidenced in the SARS outbreaks of 2003 in Asia and Canada. Infection control practices and the use of PPE seemed to be the most reliable way to interrupt disease spread and protect those most directly affected since a solid treatment for this novel virus had not been developed (CDC, n.d.). These practices would need to be employed for any major outbreak. Proper PPE and infection control precautions would naturally need to be applied to any mass casualty response.

In the event of a pandemic or other emerging infectious disease outbreak, it is likely that a surge in caseload will quickly overwhelm the public health system. For example, clinic and hospital settings are expected to be swamped with both ill patients, as well as the "worried-well." LHDs will not necessarily see patients in their offices and clinics, but mass medication and vaccination campaigns will require immense staffing demands. To address the need for medical materials, public health officials have been working to stockpile resources, both in the aforementioned SNS and in state and local caches. However, to prepare for the need for additional personnel, teams of volunteer health professionals must be ready to augment the public health emergency response.

Similarly, an influenza pandemic or other infectious disease outbreak will weigh heavily on the medical community and especially on hospitals (Buehler et al., 2006). The National Response Plan speaks specifically to this issue, and a pandemic scenario is prioritized via the list of National Planning Scenarios. History has taught us about the need for this type of plan: The 1918 pandemic was characterized by such an exceptional surge on the medical system that many lay persons were conscripted to assist with the medical response and received a crash course in medical therapy. These individuals worked closely alongside the few nurses who were healthy and available, taking direction from the nursing staff and supporting medical and nursing care in what ways they could. This particular emergency illustrates the expandable role of the disaster nurse responder. Depending on the severity of the response, nurses may be asked to fill nontraditional roles.

EMAC, briefly mentioned earlier, is a mutual aid agreement, adopted by all 50 states. This agreement allows for rapid resource sharing and state assistance among states during governor-declared emergencies. Through EMAC, states are allowed to request anything they need, for any specific response; the requesting state pays for the response costs of the responding state (National Emergency Management Agency, 1995–2007). Previously, IMERT's response and deployment to Hurricane Katrina was mentioned as being a response to the EMAC agreement between Louisiana and Illinois. Once the agreement was secured with a specified response package selected by Louisiana, IMERT was deployed and Louisiana reimbursed Illinois for its response efforts.

Receiving a surge of volunteers from outside of the affected area's jurisdiction can be a challenge in itself, as was dramatically seen in the response to the World Trade Center bombings in 2001. As human resources swarm into an affected area, providing services for those individuals can be a challenge. The receiving entity must establish reception and processing centers to receive these responding teams efficiently and effectively. EMAC frees up many of the issues associated with license portability (an Illinoisan being able to use his or her Illinois nursing license to do the necessary response in an emergency capacity in Pennsylvania), credentialing, liability, and so on.

WMD and CBRNE agents need to be considered in any disaster response, including those responses that seem benign. Historically, initial attacks may be followed up with secondary devices specifically set to detonate and harm the first responders. These devices must be accounted for and considered throughout the response. Generally, volunteers should never be allowed to enter what is considered the "hot zone" or the immediately impacted area, but there are occasions where there are no highly recognizable zones or a volunteer is the first responder on the scene. These situations need to be approached with additional caution. Learning how to deal with such possibilities should be incorporated into any emergency management and disaster volunteer training curriculum.

Lastly, it is critical that during the preparedness and disaster response orientation phase that a responder, paid or volunteer, makes his or her capabilities clear to the response teams, whether volunteer or governmental. Recent disasters are filled with anecdotal evidence illustrating situations wherein individuals presented to assist with the response, but were placed into situations unfit for them based upon their experience and degree of comfort. This is especially troublesome and more probable in diverse disciplines like those of physicians and nurses. In a disaster situation, one may be compelled to assist in any way possible, but there is a huge difference in skills and knowledge between a trauma nurse specialist and a nurse who works in public health providing chronic disease preventative education. Based on the circumstances of the event, it is easy for someone to be placed in a situation that could quickly overwhelm him or her, and caution should be exercised both by the responding agency and by the volunteer when the agency is tasking individuals with response missions.

After the Response: The Recovery Phase

This period is probably the most important portion of the response, especially for the volunteer who might not regularly be exposed to disaster outcomes, including mass illness or death or exposure to body parts. Responses to these unusual and often disturbing experiences can have significant mental health repercussions, including development of post-traumatic stress disorder, substance abuse, hypertension, depression, sleep disorders, panic attacks, memory loss, and other physical, mental, and behavioral problems (Hammond & Brooks, 2001). Critical incident stress debriefing (Chapter 8) must be carefully conducted, including the timing of when the counseling is employed (Campfield & Hills, 2001). Regardless of the timing of the intervention and counseling, it is clear that critical incident stress management (CISM; Chapter 8) must be conducted, and it must be conducted by trained individuals. Without some degree of counseling, the volunteer or paid responder runs the risk of mentally reliving the disaster experience, potentially harming the person's health and livelihood over time.

As frontline responders, nurses will likely be exposed to the more gruesome effects of any disaster response. The SARS outbreak affected healthcare workers at a higher incidence than other groups, because of the proximity of the workers to the pathogen and the ways the virus was spread. As a result of situations such as the SARS outbreak, healthcare workers are in a cohort that is more likely to need counseling both immediately afterwards and long term, especially if a significant amount of healthcare personnel are injured, infected, or killed by a disaster's effects. Therefore volunteer response teams should look to include CISM into their response plans and seek ways in which this type of counseling can be provided to the volunteer team's responders. If a responder is on a team without any observable CISM program, this should be brought to the attention of the team's leadership so that it can be adequately addressed, and this important component can be provided for.

Go Forth and Volunteer

Volunteer teams are actively recruiting and lining up personnel before an emergency hits; the response goes more smoothly when volunteers are already preloaded into the response apparatus rather than showing up cold. If you have ever watched a disaster response on TV and wanted to be there on the ground helping but did not know how to get involved, you should begin exploring the types of teams that are out there and talk to the coordinators of the programs to see what role or team might be a good fit for you. Volunteering for disaster nursing teams is an old and time-honored tradition in nursing, going back in this country to Clara Barton in the Civil War and starting the American Red Cross as her response to the needs of soldiers. One never knows when a disaster will strike, but one can be prepared, as Barton wanted nurses to be, to help those caught in a disaster—those who might even include the nurse and his or her family. Being prepared means being safer and knowing what to do when disaster strikes.

References

American Medical Association and American Public Health Association. (2007). *Improving health system preparedness for terrorism and mass casualty events: Recommendations for action.* Retrieved November 28, 2007, from http://www.ama-assn.org/ama1/pub/upload/mm/415/final_summit_report.pdf

American Red Cross. (2007a). *Get prepared.* Retrieved November 28, 2007, from http://www.redcross.org/services/prepare/0,1082,0_239_,00.html

American Red Cross. (2007b). *Home.* Retrieved November 28, 2007, from http://www.redcross.org

Buehler, J. W., Craig, A. S., del Rio, C., Koplan, J. P., Stephens, D. S., & Orenstein, W. A. (2006). Critical issues in responding to pandemic influenza [conference summary]. *Emerging Infectious Diseases* [serial on the Internet]. Available at http://www.cdc.gov/ncidod/EID/vol12no07/06-0463.htm

Campfield, K. M., & Hills, A. M. (2001). Effect of timing of Critical Incident Stress Debriefing (CISD) on posttraumatic symptoms. *Traumatic Stress, 14*(2), 327–340.

Center for Health Policy. (2004). *Competency-to-curriculum toolkit: Developing curricula for public health workers.* New York: Columbia University School of Nursing and Association of Teachers of Preventative Medicine. Retrieved November 21, 2007, from http://cumc.columbia.edu/dept/nursing/chphsr/pdf/toolkit.pdf

Centers for Disease Control and Prevention. (n.d.). *Severe Acute Respiratory Syndrome (SARS).* Retrieved November 28, 2007, from http://www.cdc.gov/ncidod/sars

Federal Emergency Management Agency. (n.d.). *Citizen Corps.* Retrieved November 28, 2007, from http://www.citizencorps.gov

Hammond, J., & Brooks, J. (2001). The World Trade Center attack: Helping the helpers: The role of critical incident stress management. *Critical Care, 5,* 315–317.

Hospital Core Competency Subcommittee. (2004). *Recommended hospital staff core competencies for disaster preparedness.* Tallahassee, FL: Author. Available from http://www.emlrc.org/pdfs/disaster2005presentations/HospitalDisasterMgmtCoreCompetencies.pdf

Illinois Medical Emergency Response Team. (n.d.). *Welcome to IMERT.* Retrieved November 28, 2007, from http://www.imert.org

Illinois Nurse Volunteer Emergency Needs Team. (n.d.). *Welcome to INVENT.* Retrieved November 28, 2007, from http://www.inventrn.org

National Emergency Management Agency. (1995–2007). *EMAC.* Retrieved November 28, 2007, from http://www.emacweb.org

Nursing Emergency Preparedness Education Coalition. (2003). *Educational competencies for registered nurses responding to mass casualty incidents.* Retrieved December 12, 2007, from http://webapps.nursing.vanderbilt.edu/incmcemodules2/main.html

Office of the Surgeon General. (2007a). *MRC core competencies matrix.* Retrieved November 21, 2007, from http://www.medicalreservecorps.gov/File/MRC%20TRAIN/Core%20Competency%20Resources/Core_Competencies_Matrix_April_2007.pdf

Office of the Surgeon General. (2007b). *Medical Reserve Corps.* Retrieved November 28, 2007, from http://www.medicalreservecorps.gov/HomePage

Oklahoma City National Memorial and Museum. (2006). *Those who were killed: Rebecca Anderson.* Retrieved November 28, 2007, from http://www.oklahomacitynationalmemorial.org/secondary.php?ordering=7&view=19§ion=10&catid=24

Peterson, C. (2006). Be safe, be prepared: Emergency System for Advance Registration of Volunteer Health Professionals in Disaster Response. *OJIN: The Online Journal of Issues in Nursing, 11*(3), Manuscript 2. Available at www.nursingworld.org/ojin

State of Illinois. (2007). *Ready Illinois.* Retrieved November 28, 2007, from http://www.ready.illinois.gov/

Toner, E., Waldhorn, R., Maldin, B., Borio, L., Nuzzo, J. B., Lam, C., et al. (2006). Biosecurity and bioterrorism. *Biodefense Strategy, Practice, and Science, 4*(2), 207–217.

United States of America Freedom Corps. (n.d.). *Home.* Retrieved November 28, 2007, from http://www.freedomcorps.gov/Default.asp

United States Department of Health and Human Services. (2007). *National disaster medical system.* Retrieved November 28, 2007, from http://www.hhs.gov/aspr/opeo/ndms/index.html

United States Department of Health and Human Services. (n.d.). *PandemicFlu.gov.* Retrieved November 28, 2007, from http://www.pandemicflu.gov

United States Department of Homeland Security. (n.d.). *Ready.* Retrieved November 28, 2007, from http://www.ready.gov

chapter 3

The Varying Faces of Disaster

Sharon Druce

GOAL

The goal of this chapter is to provide an overview of organizational responses in a disaster, from preparation to recovery.

OBJECTIVES

At the completion of this chapter, the reader will:

1. Formulate a structure of organizational response in disaster response.
2. Assess organizational vulnerability and mitigation in a disaster.
3. Understand the differences between internal and external vulnerabilities in a disaster.
4. Discriminate between various organizational standards used in organizational disaster planning and response.
5. List key concepts in organizational disaster response.
6. Develop disaster drills for organizations.

Key Terms

- Organizational disaster response
- Vulnerability
- Mitigation
- Internal vulnerability
- External vulnerability
- Organizational disaster standards
- Organizational disaster planning
- Organizational disaster concepts
- Disaster drills and exercises

Organizational Response to Disasters

Healthcare organizations have a responsibility to be engaged in preparation and support of disaster response activities. During a disaster, healthcare organizations must ensure the safety of staff members, volunteers, and patients.

State and federal accreditation standards provide guidance and an additional level of expectation over that of the individual healthcare organization. These standards ensure that healthcare organizations have disaster management plans in place, including plans for assessment and mitigation of known and potential hazards, planning for possible disaster scenarios, training and practice of disaster scenarios, and evaluation of response efforts to real or practice scenarios to ensure continuous quality improvement.

In the next sections, the various parts of the disaster plan will be discussed. Each section will examine how one assesses vulnerability, what should be in the disaster plan, preparing for the different disasters historically known in the agency's geographic location, training and practice, and how to evaluate the plan and all of its components.

Assessment of Vulnerability and Mitigation

Emergency and disaster events may be confined to the facility, involve infrastructure support, or affect the entire community. Organizations must assess individual risk factors to ensure that disaster planning and training includes the most likely disaster scenarios for the agency's geographic location. However, because no one healthcare facility is usually alone in a disaster of any size, assessing the risk factor to the agency must include assessing and working with the entire community.

Disaster planning begins with an assessment of vulnerability based on risk for actual or potential events and includes a thorough evaluation of risk factors for natural and man-made disasters. This is most effective when performed collaboratively with community agencies to identify hazards as well as support available to and from the organization. A careful, thorough, and thoughtful examination of an organization's vulnerabilities should serve as a practical guide for the development of general and specific disaster management planning. An honest appraisal of an organization's incident management system and structure should be included in the assessment of hazards. This assessment enables organizations to determine their vulnerabilities and focus on their resources and planning methods. This assessment is the basis for the development of a flexible emergency response plan, enabling the organization to respond rapidly to anticipated or changing situations. Although most organizations may have similar components in their plans, the response and site-specific plans may vary from agency to agency and understanding how each agency's plan fits within the overall disaster plan for a city, region, or state will save time, energy, and redundancy in the case of an actual disaster.

Assessing Different Vulnerabilities

As described in Chapter 1, there are different types of disasters (i.e., man-made and natural). Each of these types of disasters will have some core similarities in terms of response, and each will have a unique component to the response.

External Vulnerabilities

Natural disasters include events that provide limited or no forewarning of the event as well as events that are anticipated to occur on a more frequent basis. Major earthquakes, landslides, volcanic activity, sudden flooding, or large-scale community fire events may provide limited or no forewarning of imminent disaster. Temperature extremes of heat or cold, tornadoes, blizzards, and hurricanes are relatively common events in many geographical areas, some with warning and others without. Although the event may occur with varying degrees of frequency, assessment must include an organization's risk for such events. Assessment of vulnerability for these events increases the likelihood of effective disaster planning, response, and ability to provide care.

A biological disaster caused by communicable diseases has long been recognized as an area for increasing concern. International travel, gene mutations of disease, interspecies disease transmission, and deliberate bioterrorism with infectious agents have generated increased public attention to this issue. Assessing an organization's ability to recognize, isolate, treat, and decontaminate as indicated are part of the assessment of vulnerability for healthcare organizations that is gaining increasing attention.

The potential for man-made disasters requires additional careful assessment for vulnerability. Structural instability of man-made structures in the area may precipitate disasters or hamper disaster relief efforts, transportation, and communication. Collapse of dams and large bridges may cause loss of life, major injuries, serious damage, and disruption of anticipated evacuation and exit routes. Evaluation of transport routes, including rail and air traffic, may reveal a vulnerability to transportation disasters.

Civil disasters, including riots and large strikes and demonstrations, may disrupt routine working environments and supply delivery in addition to causing injuries and deaths. Warfare and terrorist activities may involve conventional, nuclear, biological, and chemical weapons. All of these man-made events can cause significant physical and psychological injury, impair relief efforts, and further complicate the effects of the disaster.

Internal Vulnerabilities

Vulnerability to internal disasters of the organization also needs to be assessed. Radiology and laboratory biological, chemical, and nuclear materials used in diagnostics and medical treatment are a primary source of potential internal disaster concerns. Disruption, sabotage, and loss of electronic documentation or inability to access electronic medical records can severely disrupt the organization's ability to provide care within the organization or in transferring patients out of a damaged hospital to another healthcare agency.

Included in the assessment of vulnerability for natural and man-made disasters must be an assessment of the organization itself. The physical structure of the facility requires an assessment to determine structurally vulnerable areas, areas that could be converted to another use during disasters, food and supply storage, and communication ability under various scenarios. A realistic evaluation of the number and types of patients that can be cared for under varying conditions needs to be performed. Patients requiring isolation or decontamination may strain an organization's ability to provide care, as well as protect staff and patients from contamination. Disaster and evacuation plans need to be assessed on a regular basis to ensure that changes in infrastructure construction, conversion of existing areas to new uses, and equipment changes are incorporated into disaster plans.

Mitigation of all possible risk areas is not a realistic possibility. However, sufficient resources must be in place to ensure disruptions are limited. Supplies and equipment must be kept in working order and be accessible for use, and training must be provided on a regular basis for specialty equipment and procedures. Disaster procedures must become part of the culture of the organization and practiced on a frequent and regular basis. Disaster procedures must also be revised as indicated by the evaluation of the training and practice scenarios.

Emergency Preparation Standards for Healthcare Organizations

National guidelines and accreditation standards form the general framework for disaster planning and preparedness assessment within hospitals and healthcare organizations. The National Incident Management System (NIMS) provides specific guidelines for healthcare systems to prepare and respond to disaster situations (Federal Emergency Management Agency [FEMA], 2006b). These guidelines are integrated within Joint Commission accreditation standards for healthcare organizations for emergency management standards (2007). The Health Resources and Services Administration and the National Bioterrorism Preparedness Program also require hospitals to be compliant with the NIMS standards. The development of a unified and comprehensive national approach to disaster management that encompasses standards across multiple agencies, jurisdictions, and disciplines requires standardization in planning, training, communication, and collaboration. Additional regional and state organizational requirements for healthcare organizations may apply to specific situations beyond the scope of discussion for recognized national standards that impact acute care health systems.

NIMS Standards for Healthcare Systems

NIMS standards include 17 key elements for healthcare systems, the foundation of which is the directive to adopt NIMS across the organization within all relevant departments including vendors and suppliers. Using national response guidelines across organizations, agencies, and jurisdictions enhances the response capabilities. The additional NIMS standards include command and management, preparedness planning, preparedness training, preparedness exercises, resource management, and communication and information management.

Command and Management

Command and management elements of the NIMS standards include use of the Incident Command System (ICS), development of a multiagency coordination system (MAC), and implementation of a public information system. Hospital policies and procedures should reflect the integration of an ICS in the emergency operations plan that reflects the core elements of command staff, operations, planning, logistics, and finance. The ICS should be utilized to manage preplanned drills and special events, as well as emergency incidents that occur internally or externally. Hospital policies and procedures should reflect the integration of an ICS in the emergency operations plan that reflects the core elements of command staff, operations, planning, logistics, and finance. The goal of any healthcare organization ICS must be the provision of safe patient care and continuity of hospital operations despite the constraints of resources during a disaster. (For further details on communications in a disaster, see Chapter 9.)

Multiagency coordination involves the assessment of additional agencies that are integral to the support of organizational plans. Outside sources include the obvious integration with emergency support services such as public health departments, law enforcement, fire departments, and hazardous materials response teams. Additional outside agencies to consider may be medical offices, urgent and ambulatory care centers, and other community health centers including mobile healthcare resources. Organizational plans need to consider the integration and implementation of multiagency capabilities to promote effective use of services, equipment, and safety within disaster policies. Disaster drills need to be conducted that involve multiagency responses to validate expectations and communications across all agencies.

Public information system standards include Joint Information System (JIS) and a Joint Information Center (JIC). It is imperative that the JIS provides accurate, clear, timely, and coordinated information to the public during a disaster. Healthcare organizations assign this role to a public information officer who is the pipeline for media information and inquiry. Typically the person assuming this role has some expertise in public relations and communications. Working relationships with multiple agencies, through collaborative planning and disaster drills prior to a disaster event, enhance the capabilities of the healthcare system spokesperson. The JIC is a physical command area reserved for information professionals from multiple agencies to assess critical emergency information, crisis communications, and public affairs. Depending on the situation, healthcare organizations may be expected to provide physical space and utilities to support these services.

Preparedness Planning

According to the NIMS standards, healthcare system preparedness is focused on the establishment of guidelines, protocols, and standards for planning, training, exercises, personnel, equipment certification, and publication management. Preparedness planning includes expectations to track NIMS implementation standards within the healthcare system, generate a system to coordinate hospital funding to comply with the NIMS standards throughout the organization, review and revise disaster and emergency operations plans to reflect NIMS standards, and establish mutual aid agreements with public, private, and/or nongovernmental organizations.

Tracking of an organization's compliance with the NIMS standards is essential to continued validation of emergency preparedness at the level expected and required of healthcare systems. Activities must be tracked yearly with the goal of enhancing performance within the facility or organization. The ability to assign a dedicated person to this requirement will vary among organizations depending upon size and resources available. Although this role may be assigned along with other responsibilities within a job description, the expectation remains that the tracking of NIMS compliance will be performed by an individual who possesses at least a working knowledge of emergency management (including the essential phases of preparedness, prevention, mitigation, response, and recovery), hospital daily and emergency operations, and hospital command center operations.

There is an obvious need for adequate funding within healthcare systems to implement and maintain disaster preparedness activities and respond adequately to disaster events. Implementation of the NIMS standards requires the hospital or healthcare system to obtain and effectively allocate funding for disaster preparedness. Implementation of this standard requires healthcare organizations and systems to proactively identify local, regional, state, and federal funding opportunities to meet this standard. Documentation within this standard includes identification of funding received and what has been achieved with the funding. Additional documentation must include how the system met funding commitments. Strong interagency working relationships can enhance this ability to coordinate funding across multiple agencies. Healthcare organizations need to work cooperatively with their state hospital association and emergency management authority that can assist with coordination of funding and distribution.

Every healthcare organization must have emergency operation plans to support disaster activity management. These plans must be reviewed following any incident or at least annually and revised as indicated to meet NIMS and accrediting organization requirements. These plans describe how resources, including personnel and supplies, will be managed for daily operations to support the activities generated by the emergency. These plans need to be fluid and flexible to meet changing situations that impact the original disaster process. The disaster events surrounding Hurricane Katrina in 2005 provided ample proof that disaster teams need to be flexible to respond to new situations that occur. Evacuation of civilians and hospitalized patients; access to supplies and personnel; additional flooding from broken levees; the response of the civilians affected; local, state, and federal officials; and communication to the public and within responding agencies all significantly impacted previously prepared disaster plans.

Mutual aid agreements are intended as a supplement to existing disaster plans of each organization. It is unrealistic to expect mutual aid agreements to be the sole source of support during a disaster. Mutual aid agreements are voluntary arrangements between organizations and nongovernment or private sectors to provide additional personnel, supplies, services, or facilities in the event of a disaster. Mutual aid agreements are encouraged between health systems, local emergency response teams, supply vendors, and public health departments. Established mutual aid agreements need to be reviewed at least annually, included in the disaster plans, and shared with local emergency management agencies.

Preparedness Training

Personnel training is essential for disaster plan implementation. NIMS standards include completion of standardized coursework to ensure performance standards are understood; provide clear, standardized expectations; and enhance collaboration among agencies and within the organization. Specific courses are required based on expected roles of staff and leadership within the organization during a disaster. Healthcare organizations must identify the appropriate personnel to complete the required courses, and guidance can be found within the individual standards and courses. Documentation of NIMS compliance requires validation of course completion by appropriate personnel. Courses can be completed in a classroom with a qualified instructor or online through the FEMA training Web site http://training.fema.gov/IS/crslist.asp.

Multiple disaster courses are offered by FEMA, but NIMS standards identify several specific courses that must be completed by appropriate personnel based on roles they may be expected to perform during a disaster. These are minimum standards, and additional course completion is encouraged. Course *IS-700 NIMS: An Introduction* should be taken by staff who would be expected to fill a leadership role for emergency preparedness, incident management, or emergency response. *IS-800 800.B: National Response Framework: An Introduction* (formerly titled *IS-800.A NRS: An Introduction*) is for personnel who would be responsible for emergency management within the organization. *IS-100 Introduction to ICS* and *IS-200 ICS for Single Resources and Initial Action Incidents* (or their equivalents) present the foundation for understanding the ICS framework for personnel during a disaster. Similar to expectations for personnel completing *IS-700, IS-100* is especially recommended but not limited to personnel in administrative leadership roles who would be involved in emergency preparedness, incident management, or emergency response. *IS-200* is expected, at a minimum, to include personnel in middle management roles and should also include any staff that would have a role in an emergency operations center. It is important to remember that these identified courses and personnel are minimum requirements, and additional courses and completion by other staff members should be encouraged and tracked with documentation of course completion.

Preparedness Exercises

Actual practice of a healthcare organization's disaster plan is an essential standard for all healthcare organizations. Practice of the disaster plan with varied preparedness exercises will help ensure NIMS standards for training and exercises, all-hazard exercise program, and corrective actions are tested. Healthcare organizations must ensure that NIMS and ICS standards are incorporated into the preparedness exercises that include internal and external local, regional, and state emergency management exercises. Preparedness exercises for all-hazard exercises also need to involve responders from multiple disciplines and agencies. The frequency of these exercises depends on the type of exercise executed. Tabletop exercises, functional, and/or full-scale exercises may be used to meet this requirement. All-hazard drills that involve full-scale exercises are especially valuable as they provide a scenario that allows multiple agencies to test and practice with equipment and collaboration in real-life scenarios.

The goal of any preparedness exercise is to identify strengths and weaknesses within a plan. The standard of corrective actions requires a review of the preparedness exercise and preparedness plans to ensure that corrective actions are incorporated into revised plans. The corrective action standard requires healthcare organizations to identify deficient issues. For each deficiency identified, the corrective action plan must include identified actions to correct the deficiency, who will be responsible for implementing the action, due date for completion, and a revision of the plan to include the new policies or procedures. Essential elements of preparedness planning and exercises will be discussed later in this chapter.

Resource Management

Resource management includes an adequate resource inventory and resource acquisition. These standards include both an on-site inventory of appropriate supplies and mobilization of additional supplies and personnel required to support a disaster event, including communication infrastructure. This expectation must be reviewed and met within all phases of disaster management. As noted earlier, contracts with vendors, mutual aid agreements, and memorandums of understanding between agencies and organizations all supplement existing organization standards but do not substitute for basic essential organizational preparation. Consideration must be given to supplies that would be utilized in excess during a disaster event, and appropriate considerations for both on-site and easily accessible local storage should be evaluated. Many organizations use a just-in-time ordering method for supplies with frequent deliveries. During a disaster this may leave the organization with insufficient supplies to meet a surge in need.

Resource acquisition for communication and data transmission within the organization and among external agencies is considered in the resource elements. Documentation must exist within the plans to ensure communication equipment and data systems are functional with outside agencies. When existing infrastructure is not operational, alternative sources such as radios, information technology resources, and phone technology may be options to ensure clear and vital communications within the organization as well as outside agencies. Use of runners to carry written communication within a facility may be another option but will translate poorly when interagency communication is needed. Compatibility of these systems as well as their functionality must be assessed in the preparedness exercises that involve multiple agencies.

Communication and Information Management

The final element of the NIMS standards requires the use of standard and consistent terminology among agencies. Clarity in information management requires the use of plain English and avoidance of slang or code phrases that are specific to one agency. This does not prevent a healthcare organization from using established internal codes, but involvement in outside reporting to agencies requires the use of common English to ensure clarity for the event. Interagency and interdisciplinary communication must rely on common English rather than 10-codes or internal organizational codes whose meanings may vary among agencies and local, state, or national responders. (See Chapter 9 for further details on communication.)

Joint Commission Standards for Healthcare Organization Disaster Planning

The Joint Commission has published a set of accreditation standards to address healthcare organization disaster planning. The standards cover five areas defined as critical to disaster operation plans. The Joint Commission has placed a great emphasis on flexible disaster plans that emphasize planning for events that are likely to occur as well as escalating or multiple events. These emergency management standards include standards for communication, resources, and assets; safety and security; staff responsibilities; utilities management; and patient clinical and support activities (Joint Commission, 2007).

Communication

Communication standards include the surveillance, identification, and communication of emergencies to appropriate authorities. Symptoms and diseases that may represent biological emergencies, natural or man-made, must be reported to public health agencies in a timely manner. Chemical contamination must be recognized quickly, isolation and decontamination procedures initiated for patients and exposed healthcare providers, and emergency authorities notified.

Organizations are required to plan for alternative methods of communication within the organization and within the community emergency response infrastructure. Loss of phone lines, fax, and computer access can seriously disrupt an organization's ability to provide care and communicate within the infrastructure.

Batteries for cell phones and radios have limited shelf lives and length of use. Alternative sources such as messengers, amateur radio operators (ham radio), battery-powered and two-way radios must be available for rapid implementation. Staff must be trained and, in some cases, licensed in the use of these devises. Access to volunteer amateur radio operators and their role should be planned and practiced as part of the disaster planning scenarios. Use of standard terms to ensure clear communication between departments and agencies must be coordinated following the National Incident Management System guidelines for use of plain language (FEMA, 2006a). Communication with on- and off-duty staff members needs to be planned and practiced. Procedures for notifying off-duty staff through phone lists, cell phones, pagers, or media announcements need to be planned, evaluated, and adjusted. Communication with vendors for needed supplies and resources may need alternative methods.

Regulations under the Health Insurance Portability and Accountability Act of 1996 (HIPAA) require organizations to maintain access to confidential electronic healthcare records in addition to ensuring access is restricted to protect sensitive information. With the increasing trend to provide electronic documentation of healthcare services, organizations must also ensure that access can be generated quickly in a disaster situation. Failure to maintain access to medical records may negatively impact the health and safety of patients and would be a severe disruption in care.

The review of electronic record safety and accessibility follows the key steps of any disaster plan: assessment of vulnerability and mitigation of effects, planning for potential disaster scenarios, and evaluation of the plan through testing and refinement. Risk assessment for electronic services and documentation needs to include the analysis of current equipment, vendor contracts, built-in resiliency and redundancy, geographic location, and potential hazards. Included in this assessment would be the grading of loss of various services from minor (i.e., relatively minor disruptions of services, rapid repair, and resolution with minimal cost) to critical (i.e., extreme disruptions of services, significant legal or financial effects, or a threat to health and safety). Repair or recovery may be time consuming and expensive in a critical disruption. In addition to the review of services that would impact patient safety, employee human resource and payroll records must be assessed for vulnerability in the event of technology disruption.

Disaster planning for technology service disruption should be part of any facility's disaster plan integration. Included in the plan should be the people and resources available to restore services, escalation procedures, off-site storage and access for critical data, and redundancy of information storage and access in case of widespread disaster effects. Procedures to be followed for loss of electronic technology need to be clearly written and practiced to determine additional areas of vulnerability and ease of plan implementation.

Continuity of documentation provided to individual patients from initial triage to discharge is also required. Although some patients may arrive with numbered triage tags to facilitate eventual registration and coding for care during the entire hospitalization, many others may arrive by private vehicle. Identification and medical information may be limited by the victim's condition. As a result, healthcare organizations must include documentation as part of a standardized emergency response plan. Several options may be necessary depending upon the extent of the disaster, the extent of damage to internal electronic infrastructure, and resources available. Disaster planning needs to include staff and resources to integrate information and ensure that the correct information is associated with the appropriate victim.

Communication planning must include patients and family members during care and evacuation. Loss of infrastructure to support call lights may produce harm to patients if communication is lost between patients and responding staff members. Transfers of patients within the organization or as part of a larger evacuation plan must include plans to notify family members appropriately and in a timely manner. Additional resources will be required to obtain and provide information to distraught family members searching for missing relatives. Social workers, psychologists, psychiatric nurses, disaster mental health workers, and spiritual care leaders from the hospital and community may provide valuable emotional support to families. On-duty staff who are away from family members may also need to be kept informed of efforts to locate and communicate with missing family or loved ones.

Planning for media access is an essential part of disaster planning. Communication with media representatives must be implemented to maintain patient, family, and staff confidentiality while providing accurate information. Careful consideration to media access should be provided to ensure the emotional welfare of vulnerable staff, patient, and family members is not compromised. FEMA (2007) has issued mandatory guidelines for media coverage of disaster events. These policy guidelines, as part of the national response plan for federal domestic incidents, cover media roles and responsibilities during their participation in disaster coverage with disaster responders and in medical facilities. The guidelines clearly indicate that local officials are the final authority for media access.

Local authorities may need to restrict media access to some areas, and FEMA guidelines help by providing specific procedures and policies for media coverage (FEMA, 2007). Healthcare organizations and staff who are responsible for interacting with media representatives should be fully aware of FEMA's guidelines and confidentiality guidelines that must be maintained during the disaster care. Representatives of the organization who are responsible for media relations should ensure that policies are reviewed with media representatives. Media representatives must provide proof of identification and display their credentials. Media representatives who do not comply with the established guidelines may be denied access and information.

As defined by FEMA policy guidelines (2007), media and facility leadership must maintain a heightened awareness, sensitivity, and confidentiality concerning photographs and information released publicly through the media. Photographs or names of casualties require permission of state authorities. Since state authorities are responsible for notifying appropriate next of kin, release of names or identifying photographs of casualties is prohibited until verification of notification has been obtained. Photographs or names of casualties require permission of state authorities who are responsible for notifying family members. Photographs, videotapes, or audio recordings of victims must have informed consent from the person in the publication or a legal parent or guardian that clearly indicates the victim understands the photo or comments may be distributed in international media reports. The victim or the organization, acting in the best interest of the victim, may also rescind consent at any time after the photograph or comments have been collected.

Media access to disaster areas and facilities caring for disaster victims may be restricted for physical safety as well as to limit access to confidential information and to protect patient and family privacy and confidentiality. Access to locations and information may also be restricted to protect legal or classified investigations. Medical procedures must take precedence over media access. Access to various areas of the facility is at the discretion of the organization's leader responsible for media relations. Access to areas of the hospital, other than the media control center, must be with the accompaniment of designated facility leaders. Media may not wander independently within the facility. Operating room access during surgical procedures is prohibited.

Resources and Assets

Management of resources and assets during a disaster is critical to be able to provide care and services. This also requires the organization to identify the culture of the organization and its role within the community. Depending upon the scope of the emergency, resources may be strained, unavailable, or unable to reach the organization.

Disaster response plans must include open access to the community for food and shelter. Appropriate budgeting to permit storage of key equipment and additional supplies is necessary. Many organizations utilize a just-in-time ordering method of supplies with frequent deliveries. During a disaster this may leave the organization with insufficient supplies to meet a surge in need. Alternative vendors, access from other community healthcare organizations and organizational affiliates, and state or federal resources may need to be utilized. Some resources may not be available or may be dealing with a disaster themselves, and alternatives and improvisation may be needed.

Disaster management plans need to include methods for maintaining necessary pharmaceutical supplies, medical supplies, and nonmedical supplies such as food, water, and linens for patients and staff. These plans also need to include how to request, share, and offer aid to other healthcare organizations. Budgeting for disaster planning and readiness may need to include infrastructure upgrades, personal protective equipment (PPE) and PPE upgrades, disease surveillance monitoring resources, and decontamination equipment in the event of nuclear, biological, or chemical exposure.

The healthcare organization must also be able to identify when the infrastructure, in whole or part, cannot support care. Written plans for evacuation of patients with medications, supplies, and records within the organization or to another facility entirely are required as part of the resource and asset management plans.

Safety and Security

Healthcare organizations must establish plans to ensure safety and security during a disaster. In establishing plans, the safety and security of staff, patients, and volunteers and the management of resources and supplies all must be considered. The type of the disaster and the evolution of the events during and after the disaster may affect access and movement within the local area.

Security measures may be the responsibility of the organization or involve local, state, or federal agencies at various intervals. The command structure of the disaster response plan must include clear communication within the organizational security infrastructure as well as with outside agencies that need to be involved. Access to the facility and within the facility may need to be controlled for safety and security. Provisions for management, isolation, and decontamination of potential hazardous radioactive, biological, and chemical products need to be defined in the emergency plans.

Staff Responsibilities

During disasters, staff roles and expectations are determined by the emergency needs, report routes, and command infrastructure in place during the disaster. Prior to an actual disaster, staff are expected to take disaster training and disaster practice scenarios seriously to be able to provide effective care under real disaster situations. Staff must receive training for their assigned roles during a disaster although the amount of training required will vary according to the role they are expected to perform.

Basic job action sheets and checklists for jobs may be utilized as part of the flexible training process. Special job action sheets, designed for use in a disaster, should be developed and given to appropriate staff members. Staff roles and identification of care providers must be defined through some means of clear communication (e.g., vest, armband, or badge). Provision for use of volunteers and licensed staff not employed by the facility must be addressed in the emergency management policy.

Utilities Management

The disaster management plan needs to include how healthcare organizations will continue to provide essential utilities to support care. Supplies of water, fuel, electricity, waste disposal, medical gases, ventilation, and vacuum systems must be identified and include an estimate of how long care can be provided with the current resources and what may be needed depending on the type of disaster experienced. Alternative vendor sources, resource sharing, and resource management need to be addressed in the plan.

Patient Clinical and Support Activities

During a disaster, the healthcare organization's focus is to provide emergency services to protect life and to prevent further disability. The nature of the disaster and evolving events during and after the disaster will dictate how patients are managed. Basic sanitation needs must be addressed. Plans must include provision of care for special needs populations, mental health care, and mortuary services. The healthcare organization must have plans to manage patients through all phases of expected assessment, treatment, admission, discharge, transfer, or evacuation.

Key Concepts in Emergency Response Planning

Developing a chain of command and an organized emergency management command response system for use in disasters is a key administrative leadership role within any healthcare organization. Assessing the vulnerabilities of the organization; writing, reviewing, and updating policies that address the disaster response; ensuring appropriate and adequate training; and implementing functional roles within the emergency management command system are roles assumed by administrative and leadership team members. Once the plans are written, organizational leadership is responsible for ensuring that all staff members are informed, prepared, and understand the roles they play during a disaster. Emotional competence, creative thinking, ability to adapt to rapidly changing conditions, effective resource management, identifying improvements needed in the disaster response, and the ability to communicate clearly and collaborate with local, state, and federal agencies are additional key competencies required of organizational leaders. (See Chapter 4 for leadership and management in a disaster.)

Practicing and Evaluating Disaster Drills

Disaster plans provide the framework for disaster response, but, without practice and drills, these disaster plans are worthless. In healthcare organizations, the challenge to provide an effective and functional disaster response framework can be daunting. Coordinating and testing plans with multiple departments, staff who will actually respond, and outside agencies is critical to the success of disaster management. Unfortunately, plans are often created by those who have limited knowledge of clinical services and impact, are poorly distributed within the organization to cover all shifts, are poorly trained, and are reasons paper plans fail when exposed to an actual event. Disaster training should be included in all staff orientation sessions, included in annual competency updates, practiced under real-life circumstances, evaluated for changes, and plans redesigned based on lessons learned during drills to ensure continuous quality improvement.

Disaster drills should include the most expected scenarios as a basis for developing a general disaster plan framework. The more plausible the disaster scenario, the greater the feeling of urgency that will be felt among staff participating in the drill. Drills are a vital way to test new equipment and to provide additional training to staff members who might be responsible for setting up and maintaining the equipment. Disaster response drills should occur on weekends, holidays, and non-daylight hours, even though the cost of paying overtime may seem a "waste." However, disasters do not conveniently occur during daylight hours on weekdays.

The most effective drills include community agencies in the response to test coordination of care and communication between agencies that would be involved in disaster response efforts. In the most ideal situation, drills are conducted to involve staff members on evening or night shifts when administrative leadership is less accessible and others are expected to assume leadership roles initially. Plans that may work well when large numbers of leadership and senior staff are available may fail to point out deficiencies in manpower to execute the plan or inexperienced staff that are uncertain of their roles.

Staging a disaster drill may point out potential disaster plan failures that require new options to mitigate challenges. Plans that include participation of staff will point out clinical issues with hazardous material protective gear, lack of proper PPE, longer than anticipated time to set up equipment, new equipment that no longer performs in the same manner as old equipment did, construction or closure of areas that were identified in the disaster plan as response points, staffing changes in key roles, and environmental conditions such as wind or rain that interfere with planned responses.

Essential to the drill experiences are evaluators who are able to observe and record positive and negative observations of the drill itself. Evaluators should include members who are both part of and from outside of the healthcare organization. These objective evaluators may identify flaws and strong points in the disaster plan that might go unnoticed by those participating. Debriefing of participants also provides valuable insight into how well the disaster plan worked. It is important to ensure that disaster drill participants are encouraged to share their perspectives and feelings in this debriefing. Being sensitive to feelings of failure, assuring staff that their honest feedback is vital to eventual safe and effective care during a disaster, and being sensitive to emotions that may arise during a disaster drill are important skills for debriefing and follow-up from the drill leaders. If changes are made to the disaster response plan as a result of the drill and debriefing, these changes need to be clearly communicated to staff that would be impacted.

Conclusion

Regardless of the size or scope of service, all healthcare facilities must have clearly defined disaster plans in place. These plans must include the thoughtful evaluation of the most likely disaster events that will occur locally, as well as guidelines to respond quickly to unanticipated or multiple evolving events. A clearly defined chain of command, including collaboration with local community agencies is essential. The most critical elements in any disaster plan include competent leadership and practice of the proposed plans to ensure staff is competent and able to understand their own roles during a disaster.

References

Federal Emergency Management Agency (FEMA). (2006a). *NIMS Basic: Communications and information management.* Retrieved January 2, 2008, from http://www.fema.gov/pdf/nims/NIMS_basic_communications_and_information_management.pdf

Federal Emergency Management Agency (FEMA). (2006b). *NIMS implementation activities for hospitals and healthcare systems.* Retrieved February 18, 2008, from http://www.fema.gov/pdf/emergency/nims/imp_hos.pdf

Federal Emergency Management Agency (FEMA). (2007). *Specific ground rules: Media access policy and operations.* Retrieved January 6, 2008, from http://www.fema.gov/media/resources/ground_rules.shtm

Joint Commission. (2007). Emergency management standards: January 1, 2008. [Electronic version]. Oakbrook Terrace, IL: Author. Retrieved December 31, 2007, from http://www.jointcommission.org/NR/rdonlyres/2F7A3491-8D8F-4AE2-8BC7-52B2CEC3E3B7/0/sii_EM_approved_stds_0108.pdf

chapter 4

Leadership and Management in a Disaster

Sharon Druce

GOAL

The goal of this chapter is to provide an understanding of the differences between nursing leadership and nursing management in a disaster.

OBJECTIVES

At the completion of this chapter, the reader will:

1. Compare and contrast the concepts of nursing leadership and nursing management.
2. Define nursing leadership and nursing management competencies for disaster response.
3. Apply appropriate communication skills as a disaster nurse leader.
4. Explain motivational skills and needs in a disaster for effective leadership.
5. Apply lessons learned from prior disasters that showed poor leadership and management behaviors.

Key Terms

- Disaster nursing leadership
- Disaster nursing management
- Leadership competencies
- Leadership communication
- Motivation in a disaster
- Flexibility in a disaster

Leadership or Management?

Leadership is essential to successful outcomes, whether in an established organization or during periods of crisis as seen during disaster events. Management is also essential to an organization, but leadership and management skills are not the same set of competencies. Although they may be integrated competencies within one individual who chooses one set of skills and competencies over another depending on the need and the event, the two sets of competencies are separate and distinct.

Although the competencies of leaders and managers differ, the successful leader may find that a combination of techniques increases the effectiveness of a team, solves a problem, or reaches a goal. In a study of business teams, the most productive and most innovative teams derived their success from the leadership of the team. The leaders of these teams were both task- and relationship-oriented in their approach to projects. The early phases of team building were focused on the goals and individual responsibilities of each team member. Once the goals and individual accountabilities were understood, leaders of these successful teams focused on the relationships and knowledge sharing. Although leadership during a disaster may be based on roles assumed as part of an Incident Command System or other defined command structure, true leadership depends upon the successful integration of management and leadership competencies (Gratton & Erickson, 2007). Truly effective leaders will understand the differences in leadership and management competencies and make a thoughtful decision to use specific techniques in a variety of situations. The differences between leadership and management skills will be reviewed further in this chapter.

The approach to problem solving, engagement of others, and the decision-making process varies among leaders and managers. Leadership is not conferred by title or administrative position although that is still a common assumption. Leaders must have influence over others (followers) to get things done, especially those things the leader believes needs to be accomplished. Manion asserted that the work of true leadership is a process that releases the full potential of the follower (2005). The process is not dictated to the follower, but the goal and vision must be clearly described to mobilize and maintain interest and energy.

Multiple definitions of leadership have been proposed, and multiple theories of leadership exist. Debate continues as to whether leaders are born or made and whether effective leadership skills can be a learned experience through study and practice without an innate ability to inspire and lead. Character does influence the leadership quality. Innate talent for leadership may be a trait that can be honed and improved just as other talents can be strengthened through practice and study. However, the overriding expectation and commonalities within leaders all point to a motivated and motivational leader who communicates the overall organizational goal or vision to a group allowing the group to work with a purpose to achieve a common goal or mission. As will be seen, the true leader does not provide the means or process to achieve the goal. The members of the team all play varying roles in defining and deciding how this process will occur, how it will be managed, and what their roles and the roles of others will be and how they will be established, monitored, and sustained.

Effective leaders seek input and collaboration among their followers instead of relying on hierarchical organizational structure that limits contributions and creative thinking from members. Group dynamics also imply that the followers have trust and confidence in the leader to believe that the goal can be achieved with the resources available. This trust relationship also implies that the leader has clearly communicated the goal to the group and that people-oriented relationships exist or can be formed rapidly through the desire to achieve a common goal. During a disaster, leadership responsibilities are defined by the Incident Command System (ICS). However, it is important to remember that leadership must also exhibit leadership and management skills as required by the situation.

In this chapter, differences between leaders and managers will be explored, and leadership core competencies needed in a disaster will be reviewed. The leadership competencies will be evaluated in light of disaster situations, and implications for expanded and critical leadership competencies will be discussed.

Leadership and Management Differences

Leadership and *management* are discrete terms but are often used interchangeably. Authority generated by position title or election to a role does not imply automatic leadership ability or capability. The way leaders and managers approach problem identification and resolution is often the key factor in defining leadership versus management competencies. Manion identified key differences between leaders and managers in their approach to problem solving, team leading, role responsibilities, and purpose (2005). These differences will be reviewed to differentiate the approach taken by leaders and managers. Leaders look at the big picture and implications for effective and appropriate change. Leaders often ask themselves if the concept is in line with new expectations rather than relying on the same goal but a different approach to make the old goal workable (Manion).

Managers are more often involved with making the plan work or, if it is working now, looking for ways to streamline efficiency, improve the process, or make it easier for the person performing the task. Managers may not stop to consider whether the task or process really needs to be done at all. A leader will question the task itself and wonder if it promotes the best practice or merely meets the supposed needs of the organization. It is the leadership ability to question the presumed need that frequently injects change into an organization (Manion, 2005).

Leaders and managers differ in the way they process the problem. The leader must be willing to communicate clearly to followers what the broad goal is, share the vision to convince others to embrace a goal as their goal and work toward a solution, and be willing to embrace solutions that may be different or unexpected to accomplish the goal. The true leader does not dictate the process of how and why to the team, only the vision and goal. Collaboration allows the leader to step back and allow others to identify a process and make it work. Managers tend to have intimate knowledge of how to make a process work. They frequently have high levels of technical knowledge and are highly skilled practitioners. Within health care, as well as other industries, competent and skilled performers are often promoted with the expectation that their technical expertise will generate inherent trust and respect from the followers. Leadership mentoring may be limited or nonexistent, and the new leader may experience burnout and stress.

Leadership is people and relationship oriented. Effective leaders understand that relationships are the reason for their existence: Leadership does not exist in a vacuum, and people skills are an integral part of leadership. To exist in a leadership role, one must have followers to lead. The ability to work in a group situation with behaviors that empower others, while building trust and confidence, are key interpersonal skills required of leaders. Leaders exhibit courage, reliance, and strength of character with high standards. They are persuasive, have expertise and experience, and are willing to share that knowledge to increase the effectiveness of the team (McCullough, 2008).

Managers are commonly driven by organizational policy and procedure. Deviation from standard policy usually implies that the manager must investigate why the gap occurred and institute processes to prevent the recurrence. Managers may be less involved with development of strong interpersonal skills and group process skills and more concerned that the existing policies are followed.

Change, innovation, and embracing the resulting chaos are classic leadership skills (Grossman & Valiga, 2005). Leaders embrace change while understanding the chaos that may be felt as a result. The effective leader is strong enough to understand that there is always a way to improve the status quo, understands that others may have ideas that are better, and is not afraid to let others suggest or initiate new processes. The leader does not see deferring to others as a weakness because the truly effective leader embraces relationships, collaboration, and "outside-of-the-box" thinking. Effective leaders exhibit collaborative relationship building by surrounding themselves with people who know more and are more accomplished in their fields (McCullough, 2008). Problem solving and looking at systems that were involved and contributed to the failure without insisting on a strategy that facilitates the return to the old process are leadership problem-resolution styles. Managers are more interested in maintaining the status quo and finding ways to ensure that the reason for the deviance in practice is identified in order to return to the established procedures (Manion, 2005).

Measuring success in managers may be more easily identified than measuring success in leaders. Managers are concerned with adherence to policy and protocol. Measurements are easily defined in terms of productivity, work produced, and meeting deadlines within specified time frames. A collaborative, empowered, and relationship-oriented environment identifies leadership success. To achieve this success, professional employee development needs must be met through ongoing education, coaching, and mentoring. This is time intensive for the leader but builds stronger employee development, enhances collaborative relationships, and promotes confidence and trust for future interactions.

General Leadership Competencies

Although there is debate about innate ability to lead, leadership skills can be learned with opportunity, practice, coaching, and mentoring from strong leaders who understand that leaders can be developed. Character and temperament of the individual learning leadership skills may aid or abet this process. Common core competencies of leaders include emotional intelligence, strong communication skills, the ability to embrace change and chaos, ability to analyze and strategize for maximum impact and effect, and the ability to exhibit transformational leadership by shaping and sharing the vision so that others are motivated to share the long-term vision for the changes it inspires (Grossman & Valiga, 2005).

Freshman and Rubino (2002) include emotional intelligence (EI) as a major component of leadership and management competence in the workplace. EI encompasses the "self" of a leader: self-awareness, self-regulation, and self-motivation along with social awareness and social skills. Emotionally intelligent leaders understand their own strengths and weaknesses, emotions, and motivation. They are able to reflect upon and adapt to changes without becoming impulsive. Emotionally intelligent leaders have an inner motivation to be successful and gain pleasure from their professional passions. They are considerate of others' feelings and have the ability to motivate others toward achieving the desired goal.

Transformational leadership skills include the prerequisite strong verbal and written communication skills to share the vision effectively with others. Transformational leadership skills focus less on the successful completion of a task and more on how the vision of the preferred goal would appear. Although skill attainment may be a natural component of the vision, the motivation to master the skill becomes an internal desire of the follower to become part of the visions rather than attainment of the skill to meet a short-term goal of the leader (Grossman & Valiga, 2005).

Leadership Skills During a Disaster

During a disaster event, rapid changes occur and multiple events may occur simultaneously. Effective disaster plans and efforts do not view these events as separate and distinct events that can be managed by looking at each event separately. As seen in the events following Hurricane Katrina, multiple continued effects from the original primary disaster can occur simultaneously, as when the levies broke during the hurricane. Additional sociological and political events exacerbated the initial effects of physical disaster created by the hurricane. Unexpected and severe flooding from broken levees; loss of hospital infrastructures; inability to effectively evacuate prior to the event and for an extended period of time thereafter; and delayed and limited sanitation, potable water, food, and supplies all combined to create multiple layers of needed disaster response.

Leadership during disasters involves the recognition of uncertainty created during rapidly evolving events and requires flexibility and creative thinking for problem management. Leaders in such situations may influence groups of people who have not been part of the same group before the disaster and who had different expectations prior to the disaster. Inherent limitations in trust and confidence may exist normally between such groups, only to be exacerbated by the disaster.

Leadership and Communication

Although levels of command, job roles, and duties are defined by the ICS structure, leadership may arise from unexpected sources, and clear communication between all levels of authority is obligatory. Even though use of an ICS defines the roles and expectations for various command infrastructure duties, communication must pass vertically between groups and horizontally among similar groups (see Chapters 3 and 9). Leaders must also develop trust from followers by exhibiting and demonstrating attributes that inspire confidence in their leadership's ability to lead and perform.

Leadership competencies during crisis situations have been studied in combat situations. Essential competencies included leadership integrity, knowledge and experience, communicating expectations and goals, demonstration of leadership commitment to the cause, an expectation of success, avoidance of selfish agendas, relationship investment in the followers, and leadership by example (Cohen, 2000). Kolditz evaluated leadership competencies that were essential in crisis-oriented leadership. The traits that were identified build upon the common themes of people-relationship building, confidence of followers in leadership ability to analyze the situation and make goals based on information leading to strategic and creative thinking, and the ability to communicate clearly and effectively. Leadership traits that were identified as critical within crisis situations included strong communication skills, decision-making abilities, ability to motivate and inspire others, ability to plan and execute the plan, assessment skills, use of development skills to grow others, building improvements in groups, and personal growth and development (Kolditz, 2007).

Communications skills are an integral part of every leadership competency regardless of the situation. Leaders must be able to listen thoughtfully to information provided from all levels of command leadership, followers, and the environment cues. Decision-making leadership skills require use of information gathered from multiple sources and the ability to process the information utilizing sound judgment and knowledge, and then clearly communicating decisions or plans to those who will carry out the process. Strong written and verbal communication skills are integral to imparting the plan and expected outcomes throughout the groups.

Motivation and Trust

Motivation during initial disaster response is often dictated by the environment rather than transformational leadership skills. During initial disaster situations, responders are highly motivated to succeed. In some cases, the risk of self-injury, or even death if failure occurs, are extreme motivating factors for followers. In these situations, a hazardous environment will demand that the leader remain extremely focused and ensure that the hazards provide self-motivation for the followers. Intrinsic desire among responders to save and rescue is also a strong motivating influence that the leader can capitalize on. When a disaster is prolonged or rescue progresses to recovery, the leader must be able to maintain motivation and inspire followers to continue.

Trust and confidence in leadership is essential in disaster situations. Leadership gains trust and confidence from followers partially by the role assigned and training for the assigned role. However, the title and training must be supplemented by demonstrating the ability to design and execute plans that are feasible and suitable for the evolving situation. A leader who can demonstrate skills inspires confidence in the followers. Again, honest and clear communication from the leader is required to impart information to enable followers in executing a plan. Sincerity in communication and confidence in what is being communicated by the leader also inspire trust from the followers. Leaders must appear decisive, thoughtful, and confident with the information and resulting plan they present.

Flexibility

The leader must also be able to assess the plan for improvement opportunities and proceed with updated or new information. This is especially important if information was inaccurate or the first attempt with a plan failed. Failure of a plan in part or whole must be rapidly and thoroughly assessed and new goals set. Unexpected obstacles and incomplete or inaccurate information must be reassessed and improvements made. In disaster situations, thoughtful but rapid response is needed and creative thinking is essential. The ability to improvise, remain flexible and adapt to changing situations, and be creative in dealing with problems are leadership skills that are as essential among disaster leadership as coordination, collaboration, and communication skills in structured planning and response plans (Harrald, 2006).

Developing Self and Others

Development of self and others are skills that are instituted and fostered by effective leaders. The effective leader seeks continuous self-improvement and must be comfortable with change and chaos. Often leaders must embrace chaos to adapt and lead during disaster situations, which are constantly evolving events. Although common disaster scenarios can be anticipated and practiced, the real event rarely follows the same planning scenario.

Leaders in disaster situations need to realize they cannot do it all or do it alone. Harrald asserted that leaders must share decision-making and promote growth in others for emergency operations: Plans will fail if emergency managers perform in an isolated environment (Harrald, 2006). Leaders during disasters must invest time and effort to develop followers into novice leaders and novice leaders into experienced leaders. Time and resources are invested with the goal of improving group performance. Ideally, groups that respond to disaster situations have practiced together and know each other's strengths and weaknesses. When placed in unfamiliar situations by the very nature of the disaster event and response, precious time can be lost unless skills are evident and expectations are clear. By promoting leadership development among others, leaders during disasters enhance the ability of the entire group.

Leadership Lessons Learned During Disaster

The near disaster events of the Apollo 13 space flight and the disaster events of the terrorist attacks on September 11, 2001 and response to Hurricanes Katrina and Rita in 2005 provided multiple opportunities for disaster leadership lessons. These events demonstrate leadership decision-making strengths, weaknesses, and opportunities for future improvement. Each of these scenarios exemplifies the evolving nature of disaster events and the need for definitive disaster leadership competencies.

Lessons From Apollo 13

The Apollo 13 space flight in April of 1970 sustained an onboard explosion of the number 2 oxygen tank, subsequent failure of the number 1 tank, and loss of two of the three fuel cells that provided electricity. Cancellation of the planned moon landing was the least of the concerns as the disaster efforts focused on the safe return of the astronauts. During the nearly 6 days before the landing of the Apollo 13 spacecraft, NASA engineers, scientists, and employees worked together to prevent loss of life. The team that assembled to determine how to bring the astronauts home safely demonstrated many of the previously discussed leadership competencies that must be exhibited during a disaster. The team was fully committed to the cause and determined to succeed. Failure was not an option. Internal motivation was high and personal agendas were put aside. Blaming and speculation for how the disaster occurred and who was responsible were not part of the recovery agenda. Creative, positive, and flexible thinking and communication among all team members for solutions exemplified the commitment of the team to find a positive focus and the team's refusal to give up hope despite the enormous damage to the spacecraft's infrastructure.

Following the safe return of the astronauts, a full internal investigation was launched to determine what occurred and how to prevent a similar occurrence in the future. As is typical of many root cause analysis investigations, multiple areas of system process and breakdown were discovered and remediated prior to the launch of Apollo 14 (NASA, 1970). Willingness to investigate thoroughly and completely and revise plans based on the findings is characteristic of leadership activities.

Lessons From September 11, 2001

The events of September 11, 2001, demonstrated leadership skill strengths and weaknesses related to disaster planning, preparation, and execution of plans. The attack on the Word Trade Centers in New York and the Pentagon in Washington, DC, along with the aborted terrorist plans when United Airlines Flight 93 crashed in Pennsylvania, demonstrated that the United States was a vulnerable target for terrorist activities. Despite the horror and tragic loss of life, leadership skills that exemplified teamwork, interagency collaboration, creative thinking, and communication were evident. In New York City, a massive deployment of staff and supplies from New York fire and police departments, including emergency medical technicians and off-duty employees, descended upon the scene for rescue operations. Evacuation procedures were immediately implemented within the towers although the fall of the towers resulted in a large number of civilian and rescue worker deaths.

Interagency communication failures were present in New York and exemplified the need for both common English communication skills and the ability to communicate between agencies (such as between fire, police departments, and the New York Port Authority, as well as the fire department and 911 centers for communication of the situation). Malfunctioning fire department communication systems prevented timely notification to firefighters engaged in rescue operations to evacuate buildings that were ready to collapse. Based on these experiences, the critical need for communication resources, common language communication, and communication center resources and responsibilities were identified (National Commission on Terrorist Attacks Upon the United States, 2004).

Lessons From the Pentagon Attack

The attack on the Pentagon also brought disaster plans into effect at area hospitals. It was a clear reminder that disaster planning and preparation are instrumental in dealing with disaster situations. Communications at Georgetown University Hospital were stretched to their limits. Telephones and cell phones were overwhelmed and backup systems were employed to distribute information. Georgetown University Hospital leadership implemented several communication strategies to receive and provide accurate information to staff and the community regarding the events. E-mail communication with situation updates, creation of three disaster lines to facilitate communication for families looking for missing or injured members, employees who needed information about disaster plan activation activities, and one for medical staff communication were all examples of systems that needed planning for and backup if they failed. The hospital Web page was updated regularly with readiness information for the community and staff members. Personal rounds by hospital administration to all departments and regular briefing sessions for hospital management enhanced trust and confidence in hospital leadership (Johnson, 2002). Accurate communication during a disaster situation inspires confidence and personal involvement of identified leadership staff exemplifies the expectations for relationship investment in the followers and leadership by example (Cohen, 2000).

Lessons From Flight 93

The aborted terrorist attack involving Flight 93 demonstrated a group commitment to a cause and probable teamwork to achieve the end result. Messages from the passengers, received prior to the crash, seemed to indicate knowledge of the eventual outcome of further loss of life and property and a commitment and collective agreement to stop the process even if it meant their own imminent demise. Leaders in this process were not part of disaster preparation and planning scenarios. These leaders arose from among the victims to meet the situation, and they were able to convince others to do something, with the possibility of personal loss of life, to prevent further terrorist attacks. From this example, it is clear to see that leadership does not necessarily come from persons invested with official authority but can be present in individuals who respond to meet a challenge.

Learning From History

Despite calls for disaster preparedness after the 9/11 disasters, many elements of disaster planning, preparedness, and responses remained primarily theoretical and untested except in small-scale events prior to Hurricane Katrina in 2005 (Crippen, 2006). Unlike many disaster events, Hurricane Katrina was anticipated and monitored for days prior to arrival. Despite preparation and planning by multiple local, state, and federal agencies, including healthcare facilities, disaster plans proved inadequate and ineffective during the evolving crisis.

The effects of Hurricane Katrina were publicized and media documented the unfolding events to millions of homes in a way that no disaster had ever been monitored before. We clearly saw the breakdown in communication between local, state, and federal officials and agencies that delivered conflicting and inaccurate reports of the disaster potential and effects to the public, provided conflicting information for evacuation processes and locations, and that provided inaccurate reports for when supplies and additional manpower would arrive. Trust in leadership at all levels was lacking; the community felt abandoned and unprepared (U.S. House Select Bipartisan Committee, 2006a). Disaster planning and preparation also did not take into account the magnitude of psychological and sociological effects of displaced and evacuated victims and the effects on the cities that accepted them (Crippen, 2006).

Personal disaster planning by those facing Katrina, and other disasters, was and is limited in many cases. Despite disaster drill exercises in 2004 that portrayed the effects of a Category 3 hurricane in the New Orleans area, few agencies and community residents were prepared for the magnitude of such a disaster. Local, state, and federal agencies had not revised their plans despite gaps in preparation and interagency communication failures that were identified during the drill (U.S. House Select Bipartisan Committee, 2006b). Many in New Orleans were unable to evacuate safely and effectively because of a lack of accessible transportation. Those who stayed in their homes found drinking water, food, sanitation, and medical supplies and assistance in short supply and, in some cases, inaccessible owing to direct damage from Hurricane Katrina or secondary damage, such as flooding from disrupted levees, downed trees, and erosion of roads that prevented establishment of effective supply routes.

Despite the damage; lack of accurate communication; inadequate disaster planning, preparation, and response; and loss of trust in authority, Hurricane Katrina still provided an opportunity to demonstrate positive leadership competencies. Imaginative thinking was essential for responders and healthcare providers. Rescue and evacuation operations frequently required nontraditional methods of extrications by boat and helicopter. Deployment of the Louis Armstrong International Airport in New Orleans as the primary evacuation center for New Orleans required creative command strategies for a workforce that would be overwhelmed with patients and limited supplies.

Klein and Nagle (2007) described innovative procedures utilized by Disaster Medical Assistance Teams (DMATs) at the airport. Despite challenges induced by weather and limited emergency power electricity and utility systems, lack of sanitation, severely inadequate supplies to treat victims, lack of effective evacuation plans for victims and staff, and a nearly complete failure of intelligence and communication systems with the New Orleans command center, these teams managed to think creatively during the situation. Collaborative discussions among team members and identified team leadership determined that a field hospital would be established and patients treated to the best of DMAT team's ability. DMAT medical tents were erected inside the building using the skylights as a light source instead of the outside tarmac area that was heavily impacted by weather conditions and helicopter transports of evacuees. As field conditions changed, concepts were changed or abandoned to meet the evolving conditions. Staffing in various areas was adjusted based on the need of the evacuees and the ability of staff to tolerate conditions in various areas caused by overcrowding and lack of sanitation.

Rapid planning and implementation for medical care of evacuees in the Houston Astrodome and Hurricane Rita preparations immediately thereafter demonstrated many of the best practice leadership competencies, and that lessons were finally being learned. Mattox thoroughly detailed the preparation and implementation procedures for both events (Mattox, 2005). The success of the initial venture to screen Hurricane Katrina evacuees, provide a triage area for each sleeping area of 25,000 people, inspect food, and establish a fully operational clinic with most medical subspecialties and access to laboratory and radiology services provided ample background experience to rapidly prepare for Hurricane Rita evacuees. Due to previous collaborative relationships, work groups were set up rapidly, given assignments, a brief implementation time and the expectation that failure was unacceptable. Within 12 hours the clinic for Hurricane Rita victims was in place (Mattox).

Keys to the success of this program included mutual cooperation among team members to meet the goal, existing collaborative relationships and networks of the Harris County Hospital District, resources provided by area hospitals for patients whose needs exceeded the ability of the clinic resources, and vendor mutual aid to provide equipment and supplies to meet the needs of the clinic. Provisions for the care, including the mental heath of the leadership and incident command group, were included in the planning (Mattox, 2005).

This same group exemplified transformational leadership with the evacuees. From the beginning, the command staff identified that the clinic and shelter could not continue indefinitely and an exit plan was part of the strategic implementation. According to Mattox, the clinic and shelter exit plan target dates and indicators were provided to the media, collaborative partners, and, more importantly, to the evacuees (Mattox, 2005). Housing, employment, and educational opportunities were provided to assist with implementation of the exit strategy. Additional leadership best-practices included having an official member of the medical group present at all media conferences to ensure correct and accurate information was provided and misinformation from less informed personnel was minimized. Plans were changed multiple times in response to changing conditions and best-leadership practices endorsed the ability to evolve based on changing circumstances. As obstacles were identified, they were addressed and measures were undertaken in a collaborative mode to facilitate the intended outcomes.

Based on the success of the clinic at the Houston Astrodome and lessons learned from the evacuation of Gulf Coast residents during Hurricane Katrina, the Galveston-Houston area was able to revise plans and planning to meet the needs of Hurricane Rita evacuees. Public information, allocation of resources and shelters in an area already saturated with Hurricane Katrina evacuees, and realization that large volumes of people cannot be rapidly evacuated by private automobiles in less than several days, provided the foundation to adjust disaster preparations and plans as needed. Incorporating best-practices and a willingness to revise plans and actions are leadership imperatives.

Conclusion

Effective leadership skills involve relationship building, transformational leadership styles to communicate the vision, communicating clearly and effectively, flexibility to adapt as disaster conditions dictate, mentoring others in leadership opportunities, and emotional intelligence. These skills are the basis of disaster leadership. Creative problem solving, ensuring collaboration to meet identified goals, and horizontal and vertical communications strategies enhance disaster leadership. Communication skills are critical in disaster scenarios to promote positive outcomes. Communication and creativity to address and successfully mitigate problems inspire confidence in followers and communities affected by disasters.

References

Cohen, W. (2000). *The new art of the leader: Leading with integrity and honor.* Paramus, NJ: Prentice Hall.

Crippen, D. (2006). Concluding thoughts on the new nature of disaster management. *Critical Care, (10)*1, 111.

Freshman, B., & Rubino, L. (2002). Emotional intelligence: A core competency for health care administrators. *Health Care Manager, 20*(4), 1–9.

Gratton, L., & Erickson, T. (2007, November). Ways to build collaborative teams. *Harvard Business Review,* 100–109.

Grossman, S., & Valiga, T., (2005). *The new leadership challenge: Creating the future of nursing* (2nd ed.). Philadelphia: F. A. Davis.

Harrald, J. (2006). Agility and discipline: Critical success factors for disaster response. *Annals of the American Academy of Political and Social Science, 604*(2), 256–272.

Johnson, J. (2002). Leadership in a time of disaster: Being prepared for New Age threats. *Journal of Nursing Administration, 32*(9), 455–460.

Klein, K., & Nagle, N. (2007). Mass medical evacuation: Hurricane Katrina and nursing experiences at the New Orleans Airport [Electronic version]. *Disaster Management & Response, (5)*2, 56–61.

Kolditz, T. (2007). *In extremis leadership: Leading as if your life depended on it* (J-B Leader to Leader Institute/PF Drucker Foundation). San Francisco: Jossey-Bass.

Manion, J. (2005). *From management to leadership* (2nd ed.). San Francisco: Jossey-Bass.

Mattox, K. (2005). Hurricanes Katrina and Rita: Role of individuals and collaborative networks in mobilizing/coordinating societal and professional resources for major disasters. *Critical Care, 10*(1), 1–6.

McCullough, D. (2008, March). Different voice: Timeless leadership. *Harvard Business Review,* 45–49.

National Aeronautics and Space Administration (NASA). (1970). *Apollo 13 review board (Cortright Commission).* Retrieved March 3, 2008, from http://history.nasa.gov/ap13rb/ch5.pdf

National Commission on Terrorist Attacks Upon the United States. (2004). *9-11 commission report.* Retrieved March 2, 2008, from http://govinfo.library.unt.edu/911/report/911Report_Ch9.pdf

U.S. House Select Bipartisan Committee to Investigate the Preparation for and Response to Hurricane Katrina. (2006a). *A failure of initiative: The final report of the US House Select Bipartisan Committee to Investigate the Preparation for and Response to Hurricane Katrina, 109th Congress.* Retrieved March 2, 2008, from http://a257.g.akamaitech.net/7/257/2422/15feb20061230/www.gpoaccess.gov/katrinareport/communications.pdf

U.S. House Select Bipartisan Committee to Investigate the Preparation for and Response to Hurricane Katrina (2006b). *A failure of initiative: The final report of the U.S. House Select Bipartisan Committee to Investigate the Preparation for and Response to Hurricane Katrina, 109th Congress.* Retrieved March 2, 2008, from http://a257.g.akamaitech.net/7/257/2422/15feb20061230/www.gpoaccess.gov/katrinareport/hurricanepam.pdf

chapter 5

Special Populations in Disasters: The Child and Pregnant Woman

Josephine DeVito and Maryann Godshall

Key Terms

- Pregnancy
- Cardiovascular changes in pregnancy
- Pregnant women's disaster needs
- Assessing the pregnant woman in a disaster
- Assessing the fetus in a disaster
- Growth and development
- Assessing the child in a disaster
- Physiological differences between children and adults
- Communication with children
- Special pediatric disaster equipment needs
- Infectious diseases in a disaster
- Terrorism-induced trauma in children

GOAL

The goal of this chapter is to present disaster nursing knowledge and skills needed in dealing with the pregnant mother and children.

OBJECTIVES

At the completion of this chapter, the reader will:

1. Understand the special needs of the pregnant woman in a disaster situation.
2. Assess the pregnant mother in a disaster situation.
3. Describe the various physiological changes in the pregnant woman that change disaster nursing care interventions.
4. Describe pathophysiological changes in the pregnant woman that need special care in a disaster.
5. List special needs in caring for a child in a disaster.

OBJECTIVES *(continued)*

6. List physiological differences to consider in a disaster between an adult and child.
7. Define special psychological needs children dealing with disasters have.
8. Be able to adapt communication styles to various age groups.
9. Classify the different equipment needed in caring for the child in a disaster.
10. Assess for terrorism-induced trauma in a child.

Introduction

In Chapters 5 and 6, special populations and how to work with them in a disaster is presented. Special populations are groups whose needs are not fully addressed by traditional service providers or who feel they cannot comfortably or safely access and use the standard resources offered in disaster preparedness, relief, and recovery. They include, but are not limited to, those who are physically or mentally disabled (e.g., blind, deaf, hard-of-hearing, cognitive disorders, and mobility limitations), have limited or non-English speaking skills, are geographically or culturally isolated, may be medically or chemically dependent, are homeless, frail, elderly, or children. These populations all have special needs that the disaster nurse must consider when providing disaster healthcare relief.

This chapter will begin with a look at the pregnant woman and her special needs. Then children and how they respond to disasters will be addressed. Chapter 6 will cover the elderly and people with disabilities.

Pregnant Women's Disaster Needs

When a woman becomes pregnant, she goes through a spectrum of changes that are both physiological and psychological. Under the best of conditions and circumstances, pregnancy is considered both a crisis and a challenge. It is a crisis because it represents a change in lifestyle for women. For the adult pregnant woman, this may indicate an alteration in how she views herself and the world around her. Some women become more interested in the future and environmental conditions that will affect not only themselves but their unborn child. Adolescent pregnant women have their own crises to overcome as they emerge into the world of adulthood while struggling to find their identity as individuals. For both adult and adolescent pregnant women, this time is also a challenge because of the changes that will take place in their worlds, such as employment, social networking activities, and freedom to do what they want when they want to.

When a disaster occurs on top of a pregnancy, the needs and challenges for pregnancy become more complicated. Planning and management of conditions that may involve casualties or immediate action need assessing according to the specific type of disaster that may be present. For example, if a disaster occurs that involves explosives resulting in injuries caused by gases or fallout of debris (e.g., C-4, Semtex, nitroglycerin, and dynamite), this demands immediate nursing assessment (Langan & James, 2005). Organ damage may occur to the respiratory system, GI tract, and cardiovascular systems. Exposure to chemicals and gas explosions will add to the woman's already overtaxed physiology during pregnancy. Debris and bomb fragments may lead to threats to safety which include, but are not limited to, head injuries, concussions, abdominal hemorrhage, and ear or eye ruptures resulting in hearing and visual deficits.

Assessment of Pregnant Women During a Disaster

When a woman becomes pregnant, in addition to changes that occur in each body system that are needed to support as well as sustain the pregnancy, there are psychosocial adjustments the mother-to-be goes through within the three different trimesters of pregnancy. It is important that healthcare professionals know these psychological and physiological changes and document the pregnant women's responses during a disaster. The following sections will discuss some of the important issues for disaster nurses to consider when caring for the pregnant woman in a disaster.

Cardiovascular System

In the cardiovascular system, changes in heart size and position and increases in blood volume and cardiac output contribute to auscultatory changes common in pregnancy. Audible splitting of S1, S2, and even S3 heart sounds may be detected at 20 weeks gestation. Systolic and diastolic murmurs may be heard over the pulmonic areas of the heart. These changes may be transient and disappear shortly after a women gives birth. At about 20 weeks gestation, the mother's pulse increases about 15 beats and remains that fast until term. It is not uncommon, also, to detect palpations at this time. For multiple gestations, the maternal heart rate increases significantly in the third trimester (Malone & D'Alton, 2004).

Complications to the cardiovascular system of a pregnant woman that may arise from the trauma of a disaster can include hypertensive disorders of pregnancy. Hypertensive disorders normally complicate approximately 8% of all pregnancies and are the most common medical complication reported during pregnancy (Martin et al., 2005). In the United States, hypertension in pregnancy is the second leading cause of maternal and perinatal morbidity and mortality (Peters & Flack, 2004). Hypertensive disorders predispose the woman to serious complications, including abruptio placenta, thrombocytopenia, disseminated intravascular coagulation (DIC), acute renal failure, hepatic failure, pulmonary edema, respiratory distress syndrome, aspiration pneumonia, and cerebral hemorrhage (Zhang, Meikle, & Trumble, 2003). Classifications of hypertensive states of pregnancy (Lowdermilk & Perry, 2007) are shown in Table 5-1.

In the nursing assessment of the cardiovascular system, it is very important to catch any early signs of these hypertensive states and intervene accordingly. Nursing assessment includes monitoring the pregnant woman's blood pressure, watching for a systolic of 140 mmHg or higher and a diastolic of 90 mmHg or higher; checking her radial pulse; and listening to heart sounds. If possible, monitoring her intake and output is also important, in order to maintain adequate fluid levels. Other signs and symptoms to watch for include the presence of a headache that is persistent or severe; visual problems such as blurred vision, photophobia, and blind spots; irritability or changes in affect; and epigastric pain.

Supine hypotension, also known as vena cava syndrome, commonly is seen in pregnant women and occurs when there is a fall in blood pressure caused by impaired venous return when the pregnant uterus presses on the ascending vena cava. This

TABLE 5-1 CLASSIFICATIONS OF HYPERTENSIVE STATES OF PREGNANCY

Hypertensive State	Definition
Gestational hypertension	Blood pressure elevated for the first time after 20 weeks gestation without proteinuria
Transient hypertension	Gestational hypertension with no signs of preeclampsia present at the time of birth, and hypertension resolves by 12 weeks postpartum
Preeclampsia	Occurs after 20 weeks gestation and is determined by gestational hypertension plus proteinuria
Eclampsia	Occurrence of seizures in a woman with preeclampsia that cannot be attributed to other causes
Chronic hypertension	Hypertension that is present before pregnancy or diagnosed before 20 weeks gestation

Source: Adapted from Lowdermilk & Perry, 2007.

occurs when the pregnant woman is lying on her back. In addition to the drop in blood pressure, the disaster nurse may assess additional signs and symptoms of pallor, dizziness, faintness, breathlessness, tachycardia, nausea, clammy skin, and sweating (Lowdermilk & Perry, 2007). The immediate nursing action is to place the mother on her left side so the uterus is off of the ascending vena cava. This action should stabilize her vital signs and additional symptoms.

Vaginal Bleeding

When caring for the pregnant woman in a disaster, awareness of vaginal bleeding and its implications must be considered. Vaginal bleeding may indicate anything from ruptured membranes to abruptio placenta. No matter what the cause, vaginal bleeding is serious, and the pregnant woman should be transported as soon as possible to a hospital. Early pregnancy assessment of bleeding involves confirming the pregnancy; assessing the characteristics of the bleeding (i.e., Is the blood bright or dark red and is the bleeding intermittent or continuous?); defining the characteristics of any pain by type, intensity, and persistence; and checking for any other types of vaginal discharge, such as amniotic fluid.

Late pregnancy assessment of bleeding includes extra assessment techniques related to the expected date of confinement, as well as the possibility of having the mother deliver a viable fetus. As with early signs, the disaster nurse must check the bleeding for quantity and associated pain, look for other types of vaginal discharge, and check for ruptured amniotic membranes. Uterine atony is relaxation of the uterine muscle. If uterine atony is present during the postpartum assessment, the uterus will feel "boggy" instead of firm upon palpation. The disaster nurse needs to massage the uterus so that it will become firm. In addition to massage, oxytocin medications given intravenously may be indicated to assist further in contracting the uterus. This condition needs immediate attention because uterine atony can lead to postpartum hemorrhage. Abdominal pain may indicate internal abdominal organ or uterine ruptures, as well as abdominal bleeding.

The disaster nurse also needs to consider fetal status and viability, as well as caring for the mother. For example, what trimester the pregnancy is in influences the care given to the pregnant woman. The needs and concerns of a mother in the first trimester are different from a mother in the second and third trimesters. Any signs of bleeding, headaches, dizziness, and the status of uterine contractions, in addition to any decreased or absence of fetal movement, need to be observed.

As a pregnancy approaches viability, continuous fetal monitoring should be initiated, especially 2 to 6 hours after a trauma. The status of the pregnancy needs to be assessed, which can include an ultrasound to evaluate the placenta, fetus, amniotic fluid volume, and presence of intra-abdominal fluid (American Academy of Pediatrics [AAP], 2002), if these tools are available in the field. A ruptured uterus may occur in a woman who has had a previous cesarean delivery or as a result of a sustained blunt abdominal trauma. The signs and symptoms of a uterine rupture are described in Table 5-2.

An abruptio placenta is a premature separation of a normally implanted placenta from the uterine wall. It is a complication that can be enhanced by women who have experienced severe trauma (Lowdermilk & Perry, 2007). An emergency cesarean-section delivery needs to be performed for neonatal survival, a procedure that is, at the best of times, difficult and, in a disaster, a serious intervention to undertake. Symptoms of an abruptio placenta may include dark, vaginal bleeding that may be bright or absent in concealed abruption; severe abdominal pain; a firm, tender uterus; shock, with blood loss; and contractions.

Other Considerations

When pregnant, a women's susceptibility to infections is altered. Progesterone, the hormone of pregnancy, which relaxes smooth muscle, also relaxes the respiratory tract. This leads to stasis of secretions and provides an environment for increased bacterial growth in the respiratory tract (White, Henretig, & Dukes, 2002). This makes the mother more at risk for infections because of alterations in the immune system that are under the influence of the pregnancy hormones.

An additional consideration for pregnant women is vaccination. When caring for a pregnant woman after a disaster that involves a terrorist attack including biologic agents such as smallpox and anthrax, it is not recommended to immunize women during pregnancy. However, there is a debate as to whether to immunize pregnant women if a release of a biological agent is confirmed or suspected. If the

TABLE 5-2 SIGNS AND SYMPTOMS OF UTERINE RUPTURE

Assessment Area	Signs and Symptoms of Concern
Fetal heart rate (FHR)	Nonreassuring pattern as a result of: 1. Impairment of fetal oxygenation 2. Late decelerations, reduced variability, tachycardia, or bradycardia Sudden, abrupt decrease in FHR
Pain	Uterine abdominal pain Chest pain between scapulae or on inspiration as a result of irritation of blood flow below the diaphragm
Lochia discharge	"Boggy"-feeling uterus, not contracted Increased vaginal bleeding Hypovolemic shock from hemorrhage

Source: Adapted from Cunningham et al., 2001.

woman or her fetus contracts these diseases, significant morbidity and mortality to both patients can occur (Langan & James, 2005).

Previous research has documented that, during pregnancy, there is an increased susceptibility to variola infection with greater severity of illness due to changes in the mother's immune system. Maternal mortality may be as high as 50%, compared with 30% for nonpregnant women. When infection occurs during the first trimester, there is more likely to be a fetal loss. If the infection occurs during the last trimesters of pregnancy it may contribute to an increase in premature birth (White et al., 2002). Therefore, there is still some debate about the advisability of giving a pregnant woman vaccinations. Some recommendations are not in debate. For example, because smallpox is a live virus, vaccination is not recommended for pregnant women (Centers for Disease Control and Prevention [CDC], 2003). There are risks associated with this vaccine for the fetus.

Anthrax is another biological agent with very little research available for pregnant women. Recommendations by the AAP and American College of Obstetrics and Gynecology (ACOG) for pregnant women who may be exposed are to use ciprofloxacin (AAP & ACOG, 2002). If the strain of anthrax is susceptible to penicillin then amoxicillin may be used. If doxycycline is prescribed during pregnancy, the effects on the fetus are not fully understood (Langan & James, 2005). Caution also needs to be exercised in women who are breastfeeding because all of these medications are excreted in the breast milk.

Langan and James (2005) suggested recommendations for pregnant women who are involved in bioterrorism or disasters. Their suggestion was that pregnant women need to have available:

- A copy of prenatal records with updated information
- Emergency numbers for family and healthcare providers
- An emergency birth kit put together under the direction of the healthcare provider
- Ready-to-feed formula, not powdered or concentrated formulas because the water supply may be contaminated
- A disaster supply kit containing items recommended by the AAP and ACOG or American Red Cross (ARC) (AAP & ACOG, 2002; ARC, 2004)

Children and Disasters

None of us like to think about what we will need to do as nurses should a disaster occur. However, disasters, natural and man-made, do occur, and it is vital to have a plan. The focus of this section of the chapter is to examine disaster preparedness particularly for children.

Children are the most precious gifts of our life, yet are most vulnerable. This is especially so in the event of a natural or man-made disaster. Children, particularly those under 5, usually bear the brunt of the death toll associated with complex emergencies. According to a report in the JAMA of all of those who died in the 1991 Kurdish refugee crisis, two thirds were children (JAMA, 1993, as cited in Burton, 2006). The *Lancet* reported that during the 1992 Somali famine, 74% of the children under age 5 that were displaced into refugee camps died. The *Lancet* also reported that in 1996, 54% of all deaths among Rwanda and Burundi refugees who fled to eastern Zaire were under the age of 5. In today's conflicts, there is no change in that statistic. Children under 18 represented 39% of the overall population of the eight countries hardest hit by the December 2004 tsunami (Burton).

According to the National Center for Missing and Exploited Children (2006), it took 6 months to track down the 5,192 missing or displaced children reported to the center as a result of Hurricanes Katrina and Rita. In the months following Katrina, the agency received reports of 4,710 children missing or displaced in Louisiana, 339 in Mississippi, and 39 in Alabama. After Rita, another 28 children were reported missing or displaced in Louisiana; 76 were reported in Texas. The number of children reported displaced or missing from their families during Hurricane Katrina was 5,088. The good news is that all of them were reunited with their families or guardians, but it took time to find and reunite them. These are just some of the scenarios experienced by children during recent disasters. We must do better in planning for these disasters and in particular, include the children into our disaster plans.

Gaps in pediatric disaster preparedness suggested by Fox and Timm are that first responders have not been educated on how to care for children exposed to chemical agents, missing recommendations for medications and antidotes used in a disaster situation, and absence of required disaster drills and pediatric disaster life support training for first responders (Fox & Timm, 2008). This was found in the aftermath of Hurricane Katrina when the response was unorganized and inappropriate care delivery to children that was compounded by the disaster situation.

Make a Plan

Everyone has heard that the best defense is a great offense. Preparation for caring for children in a disaster is a must. Disaster checklists and entire pediatric disaster triage algorithms and tools are available online. One such tool is called the JumpSTART Pediatric MCI Triage Tool, available for free from http://www.jumpstarttriage.com. This Web site also holds training footage for initial relief workers. This is also available in other languages such as Spanish, Italian, French, and Japanese. A federally coordinated system is available at http://www.ndms.dhhs.gov. Information about setting up a kit, making a disaster plan, and staying informed is available at http://www.redcross.org. A video MP3 file is available for viewing and teaching purposes.

Disaster Planning and Children

The key to disaster planning and postdisaster care for children is to keep the plan family-centered. Family-centered care is a type of care that realizes that the family is the main force or center of a child's life and world and thereby includes the family in the care of the child. This should be the focus of caring for a child in a disaster shelter, in the hospital, or in other disaster care situations. The key is to keep the family together. This consideration must be made during a disaster, triage, and post-disaster. The triage person needs to send the family unit to a facility for care. Choosing the appropriate facility should not take time if a plan is made ahead of time. For example, if the entire family is injured, send the entire family unit to a facility that has both adult and pediatric specialties. If possible, sending the entire family with an injured child is also recommended.

Caring for the Whole Family

The family unit is the strongest unit of survival. It makes sense to keep families together. Whenever possible, shelter and evacuate families together. Because families may get separated, include reunification in the disaster plan (Romig, 2008). It is also important to consider what constitutes a "family" for each child. A family or caregiver can be a biological parent, an adopted or foster parent, a grandparent, or other relative or close neighbor. Take the time to figure out who is the central figure or caregiver in the child's life. It is also very important to keep siblings together if possible. Unique relationships are formed between siblings and, in particular, twins, triplets, or other multiple birth children. These siblings can be a source of support for each other during stressful times.

Caring for the child without caregivers can be very time- and resource-consuming. An individual will need to be assigned to each child to keep him or her safe. If cribs with side rails are not available, placing infants and children on adult stretchers, cots, or beds is very dangerous. If the family is kept together, the family can help care for and maintain safety for their children. This will free other disaster personnel for other tasks to be done and is another reason why keeping the family together makes sense.

Also consider that disaster shelters need to be family-friendly. They should be safe as well as functional. They should be smoke-, drug-, and alcohol-free. The shelter should be childproofed as much as possible. Any disaster recovery center needs communication resources, child care and/or supervision, internal and external security, and the ability to isolate children from disturbing situations (Romig, 2008).

Consider what disaster supplies are needed for children. What will they drink? What will they eat? How can foods that may be a choking hazard be avoided? How will they go to the bathroom? Are they wearing diapers? How will the diapers be disposed of and where? Some of these issues may lead to causing a secondary environmental hazard from improper disposal of human waste. Diapers, formula, bottles, and infant food need to be accounted for in the plan, including biohazard disposal.

Those who are diabetic need to dispose of their needles, lancets, or wound dressings accordingly (Romig, 2008).

Children are also dependent on daily routines. They wake up, eat breakfast, go to school, play with friends, and come home. When this routine is disrupted during a disaster they become very anxious. They will look to adults for help. How a person responds to the disaster determines how the child responds. If the adults are stressed and anxious, the child will become the same. If the adults respond with a sense of alarm, the child will become even more afraid. During a disaster a child is most fearful that the event will happen again, someone will be killed or injured, he or she will be separated from family members, or he or she will be left alone (American Red Cross, 2008). It is up to the disaster nurse to remain calm, keep children with their families, and never leave a child alone.

Children are easily bored. They will not sit quietly for prolonged periods of time. They understand life through play. Play items need to be included in disaster shelters and, if there is room, disaster pediatric jump kits. Simple items such as paper, markers, games, and toys can keep a child content for extended periods of time. Some ideas are available at the Federal Emergency Management Agency (FEMA) Web site http://www.fema.gov/kidsgames1.htm and at http://www.fema.gov/kids/littleones.htm or from the National Weather Service Office of Climate, Water, and Weather Services (NOAA) http://www.nws.noaa.gov/os/brochures.shtml. Be sure to include age-appropriate toys, and be aware of potential issues such as potential choking hazards from small toys (Romig, 2008).

Pets During a Disaster

Pets in some families are often considered a member of the family. It is very stressful for a child to leave a pet behind, so provisions must be made for pets as well. The American Veterinarian Association (AVA) suggests taking pets with the family in a disaster. Most disaster shelters will not accept pets, though helping animals are accepted. If this is the case, find out if area motels will allow pets. Pets often need to be crated to stay in disaster shelters and motels. They also need a food and water supply. The AVA has a brochure about rescuing pets when rescuing families. The brochure is available from http://www.avma.org/disaster/saving_family_brochure.pdf. Suggestions are given on how to care for small animals, amphibians, household pets, and large animals in a disaster.

Emergency Services Personnel and System

Although the emergency medical system (EMS) is composed of ambulance units and trained emergency medical personnel who are primary responders during a disaster, in some communities this system is part of a larger fire department. In other communities, it is a separate organization. Each local EMS department has a medical director who establishes protocols. This director interacts with local emergency departments and trauma centers to coordinate the care of all patients needing transport to these facilities. In 1984, the federal government enacted legislation to include children with special needs into the overall plan (Ball & Bindler, 2006).

Children are not little adults. They have different physiological needs, and their bodies respond differently to emergency situations. Developmental levels must be considered when interacting with children who are hurt and frightened. Small children cannot or will not be able to verbally communicate their past medical histories. They are entirely dependent on their caregivers to provide care for them and communicate their needs when they are in these vulnerable situations. The disaster responders and disaster nurses will be complete strangers to them making providing care in an already scary situation that much harder to deliver.

The small size of children must also be considered so that pediatric-sized equipment is available. EMS providers need additional training to assess and interact with scared children, recognize signs of injury so that proper care can be provided to the child, and use the emergency equipment properly. Plans to transport children to facilities with pediatric-trained personnel must also be considered (Ball & Bindler, 2006).

Physiological Differences in Children

Because children do not respond physiologically to healthcare problems as adults do, special considerations are needed by the disaster nurse in caring for the child (Figure 5-1). A child's head is proportionately larger than an adult's in relation to body size, which predisposes children to head injuries. The cervical area is the most frequently injured area of the neck in children, and children have thinner cranial bones. In infants, fontanels may not yet be closed, leaving them more vulnerable to head trauma. Pediatric cranial vessels are thinner than in adults, which makes children more susceptible to shearing and tearing injuries. This kind of injury was evident in the Oklahoma City bombing where the explosive trauma increased the incidence of head injury (Fendya, Vanore, & Perks, 2006).

Nerve conduction differs in children, and myelination is immature. This difference means that toxic or nerve agents that children might be exposed to would affect them differently from adults. Airways are different in children, too. The child's tongue is larger and could become an airway obstruction if it were to swell. Ventilation is different in children, because they usually breathe through their noses as compared to the nose and mouth for adults. The oxygen demand of a child is two times greater than an adult's (i.e., 6–8 L/min compared to 4 L/min). Therefore hypoxemia can happen very quickly.

A child has 80 ml/kg of circulating blood volume as compared to the 65 ml/kg of an adult; thus, hypovolemia is a frequent problem in children, but with their strong hearts they will compensate by increasing heart rate and constricting peripheral vasculature until a volume loss of 31–40% will finally cause a drop in blood pressure. The child's liver and spleen are large and essentially unprotected by the thorax. The skin is thinner and more susceptible to changes in temperature, electrolytes, and burns. Children will also suffer hypothermia more easily than adults: If the

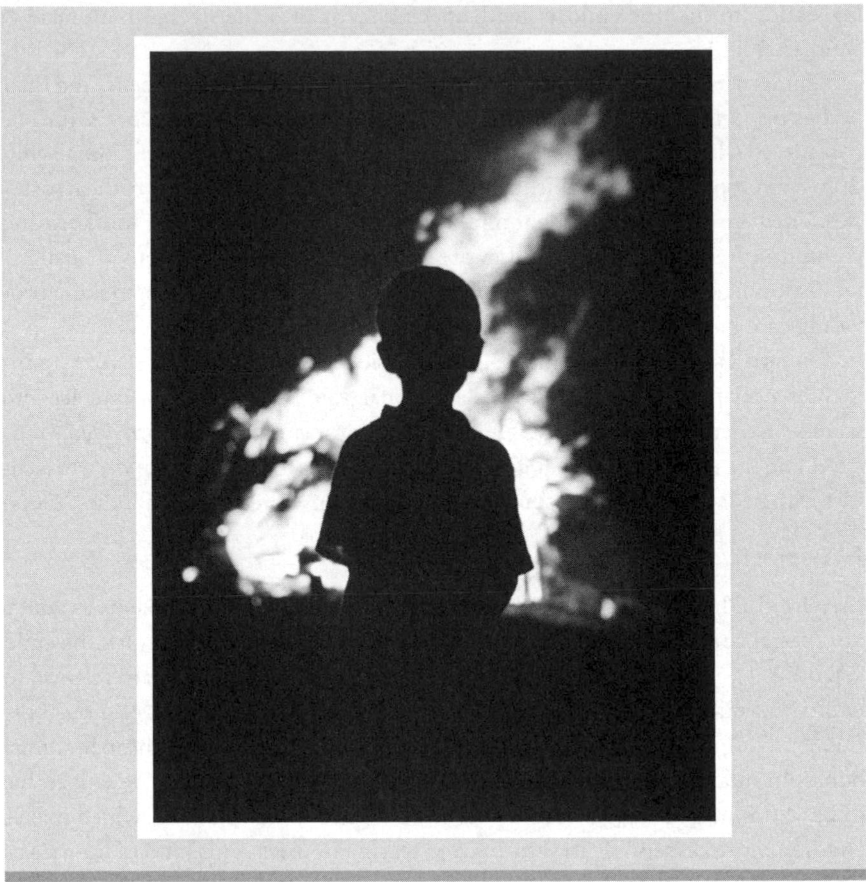

Figure 5-1 Because children do not respond physiologically to healthcare problems as adults do, special considerations are needed by the disaster nurse in caring for the child. *Source:* © Evgeni Gitlits/ShutterStock, Inc.

child is exposed to a toxic agent and needs decontamination, warm water must be used to maintain temperature. The Agency for Healthcare Research and Quality has developed a free DVD, *The Decontamination of Children*, available upon request at http://www.ahrq.gov/research/decontam.htm#Clip.

In addition to physiological differences, children seldom carry personal identification, which makes it difficult to identify a child. Children of younger ages are also noncommunicative, some may be unable to provide identification, and children who can may be too anxious or scared to do so (Ginter et al., 2006). These considerations are important when the disaster nurse provides care for the child.

Children's Responses to Disasters

There are a multitude of types of disasters that could occur each and every day. Natural disasters such as hurricanes and floods, to acts of terrorism at the local school or from an international force need to be considered. Children typically have special vulnerabilities due to their developmental ability and cognitive levels. These may interfere with their ability to both recognize danger and hamper their ability to escape from apparent danger.

Psychological Responses

Children also have unique psychological vulnerabilities. An adapted list from Ball and Bindler (2006) is provided in Table 5-3. The list contains considerations the disaster nurse must take into account when dealing with the impact of a disaster on a child's mental health.

It is also important to understand that children respond to disasters differently according to their age group. Table 5-4 is a list of responses by age group.

A child's reaction to disaster depends on basically how much destruction or loss they have seen. If a family member, friend, teacher, and/or pet has been lost, injured, or killed, or if the child's home, school, or neighborhood has been damaged, there is a greater chance that the child will experience adjustment difficulties. The other factor is the child's age. The most common reactions seen in children mirror that in other circumstances where stress and separation are present. To help children deal with a disaster, the disaster nurse must pay attention to the range of psychosocial responses. Infants, for example, will show signs of anxiety that reflect the anxiety or stress levels of the ones who care for them. Infants may also show signs of regression if they are separated from their parents. Toddlers are affected by the stress of the

TABLE 5-3 CONSIDERATIONS OF DISASTER ON CHILDREN'S MENTAL HEALTH

1. Children have fewer coping skills to help deal with witnessing injuries of others and disasters.
2. Children's understanding may be limited owing to cognitive ability and level.
3. Fear and anxiety are heightened in situations of hoaxes, actual incidents, and associated media coverage. Children feel the fear and anxiety of their parents. They become more fearful after an accident thinking that it may happen again. They fear someone will die or that they will become separated from their family and be left alone. Seeing the events again on television heightens their fear because they may actually believe the incident is happening again.
4. The disruption of normal life patterns is very fearful and stress provoking. This is especially so if the disruption is prolonged.
5. The loss of a favorite toy or security object may heighten the fear of the child.
6. Unfamiliarity with new environments may produce fear in the child. This is especially so if they are separated from their family.

Source: Adapted from Ball & Bindler, 2006.

TABLE 5-4 CHILDREN'S RESPONSES TO DISASTER BY AGE GROUP

Age Group	Reactions
Toddlers and preschoolers	- Reaction reflects that of the parent - Regressive behaviors of earlier stages of development - Withdrawal, quiet and subdued - Denial, avoidance, ignoring - Decreased appetite - Vomiting, constipation, diarrhea - Sleep disorders (insomnia, nightmares) - Ticks, shuttering, quietness, muteness - Clinging to caregiver (anxious attachment) - Reenactment by play (thematic play) - Irritability - Fears of new people, places, strangers - Post-traumatic stress disorder
School-age	- Fear, anxiety - Increased hostility with siblings, fighting - Somatic or psychosomatic complaints - Sleep disorders - School problems, inability to concentrate - Social withdrawal - Reenactment by play - Apathy - Decreased interest in peers - Post-traumatic stress disorder
Preadolescents	- Acting out behaviors, increased hostility with siblings, fighting - Displaced anger - Somatic or psychosomatic complaints - Eating disorders - Rebellion, refusal to do chores - Interpersonal difficulties, impaired socialization - Low self-esteem; self-criticism (my fault) - Post-traumatic stress disorder
Adolescents	- Decreased interest in social activity, peers, hobbies, school, which was previously their "world" - Inability to experience pleasure or have fun - Decline in responsible behaviors

(continued)

TABLE 5-4 CHILDREN'S RESPONSES TO DISASTER BY AGE GROUP (Continued)	
Age Group	Reactions
	- Rebellion, behavior problems, displaced anger - Somatic complaints - Eating disorder - Sleep disorder - Change in physical activity - Confusion, lack of concentration - Become "too old, too fast" they develop life-styles too advanced for their chronological age - Low self-esteem; self-criticism (my fault) - Risk-taking behaviors

Source: Adapted from Ball & Bindler, 2006; International Critical Incident Stress Foundation, Inc., 2001.

disaster more intensely if they are separated from their parents. Separation anxiety is most problematic in this stage and can be displayed as crying or screaming when the parent leaves. Toddlers may cling to parents. When in a state of despair, this behavior can be replaced with sadness, depression, or withdrawal. The disaster nurse needs to comfort the child as best as possible and work on reunifying the child with his or her normal caregiver. Preschoolers may regress and become passive. School-age children are better able to comprehend the nature of the events of the disaster. Children in this group fear for their own safety and may have difficulty sleeping and have nightmares. The adolescent understands on a level closer to that of an adult, but the adolescent is also vulnerable and may act out or have negative behaviors as grief reactions (Murray & Ryan-Kuntz, 2006).

When responding to disasters, the disaster nurse should recognize that despite the chaos, remaining calm and trying to maintain or return to normalcy is the key for all children. Disaster nurses need to be familiar with the special needs of children, according to age, developmental level, and cognitive development (Murray & Ryan-Kuntz, 2006). Distraction is an excellent tool. Keep children busy and playing if at all possible. Encourage family time. If children need hospitalization, be sure they are sent to pediatric facilities whenever possible. Nothing is scarier than a child stuck inside an emergency room filled with injured adults and left alone. Allow children a chance to talk about the disaster if they want to. Talking is therapeutic and an important part of healing and the recovery process for people of all ages.

There are screening and assessment tools available for the disaster nurse to use. A good tool is the Child Behavior Checklist, which can be used for children ages 6 to adolescent (Achenbach & Rescorla, 2001). An example of this form can be viewed online and can be purchased for use from http://www.aseba.org/support/SAMPLES/samples.html#forms. The Trauma Symptom Checklist for Children (TSCC) is a self-report tool available for ages 8 to 16 (Briere, 1996). Information pertaining to that scale is available at http://www.swin.edu.au/victims/resources/assessment/ptsd/tscc.html. The Trauma Events Screening Inventory—Child version (TESI-C) is a tool that has children identify and rate the severity of each traumatic event they have experienced and select the one that was most upsetting to them. This event is then used as an index for rating trauma-related symptoms (Cohen, Mannarino, & Deblinger, 2006). A vast array of tools are available; these are just a few.

Children's Understanding of Health and Illness

When caring for children, it is important for disaster nurses to understand how the children perceive health and illness. Children have certain fears that may be exacerbated during a disaster. Common fears include fear of injections, fear of human blood, and fear of being touched by strangers. The focus of nursing care needs to alleviate fears in an extremely fearful situation. Infants after 3 months of age develop a sense of object permanence, which is knowing that an object or person will continue to be there or exist even when not seen, felt, or heard.

The most common stressor for infants is separation anxiety. Infants and toddlers typically display separation anxiety, which is a loud verbal and physical protest when separated from their parent or caregiver. Infants between 6 and 18 months of age may also have stranger anxiety (Ball & Bindler, 2006). Disaster nurses *are* the stranger and remembering that the parent is the center of the infant's universe is paramount when caring for these children. For infants, the suck reflex is naturally comforting. A pacifier is a very soothing and satisfying tool for an infant. Having extra pacifiers available would be of great benefit. Rocking, stroking, and comforting the infant is also very reassuring for the infant. It is obvious that if the child's normal caregiver is not available to do this, extra staff, volunteers, or manpower will be needed to provide these basic needs.

The toddler is the most at risk and perhaps the hardest group to care for, and this is magnified in a disaster. The toddler does not yet have the cognitive ability to understand the situation or separation from the parent. Toddlers protest loudly when their normal caregiver is not present. They do not like having their world contained, and they do not like being confined to small spaces. The toddler will protest loudly if forced to lie down supine. They have fears of pain, the dark, invasive procedures, change, and mutilation (Ball & Bindler, 2006). It is important to keep the caregiver present and keep daily rituals as normal as possible for this age.

The preschooler's greatest fears are of the dark, being alone, and abandonment. They also fear bodily injury or mutilation (Ball & Bindler, 2006). They are very fearful when they wake up in an unfamiliar environment. If an intravenous line or blood studies need to be obtained, they do not like seeing their own blood. If a blood drop is on a sheet or linens, the disaster nurse should cover it, even if it is just with tape, because preschoolers view blood and other body secretions as part of themselves. For example, if their skin is not intact, they fear their body will somehow leak out. Other things the disaster nurse can do are to explain all procedures in simple terms, use topical anesthetics or procedural sedation if possible, and keep a night-light on. In an emergency, a flashlight will do, because the flashlight is something they can hold and control.

The school-age child fears loss of control related to body functions, privacy issues, bodily injury and pain, and has concerns related to death. They fear separation from friends as well as family (Ball & Bindler, 2006). With this group, the disaster nurse should encourage independence and give the child control of any procedures and situations, if possible. Encourage these children to meet and relate to other children.

The adolescent has a preoccupation with body image and appearance. They fear bodily injury or changes in body image, disability, pain, and even death. Loss of control, privacy, and independence are major stressors. The adolescent wants privacy and independence (Ball & Bindler, 2006). The disaster nurse caring for adolescents should allow them to make choices where possible, include them in their plan of care, always explain all procedures, and be truthful. Since peers are important to the adolescent, encourage them to meet others their own age and encourage them to talk about feelings and concerns. Sometimes during a disaster, the adolescent is forced into the role of the adult and they are usually unprepared to deal with that. Remembering that these children are still adolescents and offering them independence will help alleviate their fears and not overwhelm them with responsibility.

Children of all ages need to be protected from traumatic situations and sights. Whenever possible shield them from what is going on around them. All children fear being separated from their parent or caregiver. The support system in place must be maintained whenever possible. Loss of control and privacy is worrisome as well as a fear of pain or invasive procedures. Lastly, fear of bodily injury and disfigurement as well as possible death is real to all children.

How to Communicate with Children

One of the most difficult things for disaster responders and disaster nurses to do is communicate with children when they are not used to working with them. Good communication will foster a sense of trust. It is important to consider the human growth and developmental level of each child when talking with children. Table 5-5 has tips for communicating with children at the appropriate developmental level.

For all children, take time to speak to them. This may be difficult in a disaster situation, but a few minutes of sitting down to speak at the child's eye level and

TABLE 5-5 COMMUNICATION PRINCIPLES BASED ON DEVELOPMENTAL LEVEL

Chronological Age	Interventions for Caring
Infant	• Allow the infant time to warm up to strangers. • Respond to the infant's cries in a timely manner. Use a soft calming voice. • Talk to the infant directly. • Make facial contact.
Toddler	• Approach the toddler slowly and carefully. The child may be fearful. • Integrate the toddler's words for familiar objects of activities into your care. • Prepare for procedures to be done to the toddler right before it happens. • Integrate dolls, storytelling, and picture books into conversation.
Preschooler	• Allow choices as appropriate. • Use play, storytelling, puppets, and third parties. • Speak honestly, use simple language, and be concise.
School-age	• Use books, diagrams, and videos in preparing for the procedure. • Prepare for procedures several days in advance. • Allow for honest expression of feelings and enough time for questions to be answered.
Adolescents	• Prepare the child in advance of treatments. • Respect the adolescent's need for privacy. • Use appropriate yet understandable medical terminology. • Use or create methods to explain experiences and procedures in terms the child will understand. • Show an interest in their interests; talk about things the child is interested in.

Source: Adapted from Potts & Mandleco, 2002.

conveying a real sense of care and interest will go a long way to gain their trust. Answer the child's questions such as "Will that hurt?", or "Why do they have to do that test?", and explain procedures, being honest about pain. Never lie ever to any child of any age. Do not forget to communicate with caregivers as well as the child. Keeping caregivers informed during a stressful time will be beneficial and decrease stress levels.

Communicating When the Child Will Not

What does the disaster nurse do if the child is quiet and will not communicate? Utilize their toys to do the talking. Talk to the security objects or stuffed animals they have with them. For example: "Hi, Mr. Teddy Bear. How are you? My name is______. What is your name?" Try to get the child to share the name of his or her bear or favorite stuffed animal or toy (Potts & Mandleco, 2002). This is a good way to break the ice with the child. It is possible to elicit information from the child through the toy, also. For example, say to the bear "Mr. Bear, do you know we just had a hurricane? Are you scared Mr. Bear?" Hold the bear to your ear and pretend he is talking to you. Then say to the child, "Mr. Bear told me he is very scared. Are you scared?" When a child sees you using play to communicate, they are more apt to communicate with you.

The disaster nurse can also try to initiate communication with the child by asking if the family has any pets. Most children know something about animals, and this may be a good area to connect to them with. Ask the child what he or she likes to play, watch on television, or what his or her favorite color is or toy. Lastly, smile. A friendly warm smile can go a long way to put a child at ease in a difficult situation. Also, acknowledge that the situation may be a little scary right now, but the disaster responders are there to help make it better. Reassure the child that he or she will be all right and are now safe, if that is the case. As before, never lie to a child, so, if you are not sure the child is safe, do not tell the child he or she is.

It is also important to remember a child's cultural belief system. Culture can affect the way children respond to both the disaster nurse and the parents or caregiver. Be sure to ask about any cultural or religious practices and abide by these, if at all possible, and respect them.

Once the immediate disaster is over, reassure children that the event is over and that they are now safe. Repeat to them that you are "a helper" and here to help them. Tell the child everything you are doing. Tell the child your name and the names of people and things around them. Explain to them about physical sensations they may feel, smells, or sounds. Warn them of painful procedures and be honest. Answer the child's questions honestly and truthfully. Do not allow the child to hear stories of other disasters or cases you are caring for (Peterson, 2008). This goes beyond HIPAA privacies, as sharing such stories may be scary to children who do not understand.

Factors Increasing Trauma and Decreasing Communication

Lubit, Rovine, Defrancisci, and Eth (2003) described factors that increased the impact trauma had on children. By knowing which factors increase the impact of trauma on children and avoiding them, we can lessen that impact. Factors that impacted trauma on children were separation of the child from the parents during or after the trauma, the parent's level of stress and ability to respond to their children's needs, how quickly the child was brought to a safe place, the parent's ability to maintain normalcy of rules and routines, what the child saw (death or grotesque images), whether the disaster was an act of nature or man-made, if the child heard unanswered screams for help, and whether the child felt his or her life or that of a loved one was in danger.

How to Talk to Children After a Disaster

What to say about a disaster can be problematic for some families. According to the International Critical Incident Stress Foundation (2001), healthcare providers, teachers, and family members should be encouraged to:

1. Talk to and support the children:
   - Tell the child the facts (appropriate to age).
   - Listen to what the child has to say.
   - Be honest—even if you do not know certain facts, tell the child what you do know.
   - Tell the child honestly how you feel.
   - Provide reassurance of safety to the child; touch or hold the child if indicated.
   - Allow the child to grieve and mourn.
   - Validate normalcy of reaction.
   - Reaffirm life direction.
2. Support each other as a family:
   - In times like these, families often reunite; use the opportunity.
   - Talk to each other as indicated above.
3. Provide a supportive climate in all classrooms, and reach out to homes that are experiencing a crisis.
4. By recognizing and monitoring the distress signals that a child exhibits and by being supportive, we facilitate the normal recovery process.
5. Know that if abnormal behaviors persist for longer than 3 weeks, the child should be referred to a disaster mental health professional for help.
6. Teachers can help by taking extra care immediately to help prevent behavior and performance problems later.

Grade-specific interventions are important for preschool and older children. For the preschool to 2nd-grade child, routine is critical, as it conveys security. Children of these ages look to adults to figure out how serious things are and to protect them. The disaster nurse should project a calm attitude and, as much as possible, ensure a calm atmosphere for the child's environment. For 3rd to 7th graders, consider relaxing performance demands upon the child temporarily. Children's self-esteem is tied to their feelings about their performance. With the added stress of a disaster, a child may regress to an earlier developmental level and too much demand on the child of this age may increase negative responses and behaviors. For children in 8th to 12th grades, look for self-medication, acting out behaviors, and, with older children, identity issues. Provide guidance and stress management support.

Stress Management

A study done by Flannery describes critical incident stress management (CISM) (Flannery, 1999). He pointed out that CISM is vital for helping people deal with a disaster, particularly the family survivors of mass casualty situations. He described CISM as a serious stress reaction that can occur in either the disaster victim or in the person who witnesses the event, as well as in disaster responders. Most victims develop an acute stress disorder. This is characterized by disruptions in usual mastery, caring attachments, and meaningful purpose in life. Some of the symptoms exhibited are hypervigilance, an exaggerated startle response, intrusive memories of the event, and a tendency to avoid situations by withdrawing from them physically and psychologically. (See Chapter 8 for more on the psychology of disasters.)

In a child, stress from a disaster situation can be seen in his or her not wanting to play. Having family members missing may intensify this stress response. Important to note is that if this stress response does not resolve in approximately 30 days, the individual could go on to develop post-traumatic stress disorder (PTSD).

Fairbrother, Stuber, Galea, Pfefferbaum, and Fleischman (2004), following the September 11th tragedies, found the intensity of parental reactions and poor parental functioning were associated with children developing psychiatric symptoms after a disaster. Associated findings also showed that family vulnerability, such as single parent households and minority status, was associated with the need for services. The study urges nurses to be involved in screening and referring children with any signs of post-traumatic stress disorder to the appropriate mental healthcare provider. School-based screening is a logical place also for this to happen. The disaster nurse must realize that 60–70% of children visit a pediatrician annually, so all nurses who might care for or do care for children must be on the look out for children at risk. Identifying these children and getting them help is a key task for nursing.

The Personnel Who Respond

Equipment Needed

When planning for the pediatric aspects of a disaster, the disaster nurse needs to plan who will staff pediatric disaster shelters, as well as plan for those pediatric patients with special needs. Such questions as what is the criterion for each shelter, what training will be needed, and what are the appropriate supplies and reference materials needed should be answered. Pediatric protocols should be in place. One tool available is the Broselow tape. This is a tape that can be laid down next to an injured child according to their height. A foldout card identifies what size pediatric equipment and medication doses are needed for that child. The card is color-coded by weight. This tape is available at http://www.armstrongmedical.com.

There is also now a Broselow Pediatric Antidotes for Chemical Warfare Tape that gives precalculated antidote dosages for common chemical warfare antidotes, including such medications as auto-injectors of atropine. This tape is called the

SANDELL tape. The tape was designed to meet the needs of paramedics in the United Kingdom. Also available is a SMART tape that can be used during a mass casualty situation. It helps to provide rapid, safe triage of injured children. Both tapes are located at www.sandelltape.com/about_sandell_tape.php.

For those who have not considered pediatrics in their disaster plan, tools can be obtained for free online at www.jumpstarttriage.com. There is also another triage tool available: the Sacco Triage Method developed by Sacco. It is evidence-based and outcomes driven. This method uses a physiological score that predicts survival. This system is available online at www.sharpthinkers.com. Lastly, there is the Israeli approach. The Israelis have long experience with mass casualty situations. Their philosophy is little to no triage and treatment on scene. Triage is done by physicians at the hospital. In the case of children, triage could then be done by pediatricians in a hospital system (Romig, 2008).

Assessing the Child in a Disaster

For those disaster nurses who typically do not work with children, the first thing to do is remain calm. A child can quickly sense increased stress levels in adults by how they talk. These tips will help the disaster nurse with little to no pediatric experience: Assess the child in an unhurried manner. Ease into the exam slowly. Do not quickly start assessing a child as one would an adult. This will scare them, and they will begin to cry. Many times, respirations can be counted from a few feet away.

Make friends with the child. If the child has a favorite toy, comment on it, and ask the child about the toy. Talk to parents or other caregivers. If the child sees that his or her parent trusts the disaster nurse, the child will, too. Gently allow the child to see any medical equipment that may be used, such as a stethoscope. Allow them to touch it. Make the assessment a game if possible. A good example would be to listen to the child's heart and then let the child listen. The initial assessment should include the Pediatric Assessment Triangle (PAT) from the American Academy of Pediatrics Education for Prehospital Professionals (PEPP). The PEPP course is available at http://www.PEPPsite.com. A free lecture is also available at www.jumpstarttriage.com/uploads/PATnopix.ppt.

The cornerstone of the initial assessment is general appearance, work of breathing, and circulation to the skin. The general appearance of the child can provide much information: Does the child look good? Is the child alert and aware of what is going on around him or her? The second thing is to ascertain his or her respiratory status: Is the child using much effort to breathe or breathing comfortably? The last thing is to observe circulation to the skin. How is the capillary refill and skin color? There are subtle differences particularly in infants (Romig, 2008).

Another thing to be aware of is temperature. Infants who are cold will demonstrate bradycardia and apnea, just from being cold. If warmed up, these signs disappear. This is called cold stress. In further exploring the appearance of the child, is the child consolable? What is the child's speech or cry effort like (Romig, 2008)? Is there audible wheezing, stridor, or grunting, a sound that infants make to maintain positive end-expiratory pressure when in respiratory distress? Are there retractions and where? Upper retractions (suprasternal and supraclavicular) usually indicate an upper airway obstruction. Listen to air flow on each side. Retractions that are substernal, subcostal, or intercostal are signs of a lower airway obstruction or problem. One last sign of respiratory distress in children is nasal flaring. Do their nares open outward with each breath? Do they flare? If so, the child is using more effort than normal to breathe and is experiencing respiratory distress. In examining circulation to the skin, temperature, strength of pulses, and capillary refill will be most important (Romig, 2008). The skin may appear mottled, with a pale and marble-like appearance. Mottling occurs when an infant or child is cold or the skin is not perfusing well.

Also remember the A, B, C, D, and E of breathing:

1. Airway: Is it maintainable or not?
2. Breathing: Is it effective or not? What is the respiratory rate, oxygen saturation, and lung sounds?
3. Circulation: What is the heart rate? With infants, listen 1 full minute apically. Blood pressure is not a good indicator of cardiac output. The normal child's circulating blood volume is 80 ml/kg of body weight. A child could lose up to half its blood volume (40 ml/kg) and not experience a change in blood pressure. This is because the heart compensates by beating faster. When a blood pressure drop occurs, this is a late sign, and quick action is needed to maintain the child's life.
4. Disability: Use the AVPU scale to determine the child's level of disability.
   a. A = alert
   b. V = verbal response
   c. P = painful
   d. U = unresponsive
5. Exposure: Be sure to limit exposure and maintain temperature. Children will compensate a long time, but when they deteriorate, they do so quickly.

Typical Pediatric Problems Expected

In this section, each area of the body will be addressed for typical pediatric responses to disasters. Advice will be presented for how to deal with the issues one finds in children during and after a disaster.

The pulmonary system is usually the first system of concern for the disaster nurse. Bronchospasm is common for children with or without asthma. Children who are bad asthmatics will present early due to stress, environmental triggers, and lack of medications. Stable asthmatics will present later as triggers increase or medications run out. Supplies needed to treat children with pulmonary problems are premixed beta-agonists for nebulizers, nebulizers with and without oxygen, oral and intravenous steroids, and peak flow monitoring equipment. Consider using metered dose inhalers (MDIs) with spacers for ease in use by children. Teach children and families about allergen and environmental exposure that could exacerbate their disorder (Romig, 2008).

Close living quarters will yield ease of transmission of gastrointestinal viral illnesses. Limited water and facilities for washing hands as well as limited supplies for diaper care and hygiene in disaster shelters will increase this problem. There may be inadequate sanitation in kitchen or food distribution centers. Consider oral bottle rehydration options (e.g., Pedialyte) if available. If dehydration is severe, and if staff and intravenous fluids are available, consider that route for rehydration. Limit the use of antiemetics and antidiarrheals in children. They can be toxic. Try not to switch infant formula types, and pay attention to unusual electrolyte abnormalities in dehydrated children.

Assessing pain in an infant who is unable to communicate is important. Use of a pediatric pain scale can help. Three common scales are provided. The first is the FLACC pain scale. This pain scale is appropriate for infants to children 3 years of age. FLACC stands for *face, legs, activity, cry,* and *consolability.* The disaster nurse rates each item from 0 to 2. The scale allows the disaster nurse caring for a child to assess each of these areas by matching the child's behaviors to the descriptors in the scale. The FACES pain scale is appropriate for children 3 to 10 years of age. This scale allows the child to point to which face they most feel like. From the child's choice, a determination of the pain's intensity can be made. (See Figure 5-2.)

The last method is a 0 to 10 pain scale. This scale can be used for children 5 and up provided the child is able to understand and use this scale, especially when anxious or under stress. The scale simply asks the child to rate his or her pain on a scale with 0 being no pain, 10 being the worst pain, and 5 about medium pain. Have the child say or point to a number.

This scale is available in numerous languages with lifelike pictures in several cultural backgrounds. The scale is easy to construct by simply drawing a line on a piece of paper, putting the numbers 0 to 10 on it, and presenting it to the child, as seen in the representation in Figure 5-3.

Another thing to consider is to ask the child to point to where it hurts. Frequently, children cannot describe where pain is and may just say "my belly." By having the child point to where it hurts, this will guide the disaster nurse in determining better where a problem may be. If needed, give the child pain medicine. Children experience pain the same as adults. So, if they are in pain, medicate them for it.

Children with Special Needs

Children with special needs or who have a chronic illness need special attention in disaster planning. A good example of the disaster nurse's chances of caring for such

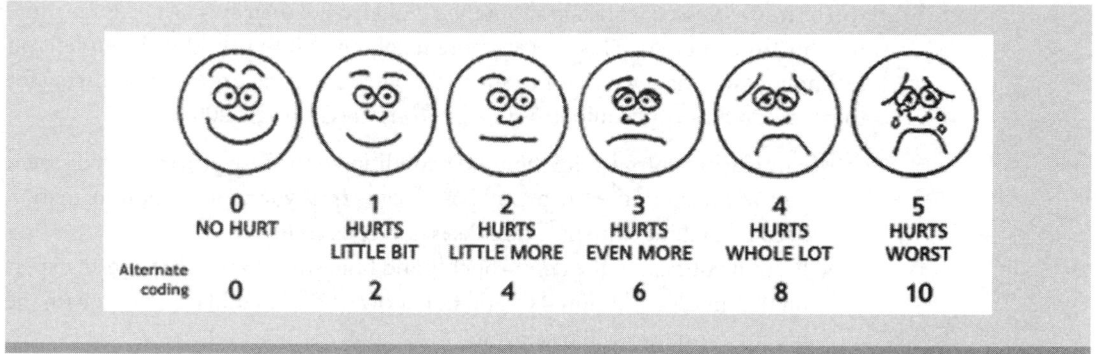

Figure 5-2 The Wong-Baker FACES Scale. *Source:* From Hockenberry, M. J., Wilson, D., & Winkelstein, M. L. (2005). *Wong's essentials of pediatric nursing* (7th ed., p. 1259). St. Louis, MO: Mosby. Used with permission.

a child can be seen in Hurricane Katrina where 34% of Gulf Coast children living in FEMA housing had at least one diagnosed chronic condition (Abramson & Garfield, 2006). A child with special healthcare needs (CSHCN) is defined as "a child who has or is at risk for a chronic physical, developmental, behavioral, or emotional condition and who also requires health and related services of a type or amount beyond that required by children normally" (Ball & Bindler, 2006, p. 648).

Children with special needs should have health records and a list of medications kept with them. Special provisions must be made for those who are technology dependent on electrical power; generators, battery, and power backups must be available in both the home and in a designated shelter (Ball & Bindler, 2006). Included is a suggested emergency information form for all children with special needs. This form can be downloaded at http://www.aap.org/advocacy/eif.doc. Plans for children with special needs need to be developed in combination with pediatricians and local healthcare response teams. The American Academy of Pediatrics has a Web page devoted to this topic. It can be accessed at http://www.aap.org/advocacy/emergprep.htm.

It is vital in a disaster for the disaster nurse to try to establish a therapeutic relationship with both the child with special needs and the parent who undoubtedly

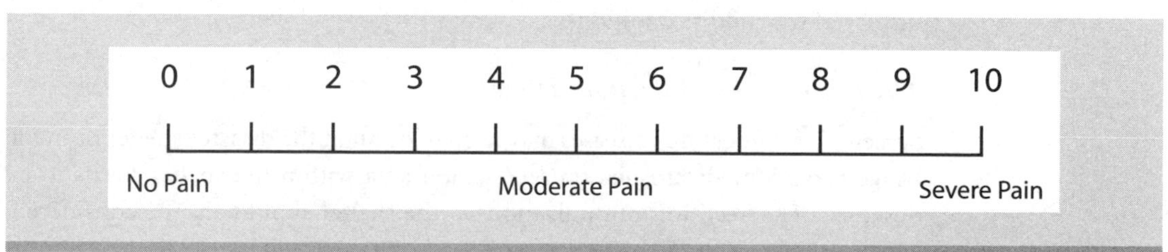

Figure 5-3 A 0 to 10 pain scale.

will be more stressed worrying about their child having their special needs met during this time of crisis. This is even more heightened if the child is dependent on technology such as a ventilator to survive. Follow the same principles in caring for these children as you would in a time of no crisis (Godshall, 2003):

- Familiarize yourself with the child's condition or disease process. In a disaster, you will need to use the parents or caregivers as your source of information because looking it up in textbooks is not a possibility.
- Present yourself to the family openly and honestly. Do not try to be an expert on the child's condition if you do not know what the child has. Work with the parents, and they will teach you.
- Include the family in the plan of care. The parent will be vital to this child's survival. They know the child best and their needs. Assist the parent to anticipate the child's needs ahead of time so that you can attempt to procure supplies needed if the parent does not have them.
- Take time to listen. Listen to the child and the caregiver. In a disaster, it is natural to rush. Try to take time to listen to what the caregivers are telling you. They are very good at anticipating changes in the child's condition. Work with them as a team. Remember, the ultimate goal is the survival and health of the child, not who is leading the team. The caregiver is the child's best advocate.
- Treat the child as an individual, and do not call the child by a diagnosis. It is easy in an emergent situation to call a child "the kid with the vent over there" or the "kid with muscular dystrophy." Try to avoid labels, and attempt to find out the child's name. It is perfectly acceptable to write it on a piece of tape and tape it to the child's shirt. This will go a long way to prove to the parents and child that you care.
- Do not panic. Do not show your fear. Do not avoid the child, triage them last, and let them sit in the corner. If you do not know how to perform a procedure like suctioning a tracheostomy, tell the caregiver honestly. They will be most appreciative of your honesty and happily show you what to do.
- Ask parents what are typical responses of the child to treatment.

Keeping the caregiver with the child is vital, especially for special needs children. One of the most important things the disaster nurse can do is obtain an accurate history of the child's condition(s).

The Emergence of Infectious Diseases

Screening for infectious diseases may need to occur at the disaster shelter or in the triage area. A medical isolation/segregation area within the shelter needs to be designed. The need for immunizations at the shelter should also be considered. Most of the individuals, particularly pediatric patients, will not recall their immunization status (Romig, 2008). They will also not typically have documentation of immunizations. For the local hospital, especially in the event of chemical warfare, attention needs to be paid to maintaining an appropriate supply of medications that may be needed.

Isolation/segregation of infected individuals is a must. Treat all open or penetrating wounds promptly to avoid infections. Provide a list of open pharmacies or where medications can be obtained. Contact local public health or hospital officials. Cooperate with public health officials in monitoring outbreaks and treatment efforts. Prescribe antibiotics judiciously. Consider handing out starter dosages of medications. Consider family environment and mobility when making decisions about admission, treatment, and rechecks. You may need to send and admit children to a hospital if they have highly contagious diseases to keep them from exposing others in a crowded environment. Consider sending children out of the area if a higher level of care or more appropriate shelter is available (Romig, 2008).

Treating Terrorism-Induced Trauma in Children

Bioterrorism Considerations with Children

It is important to recognize the different responses children have with regards to bioterrorism. Illness due to or symptoms related to bioterrorism can be hard to detect initially because all agents have varied incubation periods that can range from a few days to months. However, children who are exposed to bioterrorism may present sooner to healthcare institutions because incubation periods of some agents appear even shorter in children, thus allowing for earlier identification of a bioterrorism event. With aerosolized agents such as sarin, chlorine, or anthrax, the higher number of respirations per minute in children results in exposure to a relatively greater dosage than adults. The high vapor density of some gasses, such as sarin and chlorine, places their highest concentration closest to the ground. That is right at the breathing level of most children. The skin of infants and children with a larger surface area-to-mass ratio will result in a greater exposure of transdermally absorbed toxins (American Academy of Pediatrics, 2000).

It is important to remember that some medications, such as ciprofloxacin used to treat inhaled anthrax, may not have been tested in children or there may be limited research in children under 12 years of age. This is also true of vaccines for anthrax, plague, smallpox, botulism, and others. Only infant botulism and the smallpox vaccine are approved for use in children above 1 year of age (Chung & Shannon, 2005). Also important to consider is that children who are exposed to chemical agents may present with different symptoms than adults.

Techniques to decontaminate children must be examined closely. Given that most decontamination areas are outside a given hospital facility, they need to be divided into hot, warm, and cold zones (temperature of water). It is known that by removing clothing from patients accomplishes 85–95% of decontamination. These clothes must be placed in appropriate biohazard containers (Chung & Shannon, 2005) or in storage bags, labeled, and stored, because the clothes are now part of a crime scene (Shannon, 2005). Since clothing is removed, appropriate-sized clothes must be kept available for children as well as adults. For more on hazardous materials and decontamination, see Chapter 13.

Nuclear Terrorism

Children who are exposed to radiation are at an increased risk of developing radiation-induced cancers such as thyroid cancer. Children have higher minute ventilation and are at risk of greater exposure to radioactive gas of all types. Radioactive iodine released by a nuclear bomb or power plant can be absorbed and secreted in human breast milk. This must be considered for infants who are breastfed. An alternate source of feeding these infants will need to be available. In thinking of treatment after exposure to radioactive iodine, potassium iodide (KI) is the recommended antidote, especially for children. KI is taken up by the thyroid, which then prevents the incorporation of inhaled or ingested radioiodine. To achieve maximum effect, this medication should be taken within 8 hours after exposure. There is usually a limited supply of the liquid version for children available in most communities. The adult form of a tablet may need to be crushed. A side effect of KI in small children is hypothyroidism (Chung & Shannon, 2005).

Perhaps the biggest challenges that face hospitals are the lack of pediatric protocols for decontaminating children and lack of protocols for drug and vaccine administration. All medication dosages for children are weight based (in kilograms). Thus, it is importance to have a child's actual weight and to know what to do or give when the antidotes for these situations have not been tested before or given to children.

Thermomechanical Terrorism

Since the destruction of the World Trade Center towers in New York City on September 11, 2001, another lesson learned is the need for plans to care for specialized burn victims. If these victims are children, how close is the nearest pediatric burn center? Is the burn center a nationally accredited pediatric burn center? Before trying to care for a child who suffers from these types of burns, answers to these questions are needed. All children who suffer burns should ideally be seen in a pediatric burn center. There is a specific criterion developed by the American College of Surgeons (1999) that determines where burn victims should be treated. They are as follows:

1. Partial thickness burns greater than 10% total body surface area (TBSA)
2. Burns that involve the face, hands, feet, genitalia, perineum, or major joints
3. Third-degree burns in any age group
4. Electrical burns, including lightning injury
5. Chemical burns
6. Inhalation injury

7. Burn injury in patients with preexisting medical disorders that could complicate management, prolong recovery, or affect mortality
8. Any patients with burns and concomitant trauma (such as fractures) in which the burn injury poses the greatest risk of morbidity or mortality. In such cases, if the trauma poses the greater immediate risk, the patient may be initially stabilized in a trauma center before being transferred to a burn unit. Physician judgment will be necessary in such situations and should be in concert with the regional medical control plan and triage protocols.
9. Burned children in hospitals without qualified personnel or equipment for the care of children
10. Burn injury in patients who will require special social, emotional, or long-term rehabilitative intervention (pp. 55–62)

In children who are burned, the injury is more serious than in adults, related to their large body surface area. Children's skin is thinner, and therefore the burn may be deeper given the same exposure or circumstance of an adult. It is important to assess the burn properly using a formula such as the Rule of Nines or the Lund and Browder method to assess the total burn surface area. Then treatments must begin with the assessment of airway, breathing, and circulation followed by the determination of burn depth, the total burn surface area, and the involved body parts. It is important to pay attention to any burn that is circumferential. These burns may require escharotomy as swelling ensues and cuts off circulation to the tissue. Circumferential burns to the chest may interfere with the patient's ability to breathe and need to be watched closely.

Steps in care of children suffering from burn injuries thereafter are the immediate removal of all clothing and cleansing any area that may have been exposed to chemicals to prevent further damage to the skin. Careful attention needs to be paid to prevent hypothermia by overexposing the child. To decrease burn pain, apply cool saline-soaked gauze to the burned skin. Applying ice or placing the patient in ice water should be avoided because it causes hypothermia and additional trauma to the skin.

Any significant burn will result in a large amount of fluid loss, especially for children. A burn that is 15–20% of TBSA will produce hypovolemic shock. For the initial resuscitation phase, isotonic saline or more commonly lactated Ringers solution is recommended for fluid resuscitation in the first 24 hours. Remember that large volumes of fluid are needed for burn resuscitation since only 20–30% of the isotonic fluid given will remain in the intravascular space. Proper attention to fluid management is essential.

Pain control is also important, and appropriate pain medications need to be given. This includes the use of narcotics. Remember, if the burn is third-degree, nerve endings were destroyed and pain may be less than with a first- or second-degree burn. As soon as possible, each burn should be cleaned with mild soap and water while avoiding the use of extremely cold water. Avoid popping any blisters as long as they do not interfere with wound care or movement of a joint of the body as these blisters actually cushion the burned area, decreasing pain.

Burns should be dressed as per burn protocols of the institution or the disaster shelter or treatment shelter physician's orders. Burn centers have other synthetic dressings available that ease in scar formation. The disaster nurse also needs to monitor for any signs of infection as well as evaluate the patient for the status of their tetanus vaccination. If it has been longer than 5 years since the last vaccination, then the patient needs a booster (Reed & Pomerantz, 2005). For those 7 years and younger, the DTap (acellular pertussis vaccine and tetanus toxoid) should be given and, for those older than 7 years, the Tdap should be given (Children's Hospital of Philadelphia, 2008).

Conclusion

Even under conditions of biochemical attacks or disasters, effective and careful care of the pregnant and pediatric patient is paramount. Nursing assessments of physical and psychological needs of children and pregnant women should be ongoing and take into consideration the most optimal care available for the mother and unborn child.

References

Abramson, D., & Garfield, R. (2006). *On the edge: Children and families displaced by Hurricanes Katrina and Rita face a looming medical and mental health crisis.* Retrieved September 22, 2008, from http://www.ncdp.mailman.columbia.edu/files/LCAFH.pdf

Achenbach, T., & Rescorla, L. (2001). *Manual for the ASEBA school-age forms & profiles: An integrated system of multi-informant assessment.* Burlington, VT: University of Vermont, Research Center for Children, Youth & Families Publishers. (Sample of form also available on-line at http://www.aseba.org/support/SAMPLES/samples.html#forms.)

American Academy of Pediatrics. (2000). Chemical-biological terrorism and its impact on children: A subject review. *Pediatrics, 105*(3), 662–670.

American Academy of Pediatrics & American College of Obstetrics and Gynecology. (2002). *Guidelines for perinatal care* (5th ed.). Chicago: American Academy of Pediatrics.

American College of Surgeons. (1999). *Guidelines for the operations of burn units.* Retrieved March 25, 2008, from http://www.ameriburn.org/BurnUnitReferral.pdf

American Red Cross. (2004). *Disaster preparedness for people with disabilities and special populations.* Retrieved February 19, 2008, from http://www.redcross.org/services/disaster/beprepared/seniors.html

American Red Cross. (2008). *Children and disasters.* Retrieved March 25, 2006, from http://www.redcross.org/services/disaster/0,1082,0_602_,00.html

Ball, J. W., & Bindler, R. C. (2006). *Child health nursing: Partnering with children and families.* Upper Saddle River, NJ: Pearson Prentice Hall.

Briere, J. (1996). Trauma Symptom Checklist for Children (TSCC). *Victims Web.* Retrieved March 25, 2008, from http://www.swin.edu.au/victims/resources/assessment/ptsd/tscc.html

Burton, A. (2006). Caring for children amidst chaos: Guidelines to maintain health. *Environmental Health Perspectives, 114*(10), A584–A591.

Centers for Disease Control and Prevention (CDC). (2003). Women with smallpox vaccine exposure during pregnancy reported to the National Smallpox Vaccine in Pregnancy Registry—United States, 2003. *Morbidity and Mortality Weekly Report, 52*(17), 386–388.

Center for Drug Evaluations and Research. (2007). *Cipro (ciprofloxacin hydrochloride) for inhalation anthrax.* Retrieved February 10, 2004, from http://www.fda.gov/cder/drug/infopage/cipro/cipro message.htm

Children's Hospital of Philadelphia. (2008). *Vaccine education center.* Retrieved March 25, 2008, from http://www.chop.edu/consumer/jsp/division/generic.jsp?id=75701#Tdap

Chung, S., & Shannon, M. (2005). Hospital planning for acts of terrorism and other public health emergencies involving children. *Archives of Disease in Childhood, 90,* 1300–1307

Cohen, J. A., Mannarino, A. P., & Deblinger, E. (2006). *Treating trauma and traumatic grief in children and adolescents.* New York: Guilford Press.

Cunningham, F. G., Mac Donald, P. C., Gant, N. F., Leveno, K. J., Gilstrap, L. C., Hankins, G. D., et al. (2001). *Williams obstetrics* (21st ed.). Stamford, CT: Appleton & Lange.

Fairbrother, G., Stuber, J., Galea, S., Pfefferbaum, B., & Fleischman, A. R. (2004). Unmet need for counseling services by children in New York City after the September 11th attacks on the World Trade Center: Implications for practice. *Pediatrics, 113*(5), 1367–1374.

Fendya, D. G., Vanore, M. L., & Perks, D. H. (2006). When disaster strikes: Care considerations for pediatric patients. *Journal of Trauma Nursing, 13*(4), 161–165.

Flannery, R. B. (1999). Treating family survivors of mass casualties: A CISM family crisis intervention approach. *International Journal of Emergency Mental Health, 1*(4), 243–250.

Fox, L. & Timm, N. (2008). Pediatric issues in disaster preparedness: Meeting the educational needs of nurses: Are we there yet? *Journal of Pediatric Nursing, 23*(3), 145–151.

Ginter, P. M., Wingate, M. S., Rucks, A. C., Vasconex, R. D., McCormick, L. C., Baldwin, S., & Fargason, C. A. (2006). Creating a regional pediatric medical disaster preparedness network: Imperative and Issues. *Maternal Child Health Journal, 10,* 391–396.

Godshall, M. (2003). Caring for the families of chronically ill kids. *RN, 66*(2), 30–35.

International Critical Incident Stress Foundation, Inc. (2001, September). *Children's reactions and needs after disaster.* Retrieved March 25, 2008, from http://www.icisf.org/articles/Acrobat%20Documents/TerrorismIncident/Children_and_terroristattack.html

Langan, J., & James, D. (2005). Preparing nurses for disaster management. Upper Saddle River, NJ: Pearson Prentice Hall.

Lowdermilk, D., & Perry, S. (2007). *Maternity and women's health care* (9th ed.). St. Louis, MO: Mosby Elsevier.

Lubit, R., Rovine, D., Defrancisci, L., & Eth, S. (2003). Impact of trauma on children. *Journal of Psychiatric Practice, 9*(2), 128–138.

Malone, F., & D'Alton, M. (2004). Multiple gestation: Clinical characteristics and management. In R. Creasy, R. Resnik, & J. Iams (Eds.), *Maternal-fetal medicine: Principles and practice* (5th ed.). Philadelphia: Saunders.

Martin, J., Hamilton, B., Sutton, P., Venturea, S., Menacker, F., & Munson, M. (2005). Births: Final data for 2003. *National Vital Statistics Reports, 54*(2), 1–116.

Murray, J. S., & Ryan-Kuntz, K. (2006). Addressing the psychosocial needs of children following disasters. *Journal for Specialists in Pediatric Nursing, 11*(2), 133–137.

National Center for Missing and Exploited Children. (2006). National Center for Missing and Exploited Children reunites last missing child separated by Hurricane Katrina and

Rita. Retrieved March 25, 2008, from http://www.missingkids.com/missingkids/servlet/NewsEventServlet?LanguageCountry=en_US&PageId=2317

Peters, R., & Flack, J. (2004). Hypertensive disorders of pregnancy. *Journal of Obstetrics, Gynecologic, and Neonatal Nursing, 33*(2), 209–219.

Peterson, C. A. (2008). Calming the injured child. *The child advocate injury page.* Retrieved March 25, 2008, from http://www.childadvocate.net/index.htm

Potts, N. L., & Mandleco, B. L. (2002). *Pediatric nursing: Caring for children and their families.* New York: Delmar Thomson Learning.

Reed, J. L., & Pomerantz, W. J. (2005). Emergency management of pediatric burns. *Pediatric Emergency Care, 21*(2), 118–129.

Romig, L. E. (2008). Working kids into your disaster planning. Presented March 7, 2008, at the John M. Templeton Pediatric Trauma Symposium, The Union League, Philadelphia, PA.

Shannon, M. (2005). *The decontamination of children* [DVD]. Rockville, MD: Agency for Healthcare Research and Quality.

White, S. R., Henretig, F. M., & Dukes, R. G. (2002). Medical management of vulnerable populations and co-morbid conditions of victims of bioterrorism. *Emergency Medical Clinics of North America, 20*(2), 365–395.

Zhang, C., Meikle, S., & Trumble, A. (2003). Severe maternal morbidity associated with hypertensive disorders in pregnancy in the United States. *Hypertension in Pregnancy, 22*(2), 203–212.

chapter 6

Special Populations in Disasters: The Elderly and Disabled

Timothy J. Legg and Deborah S. Adelman

GOAL

The goal of this chapter is to present special considerations in caring for the elderly and disabled person in a disaster.

OBJECTIVES

At the completion of this chapter, the reader will:

1. Define demographics related to the elderly that impinge on disaster nursing care.
2. Apply concepts related to aging through a psychosocial lens in a disaster.
3. Assess age-related physiological changes in the elderly applicable to the disaster situation.
4. Define the concept of disability.
5. Explain federal laws relating to disability.
6. Develop plans for a disaster shelter that incorporate caring for the disabled person.
7. Learn to work with primary caregivers in caring for the disabled person.
8. Understand handling and care of service animals in a disaster.

Key Terms

- Elderly
- Psychological changes in the elderly
- Age-related changes in the elderly
- Aging body systems
- Disaster care across a continuum
- Disability
- Americans with Disabilities Act
- Special needs in a disaster shelter
- Service animals

The Elderly in a Disaster

Older adults represent a particularly vulnerable population. For example, during Hurricane Katrina in 2005, approximately 71% of the victims were age 60 and above, and 47% of the victims were over the age of 75 (American Association of Retired Persons [AARP], 2006). Many older adults have faced multiple losses throughout the course of their life, and a disaster can add to that sense of loss. The decreased physical reserve of older adults may make their ability to tolerate the physical demands associated with disasters precarious.

The disaster nurse must understand the unique needs of the older adult in order to plan effective care during a disaster situation. To understand the impact of disasters on the older adult, the disaster nurse needs to be aware of the needs of the older adult in general, then be able to discern between normal aging and pathological changes that may be manifested in the older adult. This chapter offers a brief overview of this special population before proceeding to the special needs attendant in caring for the older disaster victim.

Older Adults

Although the question of what is old seems ridiculous, it is one that needs to be addressed in order to define this special needs population. Travis described three categories of old: The "young-old" consists of individuals aged 65–74, the "old-old" group includes those aged 75–84 years, and, finally, the "oldest-old" encompasses those individuals aged 85 years and older (Travis, 1998). These delineations were selected by Travis and others who continue to use them because each are associated with changes in health, physical functioning, and dependency.

Demographics

Regardless of specialty (with the obvious exception of pediatrics and obstetrics), disaster nurses will interface with older adults. Improved immunizations, water, food, sanitation, disease prevention, and other advances in science and public health efforts have resulted in an increased life span. The older adult population is expected to increase significantly in years to come; in fact, it has been projected that the older population will more than double over the next 2 decades. The fastest growing segment of this population is the oldest-old, whose ranks will increase to approximately 9.6 million by 2030 and to almost 20 million by 2050 (Lach, 2007).

It is essential for the disaster nurse to understand that older adulthood does not necessarily equate to frailty. Despite many beliefs about the inevitability of nursing home placement and aging, only small percentages (4.5%) of older adults live in nursing homes. However, this percentage does increase with age (4.7% for the "old-old as compared to 18.2% for the oldest-old). An additional 5% of older adults were reported living in senior housing that provides varying degrees of support services to their residents (Administration on Aging [AOA], 2006).

These demographics all point to a few essential facts for the disaster nursing professional. First, the older adult population is expanding at an incredible rate. Second, the vast number of older adults will be found living in the community. Third, in order to be successful in meeting the needs of this population, the professional nurse needs at least a cursory understanding of this group.

Aging Through a Developmental Lens

There has been a great deal written about the psychology and sociology of aging. In-depth discussion of this subject is well beyond the scope of this work, but a brief look at the topic is in order: In this section, we will briefly examine the developmental and social aspects of the older adult.

Erikson's work as a developmentalist is perhaps the most widely known by nurses. According to Erikson, the older adulthood stage presents the older adult with the task of "ego integrity versus despair." According to Erikson, ego integrity was achieved when one was able to accept oneself and the life that one has lived. Despair resulted when the person had an inherent dissatisfaction with the lived experience and longed to "go back" and do things differently in an effort to give meaning to life. The latter resolution is believed to lead to anger, bitterness, feelings of inadequacy, and depression (Berk, 2001). An understanding of developmental stages of the older adult may help the disaster nurse in understanding the disaster victim in terms of his or her behavior.

Prioritization of the needs of older adults in times of disaster is essential. When the nurse is confronted with competing needs, the nurse should consider the work of Maslow and its relevance to the disaster situation. Maslow believed that a hierarchy of needs motivates all human behavior and that "lower needs" of the hierarchy had to be met before one is sufficiently motivated to reach the next hierarchical level. Maslow's theory is often depicted as a pyramid with the lowest level needs (e.g., ventilation, food, and water) serving as the base of the pyramid. Once these basic physiological needs are met, the individual attempts to meet safety and security needs; then love and belonging, trust, self-esteem, and, finally, self-actualization. Self-actualization served as the pinnacle of the pyramid and is where those persons who are doing their personal best strive for fulfillment (Engler, 2003). Maslow's hierarchy continues to be relevant to the work of disaster nurses in that the lowest level needs must be met before attempting to achieve higher level needs. Clearly, the disaster nurse seeks to enhance the patient's feeling of esteem, but in an unsafe environment, esteem needs are not a priority.

Age-Related Changes and Their Significance in Times of Disaster

The disaster nurse must appreciate the normal physiological changes associated with aging and apply this to the disaster situation. Some of the changes associated with normal aging make the older adult more susceptible to illness or injury under the stressful conditions of a disaster. The next sections examine some of these changes and their potential impact on the disaster situation.

Body Composition

The older adult experiences several changes in body composition. There is an overall decrease in lean muscle mass with an increase in body fat. The decrease in muscle mass may result in decreased strength of the older adult. Decreases in bone mass can render the older adult more susceptible to fracture. Body water concentration also decreases via a generalized decrease in both intracellular and extracellular fluids. Coupled with age-related changes of the skin, the older adult is at increased risk for hyperthermia.

The Aging Skin

The older adult's most obvious changes are found in the skin. The dermis becomes thinner, and the epidermis takes longer to renew resulting in delayed wound healing. Loss of subcutaneous fat can result in impaired insulation and resultant intol-

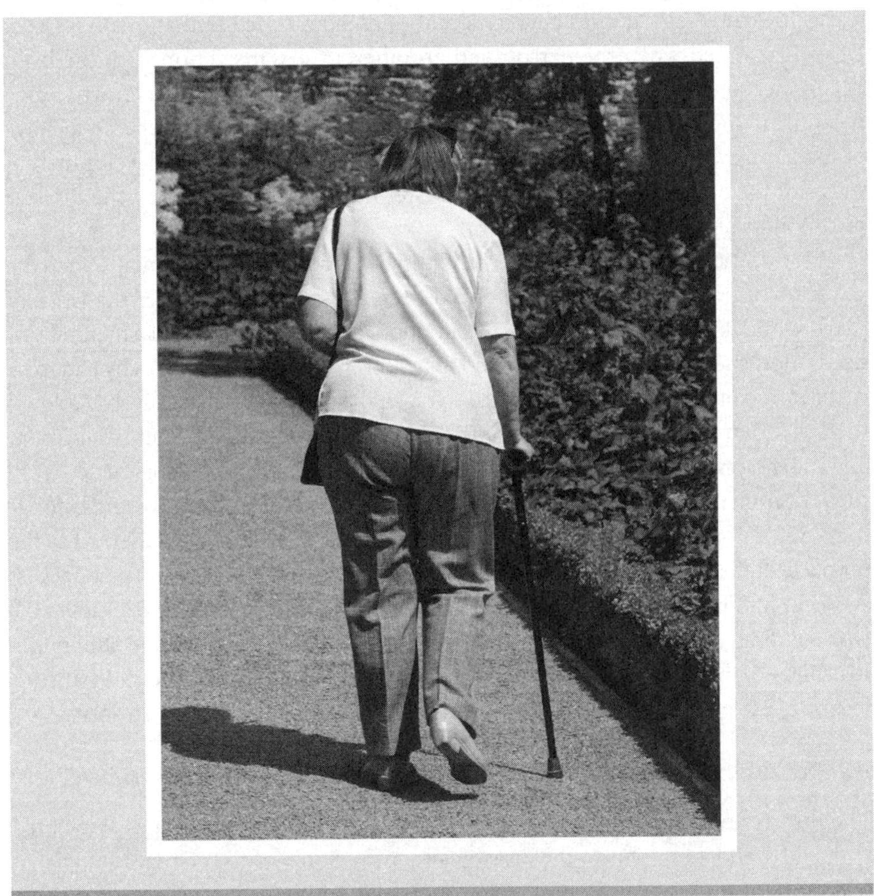

Figure 6-1 The older adult experiences several changes in body composition. *Source:* ©marilyn barbone/ShutterStock, Inc.

erance of cold. Loss of elasticity of collagen fibers results in generalized fragility of the aging skin. There is also a decrease in the overall number of sweat glands in the older adult.

The disaster nurse responding to the needs of older adults in disaster situations needs to remember that these age-related changes can impact the older adult in a variety of ways: Simple trauma to the skin can result in significant skin tears or bruising, along with increased susceptibility to hypothermia, hyperthermia, or hypothermia without sweating due to age-related changes. The disaster nurse should be cognizant of environmental temperature and offer the older adult client fluids liberally (unless contraindicated) to prevent dehydration.

The Aging Eye

Visual changes also accompany aging. Some of these changes include a decrease in night vision, which may result in night blindness. The ocular lens of the eye begins to become opaque and, if this becomes severe enough, the result is a cataract, resulting in decreased vision. The lens of the eye also yellows resulting in decreased perception of blues and greens. The disaster nurse should keep these visual changes in mind as these can result in injury to the older adult. Although glaucoma is not a normal age-related change, the disaster nurse should also be aware of older clients who may suffer from it. Glaucoma results in loss of peripheral vision, further placing the older adult client at risk for injury in disaster situations.

The Aging Ear

Presbycusis is the term applied to the totality of age-related changes of hearing. There is increased cerumen, ossicular calcification, and a decrease in neuronal function resulting in gradual loss of sound. The disaster nurse should keep these changes in mind and use some modified communication techniques when working with older adults who may be hearing impaired: Face the person when speaking; give clear, concise, and precise instructions; and pronounce and enunciate words clearly. Establishing effective communication is essential to elicit the cooperation of the older adult in times of disaster and/or evacuation.

The Sense of Smell

Aging is accompanied by a decrease in the number of olfactory cells. In evolving disaster situations, this normal, age-related change places the older client at great risk as the older adult may not be able to smell smoke or other noxious odors. Be certain to explain to the older adult any odors in the environment, the potential danger associated with the odors, and assist them to evacuate as appropriate.

The Sense of Taste

With aging, taste buds decrease in the size and number. The older adult may not be able to distinguish easily between sweet, sour, bitter, and salt. Coupled with changes in the sense of smell, this may place the older adult at risk for consumption of tainted food. When providing services to older adults, consider food supplies related to the nature of the disaster. For example, if power was interrupted, check the older adults' refrigerator/freezer to evaluate spoilage of food. This simple task can avoid considerable trouble for the older adult.

The Sense of Touch and the Nervous System

The feeling of touch diminishes with age. Proprioception (the sense of body position) may also be altered. Decreased nerve conduction velocity results in slow or delayed responses to environmental stimuli. These age-related changes may place the older adult at risk for a plethora of injuries, including falls and thermal injuries. Superimposed disease processes such as diabetic peripheral neuropathy and cerebral vascular accident with resultant hemiparesis places the older adult at even greater risk for injury. The disaster nurse needs to be aware of these age-related changes and provide additional assistance and instruction to the older adult client during disaster situations and evacuations.

The Aging Heart

Decreased resting heart rate, decreased cardiac output (both at rest and with exercise), and decreased ventricular contractility as well as decreased baroreceptor sensitivity place the older adult at risk for activity intolerance with exertion. These age-related changes should be kept in mind during a disaster, especially during evacuation. Nursing assessment should focus on the older adults' tolerance of the evacuation. If indicated, use a wheelchair or stretcher to evacuate the older adult.

The Aging Lungs

Age-related changes of the lungs include decreased effectiveness of the mucociliary escalator resulting in decreased ability of the older adult to clear secretions. Osteoporosis and calcification of the thoracic cavity results in decreased chest wall compliance. Limited thoracic movement results in decreased breathing efficiency. Decreased muscle strength also results in increased breathing effort and possible use of accessory muscles. Decreased numbers of alveoli result in decreased surface area available for gas exchange. Loss of elastic recoil of the alveoli further results in stiffness of the lung.

These changes can place the older adult at increased risk during disaster situations. The older adult is at risk for hypoxia, which may manifest itself as acute confusion. The disaster nurse should not assume that the older adult behaving irrationally is demented and, instead, should consider potential hypoxia and treat it as the medical emergency that it is. Remember that normal pulse oxygen saturation can be misleading, especially if the older adult was exposed to carbon monoxide, which is 200 times more readily absorbed by hemoglobin than oxygen. Therefore, pulse oximetry may yield a normal reading from the hemoglobin being saturated, but not with oxygen (Smeltzer & Bare, 2004).

The Genitourinary System

The older adult has a decreased bladder capacity. At night, urine production may increase resulting in nocturia. Weakening of the pelvic muscles and decreased muscle tone may result in decreased ability to empty the bladder fully resulting in urinary retention. The disaster nurse should keep these age-related changes in mind and be aware that the older adult may need to access toileting facilities more frequently than the younger disaster victim. If possible, consider placing the older adult's cot near the bathroom facilities in a disaster shelter. Incontinence of bladder is indicative of other pathology and is not a part of normal aging.

Cognition

Age-related alterations in cognition are neither consistent nor predictable. In general, there may be some decreases in short-term memory abilities (i.e., ability to recall something recently learned), whereas long-term memory is generally intact. Retrieval processes can be slowed and can be slowed even further by stressful situations and events. The disaster nurse should remember this and afford the older adult ample opportunity to respond to questions asked. Try to proceed with any questioning in an unrushed manner if circumstances permit. Most important, recall that confusion is not a part of normal aging.

Providing Care Across a Continuum of Settings

The disaster nurse may need to provide care across a wide range of settings, and actions taken in times of disaster are often contingent upon the setting in which he or she practices. Nurses in all care settings, not just disaster nurses, should be aware of the content of their organization's emergency preparedness plan and take part in disaster drills, which are now a prescribed part of all healthcare accrediting bodies. Chapter 12 discusses disaster nursing education in more detail.

Unless the hospital or medical center is directly involved or affected by the disaster, the acute care setting is usually the setting where older adults are evacuated to. Once the older adult disaster victim has been stabilized, important care considerations include assisting the older adult with basic physical care as necessary, management of medications, and ongoing assessment of chronic conditions. In the long-term care setting, the disaster nurse may need to evacuate the older adult to other long-term care facilities or may accept older adults from other facilities affected by the disaster. During this time, family members may also be quite concerned about their loved ones who have been evacuated. The disaster nurse can facilitate psychological adjustment by answering the older adults' questions about the disaster in an honest and straightforward manner.

The disaster nurse may also be responsible for caring for older adults with dementia. Dementing illness, by its very nature, prohibits learning of new information. The older adult with dementia will not be able to comprehend the unfolding disaster and reason in terms of the disaster's implications. The older adult with dementia may physically act out or display apathy toward the situation. The disaster nurse should inquire of nursing staff or family members the best way to work with this individual, if at all possible.

Nurses who care for clients in the home environment may care for a wide range of ages, including older adults, across a wide geographic range. When disaster strikes, the home care nurse may be miles away from the older adult. In this care setting, having an emergency plan is essential. The professional nurse should counsel his or her clients to have an emergency preparedness plan that includes an evacuation plan and an evacuation kit. The evacuation plan should include an evacuation location to where the client will go in the event of an emergency. The evacuation kit should include key documents (e.g., advance directives), medications, special treatment supplies, and important contacts (e.g., names and phone numbers of family members and physicians).

Conclusion

The older adult population represents a particularly vulnerable population. Age-related changes may make the older adult more vulnerable to physical injury. Nurses in all care settings should have a basic knowledge of the unique care needs of the older adult and further, should be capable of planning care for members of this population in times of disaster.

Caring for People with Disabilities in a Disaster

Persons with disabilities represent another special population that requires particular attention during a disaster situation. In the months following the terrorist attacks on the World Trade Center, most of the 54 million citizens in the United States who were people with disabilities indicated that they did not feel prepared for future crises, and 58% indicated that they did not know who to contact regarding emergency planning in their community. Another 61% of people with disabilities indicated that they had no plans in place to help them evacuate their homes safely (Federal Emergency Management Agency [FEMA] & U.S. Fire Administration, 2002).

The above statistics clearly indicate that disaster nurses may need to meet the needs of a vulnerable population that may not be prepared in an emergency situation. Although the bulk of the responsibility to meet the needs of individuals with disabilities may fall on first responders, disaster nurses may be included in the ranks of first responders based on paid and volunteer activity, the nature of the disaster, and the role the disaster nurse is playing in the disaster. Furthermore, disaster nurses will be expected to assume caring for individuals with a wide range of disabilities once they have been evacuated.

Defining Disability

The term *disability* is steeped in inconsistency. Definitions have been proposed by several organizations based on the organization's interests and populations served.

Two terms used to describe persons with disabilities have emerged, both generic terms that describe a given population in a broad sense (e.g., significant disability or severe handicap) or as a second type of term that describes the specific disability (e.g., blindness, autistic, or cerebral palsy) (Schleien, Fahnestock, & Miller, 2001).

Despite various differing classification systems there are some general approaches in caring for disaster victims with a disability that disaster nurses should be cognizant of and which relate to defining and describing of persons with disabilities. First, avoid terms that have a negative connotation with respect to the individual with a disability. For example, avoid using such phrases as the individual is "suffering from" Alzheimer's disease or that the individual is "a victim of" mental retardation. Second, speak directly to the individual, if possible, even if they are accompanied by others. People with disabilities may be able to comprehend and make independent decisions. Third, ask the disaster victim how to communicate with him or her most effectively. Fourth, be mindful of tone of voice and vigilant of behaviors as a disaster nurse; it is never appropriate to "talk down" to a disaster victim because of perceived abilities and/or disabilities. Finally, do not assume that individuals with certain types of disabilities suffer less physical injury or psychological or emotional trauma because of their disability (U.S. Department of Justice, 2002).

Federal Law and Disabilities

Disasters can be responded to in a rational and organized manner by knowledgeable professionals. That is the premise of this text. Times of disaster should not result in abandonment of our ideals as a civilization. To that end, the disaster response nurse must be aware of laws applicable to disabled persons and work within these laws, even in a disaster, if at all possible.

There are two federal laws that are applicable to individuals with disabilities. These are the Americans with Disabilities Act (ADA) of 1990 and Section 504 of the Rehabilitation Act of 1973. The ADA and section 504 of the Rehabilitation Act define a person with a disability as a person who "(1) has a physical or mental impairment that substantially limits one or more major life activities; (2) has a record of such an impairment; or (3) is regarded as having such an impairment" (U.S. Department of Justice, 2002, p. 5). Both laws require that first responders ensure victims are able to participate in programs, services, and activities afforded to other nondisabled persons. The law further requires reasonable accommodations for the person with a disability. Both laws are enforced through the U.S. Department of Justice.

Case Finding

The disaster nurse responding to a disaster must be aware that it may be difficult to identify those individuals who are disabled. Although several communities may have developed emergency management plans that include names and addresses or persons who are disabled, many individuals with disabilities may not have been included in these plans either because of privacy issues or because the person with a disability may have felt he or she did not require special assistance (FEMA & U.S. Fire Administration, 2002). Therefore, the disaster nurse should actively engage in case-finding activities. A good practice is to query each individual who is rescued as to whether or not they have any issues that may require special care and if they are aware of persons with disabilities or individuals who may need special assistance to evacuate or care for. This information should be communicated to first responders who may be spearheading evacuation activities.

Care in Shelters

Preparing the Shelter

At the beginning of a disaster, if shelters are required to care for those involved in the disaster, the disaster nurse should consider the needs of individuals with varying disabilities and plan for those needs. For example, the disaster nurse should realize that some individuals may present to the shelter in wheelchairs. Federal law requires that all shelters be wheelchair accessible, and the disaster nurse should evaluate the shelter for accessibility and consider reserving a special, accessible area of the shelter for those individuals.

If there are more private or secluded areas of the shelter, the disaster nurse should reserve these for older adults who may have cognitive impairments such as Alzheimer's or other dementias knowing that excessive environmental stimulation may result in the older adult with dementia acting out or becoming violent. Not all individuals with dementia will act out in the face of extreme environmental stimulation such as can be found in a shelter, but it is a possibility, and the disaster nurse should take steps to make certain that as appropriate as possible an environment is prepared for individuals with dementia.

Special Care Needs in a Shelter

The disaster nurse should assess whether or not individuals with disabilities have any type of special needs such as electricity-dependent equipment or adaptive devices for feeding or personal care. The disaster nurse should also inquire as to whether or not the individual has brought a ready-to-go bag or kit. If the person with special needs is evacuated to a shelter without the benefit of a ready-to-go kit, after assessing for basic physiologic stability, the disaster nurse should then focus his or her assessment on the individual's special needs.

The disaster nurse should inquire if the individual has an emergency list containing important information. The list may include such information as primary care provider, emergency contact, medication names, dosage, and frequency. The list may include any equipment the person with disabilities uses. Other items that should be included are the names, addresses, and phone numbers of equipment suppliers as well as the serial numbers of any equipment. This information may be needed after the disaster is over as the disaster nurse helps the individual who is returning home or moving to another temporary shelter.

The disaster nurse should find out if the person with disabilities requires prescription medication. The disaster nurse should also inquire as to whether or not the individual has brought a sufficient supply of medication. Certain drugs such as cardiac medications, antiseizure medications, and pain medications are an essential part of the care required by the person with special needs. The disaster nurse providing care to the person with a disability should assess the person's current medication regimen. If the individual has been evacuated to a clinic without essential medications, efforts should be made to procure the needed medication. In times of disaster, however, access to medications may be limited; therefore, the disaster nurse should consider the pathological processes that may be exacerbated as a result of the lack of medication and plan care and interventions aimed at protecting the client appropriately.

Working with Primary Caregivers

Many times, the person with a disability may receive assistance from individuals who can be identified as primary caregivers. These individuals may be family members, friends, paid paraprofessionals such as aides or housekeepers, or professional help from registered nurses. The disaster nurse should continue to allow primary caregivers and members of the individual's choosing to continue to provide as much care as they are willing. It is also important for the disaster nurse to realize that, during the disaster, it is not feasible to learn each and every aspect of the care needs of the person with a disability. If primary caregivers are present, they should be encouraged to continue providing care to their loved one. This will enable the disaster nurse to provide care and services to other individuals who may be demonstrating greater need.

Accommodating Those with Special Needs

People with disabilities face a variety of challenges on a daily basis. The disaster situation adds to these challenges. The disaster nurse should be aware of these challenges so that he or she is better prepared to provide the needed assistance to the individual with special needs.

Blind or Low-Vision

Reasons for visual impairments are varied and the younger client who is blind or has low vision is different from the older adult who is blind or has low vision. When approaching a person who has vision impairments, announce your presence. Speak naturally and directly to the individual. Remember that blindness does not make the individual hard of hearing so be aware of your volume. Provide a precise description of what you need the individual to do, and ask the person directly how you can best help. If the person is accompanied by a service animal, allow the service animal to remain with the person. If the individual has no service animal offer your arm or shoulder for guidance. Never "grab" or attempt to guide the

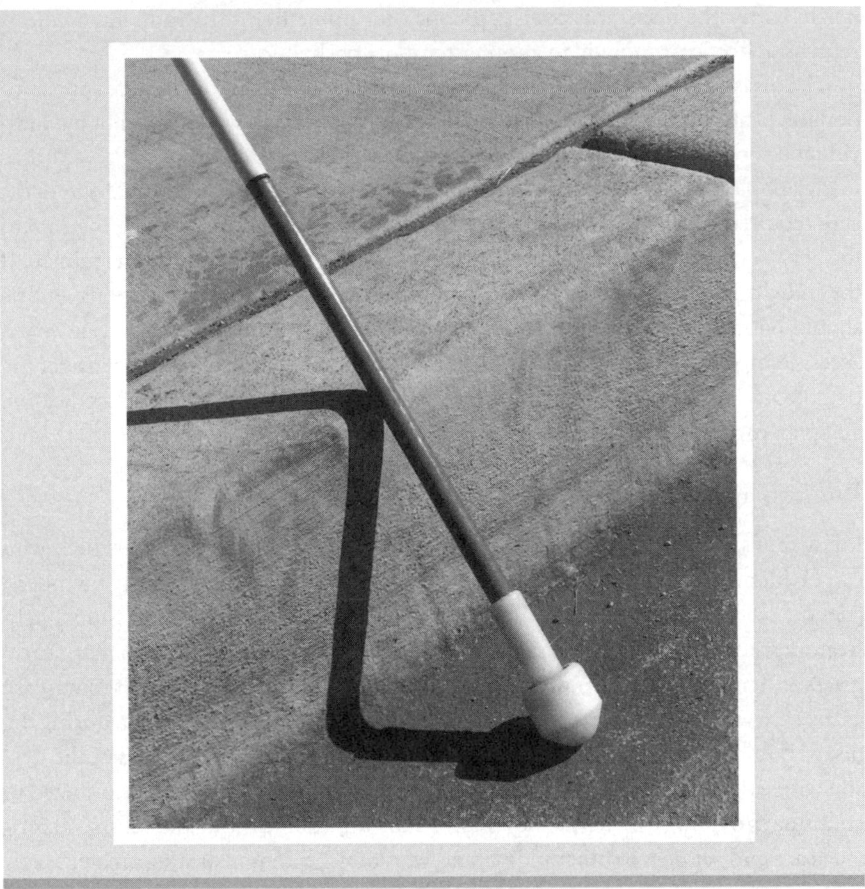

Figure 6-2 A person with visual impairment may use a white cane, which is both a mobility tool and a way to alert others to the user's impairment. *Source:* © Karin Lau/ShutterStock, Inc.

individual without first asking permission. The individual may choose to stay slightly behind you to gauge your body reactions to obstacles. Be sure to mention stairs, doorways, narrow passages, and ramps. When guiding to a seat, place the person's hand on the back of the chair. If leading several individuals at the same time, ask them to hold each other's arms (Beresford, Cahill, Pascarelli Barraza, & Carlin, 2007).

Deaf or Hard-of-Hearing Special Populations

Hearing impairments can range from mild hearing loss to an extreme of profound deafness. Do not assume because someone has hearing aids that his or her hearing is corrected or perfect. Hearing aids simply amplify sound; they do not clarify that sound. When approaching a person who is deaf or hard-of-hearing and the person does not have visual contact with the person entering the room (e.g., if you are entering a room and the person is facing away from you), the lights should be flicked on and off to draw attention to the presence of the person entering the room. When communicating with a person who is deaf or hard of hearing, do not allow others to interrupt or joke around while conveying information. Face the person when speaking, establishing eye contact even if an interpreter is present. Use facial expressions and hand gestures as visual cues. Offer the deaf or hard-of-hearing person written messages, using pen and paper, if able (Beresford et al., 2007).

Persons Who Use Wheelchairs

Persons who require a wheelchair for mobility require particular attention during a disaster. In times of disaster there is a temptation to rescue individuals without their wheelchairs, as this additional equipment may be viewed as extraneous, bulky, and hard to deal with. However, the disaster nurse acting in a first responder role should attempt to assure that the wheelchair is brought with the individual as this will aid with aftercare in a disaster shelter by allowing the individual to be more independent. If the disaster nurse is not acting as a first responder, she or he should discuss the need for first responders to evacuate with a wheelchair with the person in charge of the shelter or the incident commander.

Some general professional etiquette when working with the wheelchair-dependent client includes remembering that the chair is part of an individual's personal space. Talk directly to the individual in a wheelchair rather than through a companion. When talking with a person in a wheelchair for more than a few minutes, use a chair whenever possible. This can facilitate conversation. It will also put less strain on the individual's neck when trying to see the person speaking with him or her (FEMA & U.S. Fire Administration, 2002).

Cognitive Impairment

Individuals with cognitive impairment may have difficulty learning, problems with memory and judgment, and/or difficulty in their abilities to reason, focus, and understand. With these individuals, it is important to identify yourself clearly; use short sentences composed of simple, concrete words; and look for an identification bracelet with special health information. Shouting and frantic behaviors may scare the person and cause him or her to resist your help (Beresford et al., 2007).

Mental Illness

Mental illness encompasses a number of brain disorders that disrupt a person's mood, thought processes, memory, and interpretation of and responses to information obtained from the senses and feelings. It may limit their ability to reason and to relate to others (U.S. Department of Justice, 2002). When working with these persons, it is important to approach persons with mental illness in a calm, nonthreatening, and reassuring manner. Identify yourself clearly. Remember that the person may be confused, and the disaster nurse needs to speak slowly and in a normal speaking voice. Keep communication simple, clear, and brief. Do not use complex commands but break commands into a series of short sentences that are easy to follow. Do not argue with the individual, and be empathetic—let them know that you have heard them and care about what they have told you (Beresford et al., 2007).

Evacuation of Service Animals

There are several types of service animals people with disabilities may use. In addition to guide dogs for an individual who is blind, there are hearing dogs for people who are deaf, seizure dogs for people who have seizure disorders, assist animals for people with motor impairments, and companion animals for people with psychiatric impairments. Remember that the individual should never be separated from his or her service animal. When evacuating persons to shelters, service animals are to accompany the individual and the ADA of 1990 requires that reasonable accommodations be made.

There are no registries for service animals, nor is the individual required under law to provide proof that an animal is a service animal. If the individual tells a disaster nurse or responder that he or she has a disability and that an animal is a service animal, then the individual should be allowed to maintain the service animal alongside at all times. If other individuals within the temporary shelter indicate that they are allergic to, do not like, or are afraid of animals, move that individual away from the person with the service animal or have the person who indicates he or she has a problem relocated to another shelter, if possible (Beresford et al., 2007).

When working with service animals, never touch or offer the animal food without the permission of the owner. When the animal is wearing its harness, the animal is considered to be working and should not be disturbed. Service animals are expected to be harnessed or on a leash, but are not required to be muzzled (Beresford et al., 2007).

Conclusion

Day-to-day activities for individuals with special needs can be challenging. Times of disaster can be overwhelming. Stress may make many medical conditions worse. During the disaster, individuals with special needs and the elderly may ask for help to do things they usually would have done independently. The disaster nurse can help to create a therapeutic atmosphere through proper planning and demonstrating competence with some of the more common type of limitations that individuals may face.

References

Administration on Aging. (2006). A profile of older Americans: 2006. Retrieved January 12, 2008, from http://www.aoa.gov/prof/Statistics/profile/2006/2006profile.pdf

American Association of Retired Persons [AARP]. (2006, September 6). *AARP offers tips to help older Americans prepare for emergencies.* Retrieved January 13, 2008, from http://www.aarp.org/research/press-center/presscurrentnews/preparing_for_emergencies.html

Beresford, M. K., Cahill, A., Pascarelli Barraza, A., & Carlin, R. S. (2007). *Tips for first responders* (2nd ed.). Albuquerque, NM: Author.

Berk, L. E. (2001). *Development through the lifespan* (2nd ed.). Boston: Allyn & Bacon.

Engler, B. (2003). *Personality theories.* New York: Houghton Mifflin Company.

Federal Emergency Management Agency & U.S. Fire Administration. (2002). *Orientation manual for first responders on the evacuation of people with disabilities.* Washington, DC: Author.

Lach, H. W. (2007). Gerontological nursing: Issues and trends in practice. In A. D. Linton & H. W. Lach (Eds.) *Matteson & McConnell's gerontological nursing* (3rd ed.). St. Louis, MO: Elsevier.

Schleien, S. J., Fahnestock, M. K., & Miller, K. D. (2001). Severe multiple disabilities. In D. R. Austin & M. E. Crawford (Eds.), *Therapeutic recreation* (3rd ed.). Boston: Allyn and Bacon.

Smeltzer, S. C., & Bare, B. (2004). *Brunner & Suddarth's textbook of medical-surgical nursing.* (10th ed.). Philadelphia: Lippincott, Williams and Wilkins.

Travis, S. (1998). Demographic trends. In A. Schmidt-Luggen, S. S. Travis, & S. Meiner (Eds.). *NGNA core curriculum for gerontological advanced practice nurses.* Thousand Oaks, CA: Sage.

U.S. Department of Justice. (2002). *First response to victims of crime who have disabilities.* Washington, DC: Author.

chapter 7

Culture and Disasters

Sharon A. Nazarchuk and Timothy J. Legg

GOAL

The goal of this chapter is to begin a dialog in a little discussed area of disaster response: culture and the disaster victim.

OBJECTIVES

At the completion of this chapter, the reader will:

1. Define the term *culture.*
2. Differentiate between cultural competence and disaster nursing response expediency.
3. Apply cultural universals in providing culturally competent disaster nursing care.
4. Evaluate models of cultural competence.
5. Apply a model of cultural competence to disaster nursing.
6. Assess the disaster victim's general cultural background.
7. Provide culturally appropriate concepts to culturally sensitive disaster situations.
8. Explore the impact of a disaster on a culture.

Key Terms

- Culture
- Cultural competence
- Cultural universals
- Models of cultural competence
- Culture and communication
- Social organization and culture
- Environmental considerations and culture in a disaster
- Culture and disasters

Introduction

Nursing professionals are seemingly inundated with mandates from multiple sources and stakeholders emphasizing the need to provide care that is culturally sensitive. The Joint Commission has included requirements in its accreditation standards for healthcare organizations that address the need to provide patients with culturally and linguistically appropriate services. Hospitals have cited many challenges associated with the implementation of this standard for a number of reasons (Wilson-Stronks & Galvez, 2007). When this standard is difficult to achieve during times of "business as usual," the challenge associated with the provision of culturally competent care during times of disaster represents an even greater challenge.

On the surface, the question of the importance of cultural competence during times of disasters seems appropriate. Should culture matter when a disaster situation is unfolding and lives are being lost or altered? It is our contention that it should for the most fundamental of reasons—our humanness and our civility. The extent to which we are able to maintain the expression of our professional values and the ability to which we are able to reach out to and address the humanness of our clients represents our dedication to the preservation of our society in general and our profession of nursing in particular. To ignore the cultural needs of our clients during a disaster experience dismisses our professional integrity, which includes our ability to provide holistic care for those in need of nursing care. Culturally sensitive care is one of the central tenets of holistic health care. Additionally, the ability to which we are able to maintain orderly expression of our professional values demonstrates the degree to which we are prepared to respond to a disaster situation. Whereas it is recognized that some social constructs will be altered during the time of disaster (e.g., ability to attend religious services at a fixed place of worship), there are some facets of our culture and the culture of our clients that should not be ignored.

The multicultural nature of the United States mandates that the nurse have at least a cursory understanding of the role of culture in health care. Whereas cultural competence is important during times of relative social stability, it is increasingly important during times of disaster because it is during these times that we are at greatest risk of forgetting the rules of society that provide us with cohesion and harmony. Acknowledging the fact that, as humans, we tend to migrate toward those experiences that are more familiar to us, we must be aware of this in our work in disaster situations. The provision of nursing care including physical and psychosocial care to members of the dominant social group because of the nurses' familiarity or ability to identify with this group may be perceived as preferential treatment by members of minority groups, resulting in members of the minority group feeling disenfranchised (Veenema, 2007).

There is a propensity to address culture as other works have in the past through a pairing of cultural group with supposed universal attributes. This approach often results in a "laundry list" of attributes assigned to members of a particular culture and ultimately has the potential to result in stereotyping (e.g., all Asians eat rice and are Buddhists). Although individuals can come from a similar dominant culture, they may be completely opposite from a cultural standpoint. This concept is best illustrated in a rather poignant example provided by Purnell (2005). In a description of how people from dominant culture vary, he describes the following situation:

> Susan Jones, age 62, is an uninsured, single, white Catholic lesbian who makes $20,000 a year and practices aromatherapy. William James, age 28, is an insured, heterosexual, married, white male with four children and makes $200,000 per year and believes strongly in high-technology health care. (p. 8)

Although these two people come from the "dominant American culture," their worldview is probably very different owing to their subcultures and primary and secondary characteristics of cultures such as age, gender, sexual orientation, marital status, parental status, and socioeconomic and insurance status.

Whereas we recognize that individual members of a particular culture may be quite different in their adherence to cultural norms and values, we also recognize that there are commonalities in every culture. In this chapter, we will examine the multiple facets of culture and the potential impact of the disaster situation on the lived experience of individuals and the resultant impact on culture.

Culture Defined

To begin our discussion of culture in disaster situations we must begin with a firm definition of culture and what it constitutes. Many authors have grappled with those attributes most central to culture. Harris, Moran, and Moran (2004, pp. 4–5) described culture as "a distinctly human means of adapting to circumstances and transmitting this coping skill and knowledge to subsequent generations." They continue by contending that culture "gives people a sense of who they are, of belonging, of how they should behave and of what they should be doing . . . it is considered the driving force behind human behavior everywhere."

Parrillo offers another perspective in that "culture consists of the physical or material objects and values, attitudes, customs, beliefs, and habits shared by members of a society and transmitted to the next generation. These cultural attributes provide a sense of peoplehood and common bonds through which members of a society can relate" (Parrillo, 2000, pp. 29–30). Purnell and Paulanka described culture as the "totality of socially transmitted behavioral patterns, arts, beliefs, values, customs, lifeways, and all other products of human work and thought characteristics of a population of people that guide their worldview and decision making" (Purnell & Paulanka, 2003, p. 3). These are but a few of the definitions of culture; it is worth noting that over 164 definitions of culture have been identified (Campinha-Bacote, 2003).

Whereas the authors cited above have done an exemplary job of defining culture and of its nuances, we have taken a more pragmatic approach to the term's definition for the purposes of disaster nursing care. We define *culture* as the totality of experiences, including aesthetics and artifacts, that hold relevance for the individual enabling them to feel a sense of connectedness to their social network and preferred peer group and associated affiliations.

Culture has been described as a double-edged sword. One edge enables individuals to live and work together effectively in groups, but the other edge creates social disharmony through the tendency to judge others based on one's own cultural background (Geissler, 1998). The tendency to judge others based on our own cultural beliefs is known as *ethnocentricity*. To avoid problems that can arise through ethnocentricity, cultural competence must be achieved. But what exactly is cultural competence?

Cultural Competence

Cultural competence is another term that the nurse responding to disaster situations should be aware of. The term has appeared in a plethora of nursing journals and books: The mandate for nurses to increase their "cultural competence" has been expressed not only in Joint Commission standards for accreditation of healthcare organizations but has also been included in multiple position statements by authoritative agencies such as the American Academy of Nursing and the American Nurses Association (Gooden, Porter, Gonzalez, & Mims, 2001). Still others have established standards for culturally and linguistically appropriate healthcare services (U.S. Department of Health and Human Services, Office of Minority Health, 2007).

Cultural competence has been defined by many authors over the years. Cross, Bazron, Dennis, and Isaacs (1989) described it as a:

> set of congruent behaviors, attitudes, and policies that come together in a system, agency, or amongst professionals and enables that system, agency or those professionals to work effectively in cross-cultural situations . . . A culturally competent system of care acknowledges and incorporates—at all levels—the importance of culture, the assessment of cross-cultural relations, vigilance towards the dynamics that result from cultural differences, the expansion of cultural knowledge, and the adaptation of services to meet culturally unique needs. (pp. iv–v)

The California Endowment Project defines cultural competence as "a set of integrated attitudes, knowledge, and skills that enable a healthcare professional or organization to care effectively for patients from diverse cultures, groups, and communities" (2003, p. 11). Purnell and Paulanka described culturally competent individuals as individuals who "value diversity and respect individual differences regardless of one's race, religious beliefs, or ethnocultural background" (2005, pp. xv–xvi).

Cultural Universals

Although it is our distinct attempt to avoid introducing a list of supposed attributes of various cultural groups that could result in stereotyping, we must acknowledge the existence of cultural universals that are common features found in all societies. Cultural universals are nothing more than commonalities that individuals within a larger culture share. Such commonalities include language, socialization of children, dealing with deviance, and so on. It has been reported that as many as 88 general categories of behavior can be found in all cultures (Hughes & Kroehler, 2008). Clearly, it would be an enormous task to attempt to define each of these categories of behavior specific to each and every cultural group that the disaster nurse may interface with during times of disaster. However, the use of a model to facilitate the acquisition of cultural competence would aid the disaster nurse in providing effective care for members of other cultures during times of disaster.

Dean (2001) posed an interesting argument in that our postmodern world reflects multiple changes in culture resulting from group and individual construction, evolution, and emergence. Dean questioned the work of Goldberg (2000, as cited in Dean) who contended that one could become "competent" in the culture of another group. Dean proposed a model that maintains an "awareness of one's lack of competence" as the goal as opposed to "the establishment of competence" (Dean, p. 624). Dean's contentions have been further supported by the work of Cole who reported the use of the LEARN model for the instruction of cross-cultural health care to medical students (Cole, 2002). This model in particular is used because "it implies that cross-cultural communication is always a work in progress" (¶ 7).

Models of Cultural Competence

Whereas Dean made an outstanding argument against the ability to acquire cultural competence, we have considered her work in relation to the remainder of the body of knowledge that contends that cultural competence can indeed be achieved (2001). It is through an attempt to temper the two competing ideologies that we have decided to undertake a reconciliation of the contentions of Dean and the remainder of the body of knowledge specific to cultural competence. Instead of attempting to become culturally competent, the disaster nurse would be better served by learning how to acquire knowledge, skills, and abilities in working with members of other cultures.

To that end, we propose the use of a model of cultural competence. Models of cultural competence provide the nurse with a framework to guide his or her study or inquiry of other cultures. Whereas it is beyond the scope of this work to provide an in-depth exploration of all models, what is provided is a cursory review of some of the more widely used models.

Several authors have written about the characteristics or aspects of culture that should be examined when working with individuals from other cultures. Multiple authors have attempted to develop models and conceptual frameworks of culture with multiple underlying assumptions and with utility among different groups of clients. Perhaps one of the most comprehensive models has been developed by Purnell (2003). This model has demonstrated utility across many disciplines and settings where health care takes place. It has been described by others as conceptually clear, logically congruent, has demonstrated clinical utility, and is easy to apply to any culture or setting (Brathwaite, 2003).

The Purnell model consists of macro and micro aspects. The macro aspects include the concept of a global society, community, family, and person. The micro aspect of the model consists of 12 domains and their related concepts. Purnell's domains include the following:

1. Overview, inhabited localities, and topography (e.g., where the people came from, where they live, economics, politics, education, and occupation)
2. Communication (e.g., dominant languages, dialects, contextual use, volume/tone, spatial distancing, eye contact, facial expressions, greetings, time, and touch)
3. Family roles and organization (e.g., head of household, gender roles, goals and priorities, developmental tasks, roles of the aged, roles of extended family members, social status, and alternative lifestyles)
4. Workforce issues (e.g., including acculturation, autonomy, and language barriers)
5. Biocultural ecology (e.g., biological variations, skin color, heredity, and ecology)
6. High-risk behaviors (e.g., tobacco and alcohol use, recreational drugs, physical activity, and safety)
7. Nutrition (e.g., meaning of food, common foods, and rituals surrounding foods)
8. Pregnancy and childrearing practices (e.g., fertility practices, views toward pregnancy, pregnancy beliefs, and birthing practices as well as beliefs about women and children in the postpartum period)
9. Death rituals (e.g., burial rites and bereavement)
10. Spirituality (e.g., religious practices, use of prayer, and the meaning of life)
11. Healthcare practices (e.g., magicoreligious beliefs, responsibility for health, rehabilitation, transplantation, transfusion, mental health, the role of pain, and the role of the sick)
12. Healthcare practitioners (e.g., perceptions of practitioners, folk practitioners and their use, gender and health care) (Purnell & Paulanka, 2003, pp. 10–11)

The complexity and comprehensiveness of the Purnell model may be a bit cumbersome for use in disaster situations. However, it should be appreciated that research would need to be conducted in order to ascertain which models are the easiest to use and most effective in times of disaster.

Leininger's Sunrise Model guides the nurse to consider cultural influences that can impact health of the client. The model encourages the nurse to consider the multiple influences of culture on the patient. Based on the contemplation of the influences, one of three outcomes can result. The first is that the nurse provides care that is not in conflict with the patient's culture. The second outcome requires cultural "accommodation or negotiation" and the last outcome results in "care that requires a repatterning or restructuring of cultural beliefs for effective care" (Cutilli, 2006, p. 218).

The Campinha-Bacote model focuses on the development of cultural competence (2002). The model is entitled "The Process of Cultural Competence in the Delivery of Healthcare Services" and is based on five assumptions:

1. Cultural competence is a process, not an event.
2. Cultural competence consists of five constructs: cultural awareness, cultural knowledge, cultural skills, cultural encounters, and cultural desires.
3. There are more variations within ethnic groups than across ethnic groups (intraethnic variations).
4. There is a direct relationship between the level of competence of healthcare providers and their ability to provide culturally responsive healthcare services.
5. Cultural competence is an essential component in rendering effective and culturally responsive services to culturally and ethnically diverse clients. (p. 181)

According to Campinha-Bacote, the goal of the healthcare provider is to continuously strive to "achieve the ability to effectively work within the cultural context of the client (individual, family, community)" (2002, p. 181). The model operates on the premise that cultural competence is a process of *becoming* as opposed to the idea that one *becomes* culturally competent. This is most congruent with the contentions of Dean (2001) who believes that cultural competence is in essence a journey and not a destination.

The Giger and Davidhizar Transcultural Assessment model (Davidhizar, Bechtel, & Newman-Giger, 1998) seeks to identify differences between people in cultural groups through the assessment of six main factors. These factors are (a) communication, (b) space, (c) time, (d) social organization, (e) environmental control, and (f) biological variations. This model provides a framework that can be used by multiple disciplines in multiple settings including acute care as well as the community. Its utility has been demonstrated in specialty areas as well and has been tested with paraprofessionals in addition to nursing and other professionals. For these reasons, we have decided to explore this model in greater detail as well as its potential implications for disaster nurses.

Communication

Communication is defined as the continuous process through which people interact using written, oral, or nonverbal language (e.g., facial expression, gestures, or other symbols). It is communication that not only preserves culture, but also transmits culture over time. When a language barrier exists, a translator may be able to interpret but subtle nuances in terms of the differences in the meaning of words can be lost in the translation resulting in miscommunication (Davidhizar, Bechtel, & Newman-Giger, 1998).

Space

We are all familiar with the concept of personal space, the area that surrounds our body that we consider an area not to be violated by just anyone. Depending upon culture, personal space may be quite close to the individual's body or it can be several feet away. Feelings of discomfort result from invasions of personal space whether intended or unintended (Davidhizar, Bechtel, & Newman-Giger, 1998). Discomfort arising from invasion of personal space may manifest itself in emergency shelters where many individuals may be occupying a relatively small area. The disaster nurse can best intervene by acknowledging the invasion of personal space and assuring the client that the situation is temporary.

Social Organization

Members of virtually every culture in the world learn their own culture in the family setting. Children learn by watching adults, making inferences about their own behavior, and receiving correction from parental figures when violations of cultural norms occur. Based on this understanding, we can easily see why the family is the most important social organization in most cultures. In times of disaster, the disaster nurse needs to ascertain the social organization of the client in terms of whether the client makes decisions based on the concept of family autonomy, in which healthcare decisions are made by the family as a whole, or based on the concept of individual autonomy in which healthcare decisions are made by the individual (Davidhizar, Bechtel, & Newman-Giger, 1998). Assessment of this concept will help the disaster nurse to provide appropriate information while respecting both the individual and family autonomy.

Time

Many authors have noted the cultural variations in terms of perceptions of time in general and the concept of *on time* in particular (Hall, 1990). In some cultures, being on time is considered appropriate, whereas other cultures view being on time as rude and pushy, and in still other cultures being late is perfectly acceptable. Temporal orientation, the way in which the past, present, and future are ordered, differs between people of different ethnic heritages. For example, Native Americans do not include expectancy in their view of time. As a result, primary prevention activities may be ignored (Davidhizar, Bechtel, & Newman-Giger, 1998).

Environmental Control

This type of control is related to the individual's ability to plan activities in his or her life. The concept encompasses not only where the individual lives, but also processes and systems that affect the individual. If the individual feels that he or she can control the environment, the individual is said to have an internal locus of control. Some members of some cultures believe that things occur by fate, including luck or chance, or that circumstances occur because of "God's will." Individuals who subscribe to these beliefs are said to have an external locus of control. Some cultures have a fatalistic view of the world and as such do not seek to find meaning in life circumstances, simply accepting situations as fate (Davidhizar, Bechtel, & Newman-Giger, 1998). An excellent example of this was seen in the Iraqi war with a video of a car making it over a bridge just before the bridge was bombed by the U.S. Air Force. The general presenting the video to the media commented that the driver was the luckiest man in the world, immediately setting off an uproar among Muslims who do not believe in fate: Had Allah meant for that driver to die, then he would have. Luck had nothing to do with it. The disaster nurse providing care to members of cultures that subscribe to a fatalistic world view should not attempt to help the individual find meaning in the disaster situation. Efforts should be focused on helping the individual cope with any anticipation of "what's next."

Biological Variations

The final construct of the Giger and Davidhizar model (Davidhizar, Bechtel, & Newman-Giger, 1998) is that of biological variations. It is understood that members of different cultures may vary in terms of anatomical characteristics, skin and hair physiology, and other biological characteristics. These variations are among the least understood and recognized. Davidhizar et al. provided an excellent example of these variations:

> For example, Hispanics are at high risk for diabetes, and African-Americans have higher prevalence of cardiovascular heart disease, cancer, and diabetes. Sickle-cell anemia is found almost exclusively in African-Americans, whereas Tay-Sachs disease is most prevalent in the Jewish community. Finally, significant differences exist among members of different cultural groups in their perceptions of pain and their responses to pain management. (p. 25)

Disaster nurses should be aware of these biological variations among members of different cultures in disaster situations. Appropriate nursing assessments and interventions should be conducted to prevent complications or exacerbations of illness in an already stressful healthcare situation. In Table 7-1, three examples of how these six constructs can provide the disaster nurse with essential information about a given culture are shown.

Culture and Disasters

To this point, definitions of culture and cultural competence have been presented, and it is time to explore the impact of disaster on culture within the context of the above. To begin, one must ask: What constitutes a disaster? Although disaster has been defined elsewhere in this text, the definition offered by Landesman will be used in relation to culture. Landesman contended that "disasters are emergencies of a severity and magnitude resulting in deaths, injuries, illness, and/or property damage that cannot be effectively managed by the application of routine procedures or resources" (2001, p. 1).

TABLE 7-1 EXAMPLE OF CULTURAL COMPARISONS OF THREE DIFFERENT CULTURES USING THE GIGER AND DAVIDHIZAR MODEL CONSTRUCTS

Culture	Communication	Space	Time	Social Organization	Environmental Control	Biological Variations
People of Appalachian heritage	English is dominant language. Most are comfortable with silence.	More traditional individuals may stand at a distance to talk with people in healthcare situations.	May like to "sit a spell" and "chat" before getting down to business of collecting health information. Healthcare practitioners should be "flexible."	Large families common and can be a rich resource. Family rather than individual is often considered the basic treatment unit.	External locus of control. Strong belief in "God's will."	If of Scotch-Irish descent, with light skin tones, may be at increased risk for skin cancer.
People of Filipino heritage	More than 100 dialects are spoken. English is used for business and legal transactions. Always address Filipino adults by their title or professional affiliation until you are told that it is acceptable to do otherwise.	Greater distance can be seen when interacting with people in positions of authority. Same-gender touching is not unusual.	"Promptness" for events is determined based on the situation. Lateness for an appointment is accepted, as to arrive on time could be mistaken as a sign of "eagerness."	Father is traditionally regarded as head of household, but authority is egalitarian. Decisions about healthcare are made by family.	Some Filipinos are fatalistic and tend to accept situations that cannot be changed.	Youthful features results in difficulty "guessing age." High melanin content of the skin makes assessment of manifestations of anemia or jaundice difficult (pallor or jaundice). High incidence of lactose intolerance.

People of Mexican heritage	Great diversity exists in the Spanish language (approximately 62 dialects exist). Greet adults formally with Señor, Señora, or Señorita unless they have asked you to do otherwise.	Men and women seldom touch in public. Touch is common among individuals of the same gender. Healthcare providers should explain the need for touch.	Arriving late for appointments is acceptable. May delay seeking health care.	Concept of "machismo" is stereotypical and inaccurate of all Mexicans and Mexican-Americans. Whereas some households are patriarchal, some are matriarchal and still others are egalitarian. Specifically ask who is the decision maker for the family.	May be fatalistic and present oriented.	Darker skin tones necessitate assessment of sclera, palms of hands, buccal mucosa, and tongue for conditions such as cyanosis or jaundice. High rates of diabetes are common. Diarrheal and parasitic disease are more common among newer immigrants.

Source: Adapted from Purnell & Paulanka, 2005.

It should be understood that some disasters are geographically specific and would therefore have a stronger impact upon the cultural groups living in the defined geographic region, despite their identification or affiliation with a larger cultural group. Let us consider an example using the Midwestern state of Kansas. It would not be a surprise to learn that many members of the population of Kansas have or know how to access a tornado shelter. At the same time, the concept of a tornado shelter (e.g., having one or knowing how to access one) is relatively foreign to the inhabitant of Pennsylvania. Both groups of people are "American" citizens, but have different experiences in terms of geographic disaster preparedness.

It should also be appreciated that disasters and their resultant impact on a culture may take years to manifest. For example, cultural groups living in Sri Lanka experienced a major tsunami in 2005. The results of this disaster on the cultures of those living in Sri Lanka have yet to be fully determined. Members of some cultures may appear indifferent to a disaster situation as it may not be culturally acceptable to do otherwise. Variations in culture during a disaster situation can have the potential to lead the disaster nurse into making incorrect assumptions about the groups she or he is working with. Herein is found the importance of learning how to work with members of other cultures.

Consider the issue of feeding disaster victims. Hindus do not eat meat. Many Jews keep kosher. While it might seem self-evident that one eats what is available in a disaster, if at all possible, consideration should be given to food preferences beyond those that are medically related. An excellent example of cultural insensitivity occurred in 1992 in a small Midwestern town that experienced two tornadoes within 24 hours. Disaster relief workers from the local American Red Cross provided food for victims and disaster responders. They made sandwiches of ham and cheese, not thinking to make separate cheese sandwiches and ham sandwiches. One Jewish disaster nurse, who kept kosher, removed the ham from the sandwich and ate the bread and cheese. While even eating such a cheese sandwich was really not strictly kosher, the situation allowed for such variation from Koshrut. Had there been nothing else to eat at all, except ham, even that would have been allowed by Jewish law, but this was not the case, though all the cheese and bread had touched ham.

The disaster nurse removed the ham and threw it away, proceeding to eat the cheese and bread. The disaster relief workers who saw this and had made the sandwiches were scandalized and began talking "among themselves," but loudly enough to ensure the disaster nurse heard every word. They expressed horror at the waste they saw and debated about the ingratitude of the disaster nurse. The disaster nurse, exhausted from 12 hours of caring for tornado victims, was hurt and insulted, walking away without commenting to the others about her religious beliefs and crying in the bathroom till she could regain composure. She did report what happened to the disaster shelter manager later that day, but, to this day, she remembers that and tries not to eat around other disaster workers (D. Adelman, personal communication, March 27, 2008).

In addition to the physical injury that accompanies many disasters, loss of life is often an inevitable result of most disaster situations. The disaster nurse must develop an appreciation of bereavement across cultures. In many cultures, death is a taboo topic, one to be recoiled from, whereas in other cultures death is a celebrated part of life. The disaster nurse should follow the family's lead when attempting therapeutic intervention with individuals who have lost loved ones in the disaster situation, as dealing with death is deeply culturally embedded. If the client wishes to speak about the loss with the disaster nurse, the nurse should use appropriate therapeutic communication techniques. If the client does not wish to talk about his or her loss, the disaster nurse should respect this. There is no universally agreed upon formula for understanding or working with individuals who have lost loved ones in times of disaster.

The disaster nurse should also be familiar with some of the more important death rituals of members of the cultures that live in a particular geographic area. Times of disaster with resultant injury and loss of life are stressful enough without adding cultural insult through the improper care of the deceased. The disaster nurse needs to be aware that members of different cultures may behave differently than the disaster nurse's native culture. The disaster nurse should also be aware that members of different cultures may engage in similar practices, but for completely different reasons.

Consider the practice of sitting with the deceased. In cultures in which Buddhism is practiced, a family member or friend may remain with the body of the deceased. The purpose of this attendance of the body may be to prevent visits from cats, because Buddhists believe that cats were the only animal not in attendance at Buddha's funeral and, if a cat were to approach the deceased, the body would rise (Irish, 2000). Now, let us consider the Jewish tradition. According to Jewish tradition, "a member of the chevrah kadisha or friend of the family will perform shemirah (i.e., watching over the body from the time of death until burial)" (Clements et al., 2003, p. 22). This is done because the body is considered the repository of the soul and respect should be paid to the body.

Conclusion

It should be readily apparent that culture is not abandoned during times of disaster but is often clung to as one last normalcy of predisaster life. The disaster nurse who discounts the importance and role of culture risks placing unnecessary boundaries between the nurse and client. Cultural competence is a journey; it is not a destination. It is impossible for us to acquire all of the knowledge, skills, and abilities that would enable us to be culturally fluent. What we can do is recognize our own culture and approach others with an open mind and the innate understanding that their culture makes as much sense to them as our culture to us. By celebrating diversity in times of social order we set the stage for how we will practice in times of disaster.

References

Brathwaite, A. C. (2003). Selection of a conceptual model/framework for guiding research interventions [Electronic version]. *The Internet Journal of Advanced Nursing Practice, 6*(1). Retrieved March 26, 2008, from http://www.ispub.com/ostia/index.php?xmlFilePath=journals/ijanp/vol6n1/research.xml

California Endowment Project. (2003). Principles and recommended standards for cultural competence education of health care professionals. Retrieved March 27, 2008, from http://www.calendow.org/reference/publications/pdf/cultural/TCE0215-2003_Principles_and.pdf

Campinha-Bacote, J. (2002). The process of cultural competence in the delivery of healthcare services: A model of care. *Journal of Transcultural Nursing, 13*(3), 181–184.

Campinha-Bacote, J. (2003). Many faces: Addressing diversity in health care [Electronic version]. *Online Journal of Issues in Nursing, 8*(1). Retrieved March 22, 2008, from http://www.nursingworld.org/MainMenuCategories/ANAMarketplace/ANAPeriodicals/OJIN/TableofContents/Volume82003/Num1Jan31_2003/AddressingDiversityinHealthCare.aspx

Clements, P. T., Vigil, G. J., Manno, M. S., Henry, G. C., Wilks, J., Das, S., et al. (2003). Cultural perspectives of death, grief, and bereavement [Electronic version]. *Journal of Psychosocial Nursing & Mental Health Services, 41*(7), 18–26.

Cole, P. M. (2002). When medicine and culture intersect: Changing patient demographics means traditional approaches are inadequate [Electronic version]. *Postgraduate Medicine, 112*(4), 11.

Cross, T. L., Bazron, B. J., Dennis, K. W., & Isaacs, M. R. (1989). *Towards a culturally competent system of care.* Washington, DC: Child and Adolescent Service System Program (CASSP) Technical Assistance Center.

Cutilli, C. C. (2006). Do your patients understand? Providing culturally congruent patient education [Electronic version]. *Orthopaedic Nursing, 25*(3), 218–226.

Davidhizar, R., Bechtel, G., & Newman-Giger, J. (1998). A model to enhance culturally competent care [Electronic version]. *Hospital Topics, 76*(2), 22–26.

Dean, R. G. (2001). The myth of cross-cultural competence [Electronic version]. *Families in Society, 82*(6), 623–630.

Geissler, E. M. (1998). *Cultural assessment* (2nd ed.). St. Louis, MO: Mosby.

Gooden, M. B., Porter, C. P., Gonzalez, R. I., & Mims, B. L. (2001). Rethinking the relationship between nursing and diversity [Electronic version]. *American Journal of Nursing, 101*(1). Retrieved March 22, 2008, from http://www.nursingworld.org/DocumentVault/AJN/2001/AJNNursingandDiversity.aspx

Hall, E. T. (1990). *The silent language.* New York: Anchor Books.

Harris, P. R., Moran, R. T., & Moran, S. V. (2004). *Managing cultural differences* (6th ed.). New York: Elsevier.

Hughes, M., & Kroehler, C. J. (2008). *Sociology: The core* (8th ed.). Boston: McGraw Hill.

Irish, J. S. (2000). Mourning in rural Japan [Electronic version]. *Japan Quarterly, 47*(4), 73–81.

Landesman, L. Y. (2001). *Public health management of disasters.* Washington, DC: American Public Health Association.

Parrillo, V. N. (2000). *Strangers to these shores: Race and ethnic relations in the United States.* (6th ed.). Boston: Allyn & Bacon.

Purnell, L. (2003). Transcultural diversity and health care. In L. Purnell and B. Paulanka (Eds.), *Transcultural health care: A culturally competent approach* (2nd ed., pp. 1–7). Philadelphia: F. A. Davis.

Purnell, L. (2005). The Purnell model for cultural competence [Electronic version]. *Journal of Multicultural Nursing and Health, 11*(2), 715.

Purnell, L. D., & Paulanka, B. J. (2003). *Transcultural health care: A culturally competent approach* (2nd ed.). Philadelphia: F. A. Davis.

Purnell, L., & Paulanka B. J. (2005). *Guide to culturally competent health care.* Philadelphia: F. A. Davis.

U.S. Department of Health and Human Services, Office of Minority Health. (2007). *Culturally and linguistically appropriate services (CLAS).* Retrieved March 13, 2008, from http://www.omhrc.gov/templates/content.aspx?ID=2806

Veenema, T. G. (2007). *Disaster nursing and emergency preparedness for chemical, biological, and radiological terrorism and other hazards* (2nd ed.). New York: Singer Publishing.

Wilson-Stronks, A., & Galvez, E. (2007). *Hospitals, language, and culture: A snapshot of the nation.* The Joint Commission. Retrieved March 26, 2008, from http://www.jointcommission.org/NR/rdonlyres/E64E5E89-5734-4D1D-BB4D-C4ACD4BF8BD3/0/hlc_paper.pdf

chapter 8

The Psychology of Disasters

Carol Kleinman and Jean Rubino

GOAL

The goal of this chapter is to provide appropriate and adequate psychological support for the disaster victim and disaster responder.

OBJECTIVES

At the completion of this chapter, the reader will:

1. List the differing phases of a disaster.
2. Define the various stages of psychological response a disaster victim goes through.
3. Describe what a secondary disaster is.
4. Intervene in primary and secondary disaster situations.
5. Understand psychological responses to a disaster.
6. Modify mental health nursing care for the disaster situation.
7. Assess the disaster victim's mental health.
8. Provide appropriate mental health referrals for the disaster victim.
9. Apply concepts from psychological first aid in caring for the disaster victim.
10. Generalize the concepts of compassion fatigue in caring for self and other disaster responders.

Key Terms

- Disaster mental health
- Victim levels
- The second disaster
- Psychological responses to disasters
- PTSD/ATSD
- Special needs in a disaster
- Short- and long-term interventions
- Compassion fatigue
- Psychological first aid

Introduction

The history of nurses serving as first responders in disasters began with Florence Nightingale during the Crimean War. Since that time, nurses continue to be first responders and providers of care during and after large-scale disasters. Although nurses have a primary role in the physical management of the disaster victim, the psychosocial aspects of disaster response cannot be ignored. This chapter will present the psychological care of the disaster victim and considerations in dealing with psychological issues faced by disaster responders.

Phases of the Disaster

Disasters and disaster preparedness have been described as having several phases. Although the title of each phase differs when described by various authors, all identify several phases of the predisaster, disaster, and postdisaster period (Rao, 2006). The preevent phase involves planning and prevention and focuses on activities to develop community preparedness for a natural or man-made disaster with the primary goal of vulnerability reduction and response readiness. Disaster management in the acute phase, during the disaster, involves mitigation of the event and its consequences, with a focus on the delivery of aid, shelter, sustenance, and medical care. The focus in the response phase is on meeting basic needs until more permanent and sustainable solutions can be found. The postdisaster phase revolves around recovery activities. When the immediate needs of the population are met, the recovery phase, which is the most significant in terms of long-term outcome, begins. The recovery process must start immediately to restore normalcy and function as quickly as possible.

Disaster nurses are involved in primary, secondary, and tertiary prevention activities through the implementation of disaster nursing interventions. Interventions differ based on the type and scope of the disaster. Primary prevention involves disaster preparedness, and disaster nurses are often involved in the development of large-scale disaster plans. Secondary prevention interventions occur during the acute stage of a disaster with the goal of decreasing the effects of the disaster on individuals and the community. Tertiary prevention strategies are designed to meet the long-term needs of disaster victims after the disaster has been resolved. In all these stages, it must be remembered that a traumatic event can cause complex biologic, psychosocial, and cognitive reactions (Davidson & MacFariane, 2006; Ursano, 2002; Yahuda, 2002). Nurses are involved in providing interventions in each of these areas.

Victim Levels

Several classifications have been described that try to define the levels of response disaster victims go through. Early work has described three victim classes: the primary, secondary, and third-level victims. Recent research and analysis has further refined their work to include five or more levels of victims (Crocq, Crocq, Chiapello, & Damiani, 2005; Rao, 2006; Taylor, 1987, 1990, 1999; Ursano, McCaughey, & Fullerton, 1995).

Primary victims are those who have had maximum exposure to the event. They include the dead, the wounded, and those who are uninjured but who were directly exposed to the disaster. Secondary victims are those who have not been directly affected but are experiencing grief and mourning for a close relative who was a primary victim. Third-level victims are rescue and recover personnel such as health-care professionals, Red Cross workers, clergy persons, police, firefighters, and other first responders. These victims have intervened on the scene of the disaster and witnessed traumatizing events. Fourth-level victims are individuals in the community who were involved in the event, such as government workers or reporters, who have suffered emotionally from witnessing disaster situations and consequences. Fifth-level victims are members of the general public who were not physically present but who suffered distress when exposed to media coverage of disaster-related events (Crocq et al., 2005).

The Second Disaster

The impact of a disaster often triggers a chain of events that results in significant secondary losses that constitute what may be called a second disaster. The second disaster has an indirect effect on victims of the traumatic event as well as on those who were not involved but who subsequently experience indirect damage. For example, an initial disaster causes loss of life, damage to homes and properties, and disintegration of community life. This leads to disruption in local business activity that results in massive financial losses. These losses, in turn, result in lower income to employees in the area impacted by the disaster. People who are unable to work and meet their financial responsibilities may suffer consequences that produce psychological responses similar to the reactions of primary victims. For many, this second disaster is of even greater magnitude than the first, and interventions must be provided to minimize long-term consequences.

Psychological Responses to Trauma

Reactions to disaster are as varied as the individuals who experience them. Often, little consideration is given to the psychological trauma suffered by disaster victims as this is overshadowed by the initial primary importance of victims' physical needs and dealing with the physical disaster that is occurring or has just occurred. However, it is important to remember that, when a disaster occurs, people try to find a way to understand the experience. How they find that understanding depends on their culture, lifestyle, and previous experience with disasters on any scale.

Immediate Psychological Responses to a Disaster

According to Ruzek et al. (2007, p. 17),

> most psychological responses to trauma are relatively immediate, mild, and transient, but significant percentages of traumatized individuals experience more intense stress reactions and some develop significant mental health problems. Given the capacity of traumatic events to produce great immediate distress and sometimes overwhelm immediate coping abilities, disaster response encompasses efforts to support survivors in the immediate aftermath of disaster and to respond to their psychological needs.

When considering victims' psychological responses postdisaster, the disaster nurse must base interventions on several assumptions. First, the responses experienced by the disaster victim and the disaster responder should not be considered pathological or precursors of a subsequent psychiatric disorder. In the aftermath of a major traumatic event, many people will experience transient stress reactions that occur immediately, though these reactions may even occur years later. Most people will respond to the provision of psychological support to facilitate a return to normalcy rather than traditional psychiatric diagnosis and treatment, though some survivors may experience great distress and require clinical intervention.

Victims experience individual and subjective responses that are influenced by several factors including the immediacy of the traumatic event, its duration, proximity to the disaster, and personal injury (Ronen, 2002). Personal characteristics play a significant role in individual responses to trauma. These include age, gender, personality characteristics, culture, and ethnicity (Jordan, 2007). Other factors predispose individuals to negative responses; Wiger and Harowski (2003, p. 50–51) described factors as including "personality disorders, poor coping abilities and strategies, difficulty learning from previous experiences, low self-esteem, instable work history, lack of finances, chemical dependency, . . . and legal problems."

Many authors have described victims' psychological responses to traumatic events (Davidson & MacFariane, 2006; Fullerton & Ursano, 1997; North, McCutcheon, Spitznagel, & Smith, 1999; Schurfield, 2002; Ursano, 2002; Ursano, Fullerton, & Norwood, 2003; Yahuda, 2002). Expected reactions include anger, sadness, anxiety, fear, depression, and irritability. Other symptoms include sleeplessness, fatigue, mood swings, guilt, excessive crying, flashbacks, and panic attacks. These may be considered normal reactions to abnormal events.

Post-Traumatic Responses to a Disaster

Post-traumatic responses resemble the emotions, thoughts, and behaviors that are part of the bereavement process. Although the reactions are not predictable in their duration, they follow a developmental process. The process of coping with the experience begins with feelings of disbelief, bewilderment, and difficulty concentrating, with denial used as the primary defense. Anxiety and fear represent the next phase and are followed by varying degrees of sadness and depression.

Of greatest concern is the risk that people exposed to trauma from natural and man-made disasters are at risk for the development of a major psychiatric disorder, including aggravation or exacerbation of any preexisting psychiatric condition. These include depression, generalized anxiety disorder, panic disorder, acute and post-traumatic stress disorder, and substance abuse (Ursano et al., 2003). Research indicates that trauma alters a variety of brain regions; on a physiological level, traumatic stress significantly disturbs the homeostasis of the brain and may actually change the brain and the ways in which it responds to subsequent stressors (Weiss, 2007).

Many factors create individual vulnerability and increase the risk for developing a psychological disorder. Some of these are part of the individual's premorbid personality and behavior while others are associated with the disaster itself. Alexander (2005) identified several predisposing and post-traumatic factors. Predisposing factors include childhood sexual abuse, unresolved previous losses or traumas, substance abuse, previous psychiatric history, and the presence of multiple life stressors. Post-traumatic factors include severe psychological reactions after the event, lack of family and social support, personal loss, adverse reactions from others, and survivor guilt.

Acute and Post-Traumatic Stress Disorder

On one end of the spectrum of psychological responses to a disaster are those individuals who show little disruption in functioning. On the other are those who develop acute stress disorder or post-traumatic stress disorder. These disturbances are types of anxiety disorders that involve an extreme traumatic stressor.

According to the *DSM-IV-TR* (APA, 2000), stressors that may trigger acute stress disorder or post-traumatic stress disorder include actual or threatened death, serious injury, or any other threat to personal integrity; witnessing such a situation; or learning of such a situation happening to a relative or friend. The constellation of symptoms shared by both conditions occurs in three main categories: reliving the traumatic event through intrusive thoughts or images, nightmares, or flashbacks; avoidance of associations to the traumatic event and feelings of numbness and detachment; and increased arousal as evidenced by being jumpy, nervous, or "on alert" much of the time; difficulty sleeping; and an inability to concentrate.

When the individual experiences these symptoms within 4 weeks of the traumatic event, a diagnosis of acute stress disorder (ASD) is given. Typically, ASD resolves within 4 weeks of the event. When the symptoms emerge 4 or more weeks after the event and/or last for more than a month, the diagnosis given is post-traumatic stress disorder (PTSD). In both conditions, the individual experiences significant distress and impairment in social, occupational, and other areas of functioning (APA, 2000). According to Rosenberg et al. (2001), approximately 25% of all people exposed to a disaster or similar traumatic event will develop PTSD. Estimates of the lifetime prevalence of PTSD in the general population range from 8% to 12%.

Special Needs of Children

In much the same way as adults respond to a disaster and try to make sense of their experiences, children strive to create meaning in terms that are understandable to themselves. However, depending on their age and developmental level, children are not usually able to use logic and reason to find meaning in disaster events in the same way adults do. Instead, children may use magical thinking and believe they are the cause of the event (Timberlake & Cutler, 2001). (See Chapter 5 on pediatric disaster care and growth and developmental issues.)

The child's developmental stage influences how he or she will respond to a traumatic event. Younger children may not have reached the stage in which they can express their responses verbally and may, instead, manifest behavioral symptoms of distress. Steele (2004) observed several consistent reactions in children at various development stages. Preschool children under 5 years of age experienced generalized fears, confusion, sleep disturbance, regressive behaviors, and fantasies. School-age children from 6 to 10 years old demonstrated preoccupation, sleep disturbances, safety concerns, school dysfunction, and fears of harm or abandonment. Children older than 12 were better able to verbalize their feelings but manifested detachment, guilt, acting out, relationship issues, and a desire for revenge.

As with adults, children exposed to a traumatic event will react differently; some will develop severe psychological distress while others will not. Research after the September 11th terrorist attacks indicated that children demonstrated early symptomatic reactions to a traumatic event, as opposed to the majority of adults who did not experience stress-related symptoms immediately (Galea et al., 2003; Sadock & Sadock, 2003; Schuster et al., 2001). Children and adolescents most commonly respond with anxiety and depressive disorders, though some will develop ASD and PTSD. Most children suffer from symptoms that include anxiety, depression, sleep disturbances, preoccupation with words, and conduct problems, although most do not develop a diagnosable psychiatric condition (Cohen, Mannarino, Berlinger, & Deblinger, 2000).

Children and adolescents are particularly vulnerable during traumatic events. They are at greater risk in dangerous situations, more susceptible to injury, and psychologically more vulnerable for failing to meet developmental needs. While adults are usually overwhelmed by their own needs to cope with dramatic changes in the environment, children's needs are often overlooked following a major disaster.

Cultural Perspectives

Culture is a strong determinant of how adults, children, and entire communities will respond to a disaster or traumatic event. Attention must be paid to family and community norms and values as these will affect issues related to confidentiality, family roles, spiritual practices, and how help is sought and received. Differences in beliefs and values shape victims' willingness to engage in and sustain participation in psychological interventions. Often, people believe that tolerating distress is a sign of strength; this encourages them to minimize mental health concerns and the need for treatment. Cultural considerations include ethnicity, gender, language and literacy, immigration status, and previous exposure to violence and trauma, not an uncommon reality in other cultures from which immigrants may have come. Chapter 7 provides an in-depth look at culture and the role it plays in caring for the disaster victim.

Nursing Assessment and Intervention

Meaning of Loss

The severity of a disaster must be evaluated in ways that go beyond mere numbers and the determination of number of deaths, number of wounded, homes damaged, and other fact-based assessments. The meaning of the loss is often far more significant than the actual losses; these must be assessed for each individual and for the entire community. The impact of the disaster may be far reaching and go beyond the actual devastation. For example, family pets are often lost in a disaster, and the loss of a pet may mean far more to some than to others. The loss of a home may have vastly different meanings to different individuals. For one, it may represent the culmination of a lifetime of saving and planning and a haven in which to live out one's final years. For another, it may simply be a residence and, for that individual, the loss of the possessions within the home may have far greater meaning. Though the entire community experiences the same disaster, each individual perceives it in a unique and different way. As disaster nurses, we must learn what the loss means to each individual as only then can we assess the impact the disaster has had on the victim.

How well individuals cope with a traumatic event depends on an array of factors, such as the extent to which they directly experienced the event; their perception of threat; their level of preexisting biologic, interpersonal, and social vulnerability; and the availability of services. In a national study on coping behaviors demonstrated in response to a traumatic event, researchers found that 98% of individuals who experienced mild to severe stress reactions coped by talking to others, 60% became involved in group activities, and 30% gave monetary and other contributions to help those more in need (Schuster et al., 2001). "A psychosocial approach to disasters includes viewing them as traumatic events involving actual or threatened death or injury of people on a large scale" (Eyre, 2004, p. 23).

Psychological First Aid

A comprehensive response to disasters must attend to both the physical and mental health needs of affected groups. Mental health needs are especially important because many more individuals will report psychologically related complaints than will report physical symptoms directly stemming from the injury-causing event. Along with services to address injuries, food, and shelter, acute and basic mental health care for survivors is initially offered in the form of psychological first aid. Because large-scale emergencies overwhelm existing mental health response resources, the provision of basic psychological care in the short-term aftermath of a traumatic event is an important skill all disaster nurses should possess.

There has been a growing movement to develop a concept similar to physical first aid for coping with stressful and traumatic events in life. This strategy has been known by a number of names but is most commonly referred to as psychological first aid (PFA). PFA provides individuals with skills they can use in responding to the psychological consequences of disasters. PFA is emerging as the crisis intervention of choice in the immediate response to trauma and mass disaster.

Ruzek et al. (2007) described the psychological first aid model as "a systematic set of helping actions aimed at reducing initial post-trauma distress and supporting short- and long-term adapting functioning" (p. 17). Psychological first aid is provided within the context of a caring and compassionate relationship between caregiver and victim. The goal of the relationship is to facilitate the victim's coping in the aftermath of a disaster through the provision of necessary support, resources, and information. The use of the PFA approach is based on the premise disaster survivors' reactions are normal responses to abnormal events rather than signs of psychopathology.

Psychological first aid is as important as medical first aid. When a patient is bleeding, the disaster nurse first intervenes to stop the bleeding and then may make an appropriate referral. Similarly, a person in need of immediate psychological assistance should not be referred for psychotherapy without intervention by the disaster nurse first. Psychological responses to a disaster are best managed initially using the principles of psychological first aid before referring to a disaster mental health professional. The focus in the disaster nurse/victim relationship is on listening to whatever the victim wishes to say. The victim's needs must be assessed and all efforts made to address those needs. Victims should be encouraged to spend time with family and friends, if this is possible.

Raphael (1988, as cited in Rao, 2006, p. 502), indicated the basic care provided in psychological first aid includes:

- Comfort and consolation
- Protection from further threat and distress
- Immediate physical care and medical attention
- Helping reunite loved ones
- Linking survivors with sources of support

- Identifying those who need help
- Facilitating some sense of being in control
- Allowing for sharing of experience but not forcing it
- Provision of culturally appropriate ways of grieving for the dead
- Normalization of activity and routine as far as possible

According to Ruzek et al. (2007, p. 17), PFA is based on

> eight core actions: contact and engagement, safety and comfort, stabilization, information gathering, practical assistance, connection with social supports, information on coping support, and linkage with collaborative services. PFA for children and adolescents focuses on the same core actions, with modifications to make them developmentally appropriate.

Specific interventions, in Table 8-1, are part of the disaster relief information provided by the Substance Abuse and Mental Health Services Administration (U.S. Department of Health and Human Services, n.d.). These interventions mesh well with Raphael's (1988, as cited in Rao, 2006) basic care considerations and PFA core actions.

Nurses employing basic psychological first aid interventions must be prepared with an understanding of the following basic principles:

- The nature of traumatic crisis
- Trauma reactions and related disorders: depression, anxiety, ASD, and PTSD
- Death and grief reactions
- Knowledge of available resources
- Knowledge of social and cultural factors
- Values clarification: human rights, confidentiality, and trust
- Psychological post-trauma and crisis intervention skills
- Stress management and self-care skills for victims
- Social and cultural factors

Short-Term Interventions

Understandably, of initial primary concern to disaster victims are survival, shelter, food, and water. Once these are assured, mental health issues present themselves and generally last beyond healing of the physical trauma. Short-term interventions include psychological first aid and other primary prevention interventions designed to help victims feel safe and manage their anxiety and anger.

Critical Incident Stress Debriefing

An intervention that was originally developed to debrief first responders, critical incident stress debriefing (CISD) became so popular the approach began being provided to victims in the initial aftermath of a disaster or traumatic event. Using a team trained in the approach, victims participate in groups over a 3- to 4-hour period, ideally within 24 hours of the event or as soon as possible within the first few days.

TABLE 8-1 INTERVENTIONS FOR PSYCHOLOGICAL FIRST AID IN A DISASTER

Intervention	Actions
Communicate calmly: Use the SOLER mnemonic device	S: Sit squarely or stand using the L-stance, shoulder 90° to the other person's shoulder O: Open posture L: Lean forward E: Eye contact R: Relax
Communicate warmth	Speak in a soft tone Smile Use open and welcoming gestures Allow the person you are talking with to dictate the distance between you
Establish a relationship	Introduce yourself if they do not know you Ask the person what they would like to be called Do not shorten their name or use their first name without their permission With some cultures, it is important to always address the person as Mr. or Mrs.
Use concrete questions to help the person focus	Use closed-end questions Explain why you are asking the question
Come to an agreement on something	Establish a point of agreement that will help solidify your relationship and gain their trust Active listening will help you find a point of agreement
Speak to the person with respect	Use words such as *please* and *thank you* Do not make global statements about the person's character Lavish praise is not believable Use positive language
If the person becomes agitated, he or she may challenge or question authority	Answer questions calmly Repeat your statement calmly
If the person refuses to follow directions	Do not assert control; let the person gain control of self Remain professional Restructure your request in another way Give the person time to think of your request
If the person loses control and becomes verbally agitated	Reply calmly State that you may need assistance to help him or her
If the person becomes physically threatening	If the person becomes threatening or intimidating and does not respond to your attempts to calm them, seek immediate assistance

Source: U.S. Department of Health and Human Services, n.d.

Participants in CISD are moved through seven stages "designed to take them from a cognitive level to an emotional level, then back to a cognitive level by the close of the debriefing" (Bell, 1995, p. 37). As described by Bell, the stages include:

1. Introduction: All members are introduced and guidelines are set for the process.
2. Fact phase: Victims explain what happened during the event as they understand it.
3. Thought phase: Participants describe their thoughts at the time of the incident.
4. Reaction phase: Members describe the worst part of the event as they experienced it.
5. Symptom phase: Victims discuss the variety of reactions they have had to the event.
6. Teaching phase: Group leaders describe normal stress symptoms, assure participants that they will experience symptom reduction over time, and provide specific stress management techniques and referral resources for those who may need them.
7. Reentry phase: Final closure is provided as each member makes one final statement about the process.

In recent years, CISD has been the focus of some controversy. Questions have been raised about whether the process actually reduces the occurrence of post-traumatic stress disorder. A number of reviews of the literature on post-trauma intervention concluded there is no evidence that CISD prevents long-term negative outcomes (Bisson, 2003; Litz, Gray, Bryant, & Adler, 2002; McNally, Bryant, & Ehlers, 2003; Watson et al., 2003).

Crisis intervention is another modality that may be of use in the early stages of post-disaster mental health response. Crisis intervention can occur at any time within 6 to 8 weeks of the traumatic event, though the sooner the process is begun, the sooner the individual will experience symptom relief. The basic steps in crisis intervention involve defining the problem, providing support, examining alternative sources of support, improving coping mechanisms, and enhancing constructive thought processes. The process requires several meetings over a brief period of time and has as its goal the individual's return to his or her predisaster level of functioning. Roberts (2005) identified seven critical stages for crisis intervention workers as a guide to their work with those in crisis and through which individuals progress as they move toward crisis stabilization:

1. Complete a thorough psychosocial assessment.
2. Establish a collaborative relationship.
3. Identify the major issues.
4. Encourage expression of emotion.
5. Explore alternatives and new coping strategies.
6. Implement an action plan to facilitate restoration of functioning.
7. Plan follow up.

In an extensive review of the literature, Ruzek et al. (2007, p. 18) identified "five empirically supported intervention principles to guide intervention practices following disaster and mass violence at the early to midterm stages. These principles are (a) promoting sense of safety, (b) promoting calming, (c) promoting sense of self- and community-efficacy, (d) promoting connectedness, and (e) instilling hope."

Long-Term Interventions

There will be a certain number of victims who will require long-term intervention. The entire spectrum of mental health care must be available to those individuals whose symptoms persist and who may qualify for a psychiatric diagnosis. Individual, group, and family therapy, cognitive behavioral approaches, and medication management are all part of the services that may be needed. For the most severe cases, psychiatric hospitalization may be required.

Survivors of disaster may experience other long-term mental health consequences than anxiety and stress-related syndromes. Depression, substance abuse, and personality disorders are some of the psychiatric diagnoses that may be encountered. Grief and delayed grief reactions may occur if the victim has lost loved ones. Distinguishing between the normal grief process and pathological grief may require the skills of a mental health professional.

Cognitive behavioral approaches have proven to be effective in addressing some of the long-term consequences of the disaster experience. The survivor is encouraged to review the events repeatedly; with repetition, the memories lose their intensity and their ability to cause anxiety and pain (Monson & Friedman, 2007). Antidepressant and antianxiety medications may be a valuable aid to psychotherapeutic intervention. According to Ehrenreich (2001, p. 213),

> up to ninety per cent or even more of victims can be expected to exhibit at least some untoward psychological effects in the hours immediately following a disaster. . . . The number showing symptoms generally continues to drop, but delayed responses and responses to the later consequences of disaster continue to appear. While most victims of disasters are usually relatively free of distress by a year or two after the event, a quarter or more of the victims may still show significant symptoms while others, who had previously been free of symptoms, may first show distress a year or two after the disaster.

The Disaster Nurse

The disaster nurse plays a key role in the physical and mental well-being of disaster victims. The disaster nurse may be a victim in addition to being a caregiver as he or she may reside in the affected community or in the surrounding area and may have family and friends who are primary or secondary victims. Close contact with those impacted by the event puts disaster nurses in the category of third-level victims.

Factors that influence the disaster nurse's response to the event are related to the disaster nurse's professional role as he or she is involved in rescue or recovery efforts and the disaster nurse's personal function as a family member and friend. The closer he or she is in proximity to the disaster, the more significant the impact. Difficult working conditions, lack of necessary resources, impact on communication and organization, and isolation from colleagues are all elements that impact the disaster nurse (Jordan, 2007).

Disaster nurses are often among the first responders to a large-scale crisis. Despite professional training and socialization, disaster nurses are vulnerable to the same experiences as are disaster victims. Disaster nurses are not immune from the physical and psychological stress that accompanies a major traumatic event. They experience the same sights and sounds as the primary victims and are actually exposed to more of the horror than most victims. Disaster nurses see more than their share of death, severe injury, desperation, and destruction. Disaster nurses must have available to them the same resources afforded to victims for psychological first aid, crisis intervention, cognitive behavioral interventions, support groups, and long-term care, if necessary.

Compassion Fatigue

Also known as *donor fatigue, caregiver burnout,* or *vicarious traumatization,* compassion fatigue is brought on by indirect exposure to traumatic events (Palm, Polusny, & Folette, 2004, p. 74):

> As the nurse provider acts in response to the needs of the situation, the nurse is consciously or unconsciously taking in the human and environmental destruction all around. Symptoms associated with vicarious traumatization include, but are not limited to
>
> - Intrusive imagery and thoughts
> - Avoidance
> - Emotional numbing
> - Hyperarousal symptoms
> - Somatization
> - Physical and alcohol use problems
> - Changes in self-identity
> - Changes in worldview
> - Changes in spirituality
> - Changes in general psychological functioning
>
> The disaster nurse who experiences compassion fatigue must seek support from peers. Simple solutions include: spend time with other people, engage in activities that provide a sense of purpose, and attend to personal needs. Disaster nurses should try to maintain the personal side of their lives to provide balance.

Disaster nurses must find ways to care for themselves and minimize the impact of the forces that produce compassion fatigue. Limiting caseloads and shifts, taking breaks, meeting needs for rest and food, maintaining a support system, limiting watching media coverage of the event, and employing stress relief activities are all actions that reduce the potential for burnout. If these measures are not sufficient, recognizing the need for professional intervention requires insight and self-awareness and should not be viewed negatively.

Psychological First Aid for Disaster Nurses

The U.S. Department of Health and Human Services states:

> When you work with people during and after a disaster, you are working with people who may be having reactions of confusion, fear, hopelessness, sleeplessness, anxiety, grief, shock, guilt, shame, and loss of confidence in themselves and others. Your early contacts with them can help alleviate their painful emotions and promote hope and healing. Your goal in providing this psychological first aid is to promote an environment of safety, calm, connectedness, self-efficacy, empowerment, and hope (U.S. Department of Health and Human Services, n.d., para. 1).

Table 8-2 provides a list of dos and don'ts when caring for those suffering from compassion fatigue.

TABLE 8-2 DOs AND DON'Ts OF CARING FOR THE COMPASSION FATIGUE VICTIM

DO:

Promote Safety:

- Help people meet basic needs for food and shelter and obtain emergency medical attention.
- Provide repeated, simple, and accurate information on how to get these basic needs.

Promote Calm:

- Listen to people who wish to share their stories and emotions, and remember that there is no right or wrong way to feel.
- Be friendly and compassionate even if people are being difficult.
- Offer accurate information about the disaster or trauma and the relief efforts underway to help victims understand the situation.

Promote Connectedness:

- Help people contact friends and loved ones.
- Keep families together. Keep children with parents or other close relatives whenever possible.

Promote Self-Efficacy:

- Give practical suggestions that steer people toward helping themselves.
- Engage people in meeting their own needs.

Promote Help:

- Find out the types and locations of government and nongovernment services and direct people to those services that are available.

(continued)

TABLE 8-2 DOs AND DON'Ts OF CARING FOR THE COMPASSION FATIGUE VICTIM (Continued)

DO NOT:

- Force people to share their stories with you, especially very personal details.
- Give simple reassurances such as "Everything will be OK" or "At least you survived."
- Tell people what you think they should be feeling, thinking, or how they should have acted earlier.
- Tell people why you think they have suffered by alluding to personal behaviors or beliefs of victims.
- Make promises that may not be kept.
- Criticize existing services or relief activities in front of people in need of these services.

Source: U.S. Department of Health and Human Services, n.d.

Conclusion

Nurses play an increasingly important role in the preparation for and response to disasters. Mental health care for disaster survivors should include components of psychological processing of the disaster experience, controlling physiologic stress reactions, and reestablishing social connections and a sense of security and predictability. Disaster nurses must be sensitive to their own needs as well; they must care for themselves before they can care for others.

References

Alexander, D. A. (2005). Early mental health intervention after disasters. *Advances in Psychiatric Treatment, 17,* 12–18.

American Psychiatric Association. (2000). *Diagnostic and statistical manual of mental disorders* (IV-TR). Washington, DC: Author.

Bell, J. K. (1995). Traumatic event debriefing: Service delivery designs and the role of social work. *Social Work, 40*(1), 36–44.

Bisson, J. I. (2003). Single-session early psychological interventions following traumatic events. *Clinical Psychology Review, 23,* 481–499.

Cohen, J. A., Mannarino, A. P., Berlinger, L., & Deblinger, E. (2000). Trauma-focused cognitive-behavioral therapy for children and adolescents. *Journal of Interpersonal Violence, 15,* 1202–1223.

Crocq, L., Crocq, M., Chiapello, A., & Damiani, C. (2005). Organization of mental health services for disaster victims. In J. J. Lopez-Ibor Alino (Ed.). *Disasters and mental health.* Hoboken, NJ: John Wiley & Sons.

Davidson, J. R., & MacFariane, A. C. (2006). The extent and impact of mental health problems after disaster. *Journal of Clinical Psychology, 67*(Suppl. 2), 9–14.

Ehrenreich, J. H. (2001). *Coping with disasters: A guidebook to psychosocial intervention.* Old Westbury, NY: Center for Psychology and Society.

Eyre, E. (2004). Psychosocial aspects of recovery: Practical implications for disaster management. *Australian Journal of Emergency Management, 19*(4), 23–27.

Fullerton, C. S., & Ursano, R. J. (1997). *Post traumatic stress disorder: Acute and long term responses to trauma and disaster.* Washington, DC: American Psychiatric Association Press.

Galea, S., Vlahov, D., Resnick, H., Ahem, J., Susser, E., Gold, J., et al. (2003). Trends of probable post-traumatic stress disorder in New York City after the September 11 terrorist attacks. *American Journal of Epidemiology, 158,* 514–524.

Jordan, K. (2007). A case study: Factors to consider when doing 1:1 crisis counseling with local first responders with dual trauma after Hurricane Katrina. *Brief Treatment and Crisis Intervention, 7*(2), 91–101.

Litz, B. T., Gray, M. J., Bryant, R. A., & Adler, A. (2002). Early intervention for trauma: Current status and future directions. *Clinical Psychology: Science and Practice, 9,* 112–134.

McNally, R., Bryant, R., & Ehlers, A. (2003). Does early psychological intervention promote recovery from posttraumatic stress? *Psychological Science in the Public Interest, 4,* 45–79.

Monson, C. M., & Friedman, M. J. (2007). Back to the future of understanding trauma: Implications for cognitive behavioral theories for trauma. In V. M. Follette & J. I. Ruzak (Eds.), *Cognitive-behavioral therapies for trauma* (2nd ed.). New York: Guilford Press.

North, C. S., McCutcheon, V., Spitznagel, E. L., & Smith, E. M. (1999). Psychiatric disorders among survivors of the Oklahoma City bombing. *Journal of the American Medical Association, 282*(8), 755–762.

Rao, K. (2006). Psychosocial support in disaster-affected communities. *International Review of Psychiatry, 18*(6), 501–505.

Roberts, A. R. (2005). Bridging the past and present to the future of crisis intervention and crisis management. In A. R. Roberts (Ed.), *Crisis intervention handbook: Assessment, treatment, and research* (3rd ed.). New York: Oxford University Press.

Ronen, T. (2002). Difficulties in assessing traumatic reactions in children. *Journal of Loss and Trauma, 7,* 87–106.

Rosenberg, S. D., Mueser, K. T., Friedman, M. J., Gorman, P. G., Drake, R. E., Vidaver, R. M., et al. (2001). Developing effective treatments for posttraumatic disorders among people with severe mental illness. *Psychiatric Services, 52*(11), 1453–1461.

Ruzek, J. I., Brymer, M. J., Jacobs, A. K., Layne, C. M., Vernberg, E. M., & Watson, P. J. (2007). Psychological first aid. *Journal of Mental Health Counseling, 29*(1), 17–49.

Sadock, B. J., & Sadock, V. A. (2003). *Synopsis of psychiatry.* Philadelphia: Lippincott Williams & Wilkins.

Schurfield, R. M. (2002). Commentary about the terrorist acts of September, 11, 2001: Posttraumatic reactions and related social and policy issues. *Trauma, Violence and Abuse, 3,* 3–14.

Schuster, M. A., Stein, B. D., Jaycox, L. H., Collins, R. L., Marshall, G. N., Elliott, M. N., et al. (2001). A national survey of stress reactions after the September 11, 2001 terrorist attacks. *New England Journal of Medicine, 345*(20), 1507–1512.

Steele, W. (2004). Helping traumatized children. In S. L. A. Straussner & N. K. Phillips (Eds.), *Understanding mass violence: A social work perspective* (pp. 41–56). Boston: Pearson Education.

Taylor, A. J. W. (1987). A taxonomy of disasters and their victims. *Journal of Psychosomatic Research, 31*(4), 535–544.

Taylor, A. J. W. (1990). A pattern of disasters and victims. *Disasters: The Journal of Disaster Studies & Management, 14*(4), 291–300.

Taylor, A. J. W. (1999). Towards the classification of disasters and victims. *Traumatology, 5*(2), 12–25.

Timberlake, E. M., & Cutler, M. M. (2001). *Play therapy in clinical social work.* Boston: Allyn and Bacon.

Ursano, R. J. (2002). Post traumatic stress disorder. *New England Journal of Medicine, 346*(2), 130–131.

Ursano, R. J., Fullerton, C. S., & Norwood, A. E. (2003). Terrorism and disasters: Prevention, intervention, and recovery. In R. J. Ursano, C. S. Fullerton, & A. E. Norwood (Eds.). *Terrorism and disaster: Individual and community mental health interventions* (pp. 333–339). Cambridge, MA: Cambridge University Press.

Ursano, R. J., McCaughey, B. G., & Fullerton, C. S. (1995). *Individual and community responses to trauma and disaster: The structure of human chaos.* Cambridge, MA: Cambridge University Press.

U.S. Department of Health and Human Services. (n.d.). *Psychological first aid for first responders.* Retrieved March 27, 2008, from http://mentalhealth.samhsa.gov/Disasterrelief/pubs/manemotion.asp

Watson, P. J., Friedman, M. J., Gibson, L. E., Ruzek, J. I., Norris, F. H., & Ritchie, B. C. (2003). Early intervention for trauma-related problems. *Review of Psychiatry 22,* 97–124.

Weiss, S. J. (2007). Neurobiological alterations associated with traumatic stress. *Perspectives in Psychiatric Care, 43*(3), 114–122.

Wiger, D. E., & Harowski, K. J. (2003). *Essentials of crisis intervention and counseling.* Hoboken, NJ: John Wiley & Sons.

Yahuda, R. (2002). Post traumatic stress disorder. *New England Journal of Medicine, 346*(2), 108–114.

chapter 9

Communicating in a Disaster

Susan Sonnier

GOAL

The goal of this chapter is to identify appropriate communication in the disaster setting.

OBJECTIVES

At the completion of this chapter, the reader will:

1. Identify key communication challenges in a disaster.
2. Construct appropriate communication techniques for use in a disaster.
3. Facilitate appropriate communication in a disaster.
4. Define common terminology and language used in a disaster.
5. List technological considerations in a disaster.
6. Communicate with the media about disaster health issues arising from a disaster.
7. Establish family communication in a disaster.

Key Terms

- Communication
- Communication techniques
- Common terms and language used in a disaster
- Communicating with the media
- Communicating with families

Introduction

Disasters can affect any community or environment at any time. These catastrophic events happen daily throughout the world in a random and unpredictable manner. The uncertain dimension of disasters is detrimental in that agencies and communities may not adequately prepare themselves for a devastating event. Hurricane Rita, in 2005, on the Texas and Louisiana Gulf Coast was an example of such an event, an event that challenged all existing disaster resources and agencies.

Hurricane Katrina had ravaged the Louisiana, Mississippi, and Alabama coastal and inland areas only weeks before Rita's surprising development. Massive resource allocation and personnel had been deployed to these stricken areas already managing the massive destruction Katrina had left in her wake. Hurricane Rita did not allow anyone in the vicinity to catch their breaths as her intensity grew. She made landfall as a Category 3 storm in southeast Texas and southwestern Louisiana, destroying towns like Cameron, Louisiana, and Groves, Texas, from drenching downpours, 120 miles per hour winds, and tornadoes that typically spin off of a hurricane (Cable News Network, 2005; After Rita's damage, 2005). The ravages of the storm were coupled with unparalleled and massive evacuations in areas that were thought to be in the path of the storm. Over 2.5 million people evacuated the upper Texas and Louisiana coastal areas. Lack of gasoline, untested evacuation plans, and mixed communications wreaked havoc on large urban and rural areas alike. The crisis of both storms put significant constraints and burdens in numerous communities and taxed disaster relief efforts nationwide.

When faced with disasters such as this one or of any size, communication is a key component of rapid and effective coordination and usually the first function to fail in any major disaster. First-line responders to federal agencies must coordinate personnel, financial resources, and equipment to an impact area in a disaster. Communications must make events and processes known and transmit information, as well as exchange information between agencies and the general public for all facets of a disaster timeline: planning, preparation, response, mitigation, and recovery (Merriam-Webster, 2007; Veenema, 2007). Communication disruptions and failures are inevitable in any crisis or disaster owing to the chaos and mayhem a disaster generates. Responders and governmental and nongovernmental agencies, as well as the media and the general public, rely greatly on the ability to share information in a crisis.

Disaster nurses can play a pivotal role in communication and be a source of important knowledge for the disaster workforce as they are part of the largest single cohort in healthcare systems. Their responsibilities and skills can be beneficial in the preparedness for and delivery of emergency disaster relief. Nurses in all specialties and clinical arenas can enhance efforts to recover from disastrous events that have no predictability.

Communication Challenges in Disasters

The public has expectations that communication systems and networks are in place for unpredictable events and that conveyance of vital information will take place between disaster victims and the agencies sent to help their plight (Goolsby, Kulkarni, & Mothershead, 2006). Any form of disaster can disrupt the normal transference of communication in a community. People affected by the event and the responding agencies must be steadily engaged in disaster or crisis communications through the disaster. This information exchange is essential and vital for restoration and recovery from the disaster (Matthews, 2006; Veenema, 2007).

However, communication does not always proceed in an orderly manner in a disaster and communication challenges can emerge at any point. These challenges generally fall into two realms: people problems or technical problems (Veenema, 2007). Table 9-1 depicts examples of both types of challenges faced in a crisis situation.

Fostering and Facilitating Communications in a Disaster

Creating fluency and contiguous communications throughout the span of a disaster is critical to the mitigation of a disaster when it occurs. The continuum from first

TABLE 9-1 COMMUNICATION CHALLENGES IN DISASTERS

Type of Problem	Challenges
People Problems	1. Autonomous agencies that do not mesh with other agencies; failure to integrate resources 2. Lack of trust among victims, responders, and media 3. Political, cultural, governmental, or societal issues that may hinder rescue and recovery 4. Lack of knowledge about how other agencies function 5. Lack of preparedness by agencies or victims 6. Public complacency or cavalier attitudes that disasters will not impact an area 7. Use of different language and terminology for the same action or situation
Technological Problems	1. Terrestrial (land-based) communications are likely destroyed in the disaster 2. Delays in deployment of communication systems in the disaster areas 3. Technology compatibility issues among responding agencies 4. Lack of reliable redundant or back-up means of communication 5. Telephone or computer network logjams or overloaded circuits that prohibit information flow in and out of disaster area

Source: Adapted from Gunn, 2003, and Veenema, 2007.

responders to federal agencies must provide clear and accurate accounts of all facets of disaster operations in an affected area. Each disaster, large or small, brings its own unique challenges as well as opportunities to develop solutions and interventions that may be beneficial in succeeding disasters. Well-prepared and practiced policies, procedures, and protocols can make a huge difference in the outcome of any disaster.

Power outages in August 2003 caused extensive blackout conditions through New York, New Jersey, Ohio, Michigan, and Toronto. Cable News Network (CNN, 2003) reported that in 3 minutes, 21 power stations went down for several days to much of a power grid affecting these states and provinces in Canada. Many residents of these cities, especially New York, were fearful another terrorist attack had happened. People were terrified for their family members' safety and well-being because cellular networks had gone down with the power outages (K. B. Stanley, personal communication, February 9, 2008). The *New York Times* (Sorkin & Richtel, 2003) presented a critical online report on the cellular industries failure to upgrade and improve their backup technologies since September 11, 2001. The companies claimed that the length of the power failure caused backup batteries to fail, and the lack of power needed to recharge their system caused untimely delays reestablishing cellular network coverage. Fortunately, no significant loss of life or harm came to the public as a result of the lack of communications that presented itself (CNN, 2003).

Public communications serve several useful purposes that greatly affect the outcome of a disaster response. The benefits of communications from public health and disaster agencies include:

1. Increasing awareness of the disaster so that the public will take precautions to protect or save lives
2. Help in fostering reduction in anxiety in the public
3. Relief assistance being localized and efforts focusing on set populations that may require aid or assistance (Wray, Kreuter, Jacobsen, Clements, & Evans, 2004)

Common Terminology and Language in a Disaster

Acronyms, jargon, foreign languages, and professional terminology often become a garbled jumble of expression in a disaster as it evolves in a community, confusing the different types of communication that need to take place. *Internal* communications are communications that agencies must carry out within their infrastructures. *External* communications are those communications that extend outward from a given agency to other agencies, the public, and/or the media. It is easy to see how difficult communications in a disaster could be if a unified language or terminology is not used in a disaster.

There have been numerous disaster terminology lists, lexicons, dictionaries, and disaster terminology appendixes developed to define, refine, and clarify content and verbiage used in disaster management. There is no particular standard in use; however, some templates do exist to minimize the confusion that could result from the miscommunications that could present in a disaster. When these standards are used, internal and external communications are greatly enhanced (Gunn, 2003).

Standardization of disaster response became a reality in 2003 with Presidential Directive 5 (HSPD-5). This directive was issued to the Department of Homeland Security to develop the National Incident Management System (NIMS). NIMS provides a national template for all government, private, and nongovernmental organizations to work together during a domestic incident or disaster (Federal Emergency Management Agency [FEMA], 2007a; National Incident Management System, 2004). Included in these guidelines were provisions for standardizing the terminology and language used in disaster.

Even with these standards, it has proven difficult to get all responding agencies to use a common language. One of the inherent difficulties in this process is the changing nature of terms and language (Twigg, 2004). Because of this, guidelines have been adopted to augment the flow of communications in disasters. These include:

1. Terms should be defined clearly and concisely in plain language.
2. Verbiage should be simple and clear to understand and communicate.
3. Facilities and organizations should have members' roles defined and identified for simplified and streamlined incident management.
4. Ten codes (e.g., 10-4 for acknowledged) should not be used (FEMA, 2007a; National Incident Management System, 2004; Twigg, 2004).

Terminology, including words and phrases, must have specific and clear meanings to enact federal levels of disaster response to a disaster area under the Robert T. Stafford Disaster Relief and Emergency Assistance Act. This act was passed in 1988 to provide federal assistance to assist state and local efforts to mitigate a disaster through its course of events (Slepski, 2005; Veenema, 2007). The United Nations has also endorsed common terminology usage in disaster communications to facilitate "rapid and unequivocal communications among individuals and teams and involved institutions in actual disaster response activities, as well as in disaster mitigation by prevention and preparedness." The document entitled *International Strategy for Disaster Reduction* is a comprehensive report updated regularly that includes an international library of terms in various languages to promote congruent terminology for disaster mitigation (United Nations, 2006).

The use of a shared language allows many layers of disaster personnel to share their experiences and practices with others working toward the common goal of relief and recovery in a crisis situation (Twigg, 2004). Sharing among agencies and personnel provides invaluable resources and research to improve and enhance communications in disaster management.

Nursing and Communication in a Disaster

All nurses should prepare for disaster events and understand the terms and language used in disasters as they are among the primary responders in these types of incidents (Slepski, 2005; Willshire, Hassmiller, & Wodicka, n.d). Appendix A contains a listing of common disaster terms that can be useful for disaster nurses.

Participation in Disaster Preparedness and Training

Increasing occurrences of disasters of all types, from terrorism to large- and small-scale natural disasters and potential widespread outbreaks of pathogenic agents like Avian flu, have accelerated emergency preparedness and awareness to the forefront of the public's daily lives. Disaster preparedness is perhaps the single most important factor in disaster management. Planning and preparations involve countless hours of planning, practice, and evaluation for the unexpected, as well as the expected, disaster.

Disaster communications training and preparedness must be included in disaster management readiness. Systems and personnel must be ready and in place in hospitals, health agencies, and other ancillary agencies that respond to disasters. This periodic training and practice is essential to the success of preparedness. Nurses can participate at many levels of disaster preparedness and communications:

1. Personally be prepared by keeping personal and work information updated (e.g., cell phone numbers, addresses, and home or pager numbers) within the employing agency (Shover, 2007).
2. Meet minimal disaster preparation and training requirements outlined by an employer, such as an annual competency in disasters based on Joint Commission recommendations.
3. Seek volunteer opportunities and training within agencies that provide local disaster response and assistance during events that require response (see Chapter 2 for more about these volunteer organizations).
4. Take academic courses, seek advanced degrees or postgraduate certificates in public health nursing or disaster health care relief, and attend continuing education programs in disaster nursing to contribute to and form a scientific and theoretical base for disaster management (Slepski, 2005; Veenema, 2006; Weiner, 2006).

Weiner, the associate director of the International Nursing Coalition for Mass Casualty Education (INCMCE), and the INCMCE have identified 64 competencies for nurses that are necessary for disaster response. Two of the basic competencies listed are communicating "in a professional manner, recognizing that public statements will be made by staff assigned to that role" and defining "terms relative to disaster management response (such as incident command, scene assessment, quarantine, triage, emergency management systems)" (Weiner, 2006, p. 3).

Weiner emphasizes the importance of communication in a disaster for a disaster nurse even on an international scale.

Technology Considerations in Disaster Communications

The ability to communicate has been enhanced by the Internet, cell phones, and countless other gadgetry that simplify keeping in touch and being accessible. This access means that communications can take place faster and reach more people than ever before, as long as the communications systems are intact. Disasters strain, hinder, or disrupt normal communication lines. Military personnel and first-line responders (e.g., police, paramedics, firefighters) are working together to pioneer newer, more sophisticated systems that allow a network of communications to be open and free flowing throughout the course of a disaster, such as satellite technologies (Lenfant & Soder, n.d.).

The emergency operations center (EOC) is the hub of communications both for incoming and outgoing messages from the disaster location. Every county, state, and the federal government have these EOCs, as well as most major cities. Mobile commands and communications vans and trailers can be deployed with satellite and wireless technology that can withstand and work around barriers that present in a disaster. As technology advances, smaller, more portable units are being brought into more remote, less accessible areas with this mobile capability (Smith & Simpson, 2005). Colleges have set up crisis communication centers in the wake of several tragedies, like the Virginia Tech tragedy in 2007 and the Northern Illinois shootings in 2008, which utilize cell phone rosters, Internet sites, and telephone hotline information for students and their families in the event of a disaster.

Disaster communications hinge on the ability to have information conveyed freely and effectively, without impediment, between all parties involved in the disaster. Using common terminology and disaster language, training, and preparedness as well as advanced studies in disaster theory and best practices, can greatly enhance the communications facet of disaster management.

Media Communications in a Disaster

Internal communications within agencies and disaster infrastructures have been examined to this point. Communications must also flow outward in a disaster to inform the public and other agencies involved in mitigating, responding to, or recovering from a disaster. Among the many groups that need to be considered in communicating about a disaster is the media, a vital link in external communications in a crisis or disaster. The information flowing to and from the media can be enhanced and made more useful by effective communication or can become sensationalized and stir negative emotions and outcomes.

The media can benefit disaster efforts or have detrimental effects. On the plus side, when communications work well with the media, the public can be educated about the disaster; be told what to do at all levels of disaster mitigation, planning, and recovery; and aid in reporting disaster conditions to those outside of the disaster but working in response to the disaster. Negative results can occur when communications break down between the media and disaster responders. Sensationalism can result from misinformation and gossip being reported when hard facts are lacking. Differing agendas can lead to more serious outcomes when agencies are pitted against each other through false reports and rumors spread by the media (Nacos, 2007).

The media plays a vital role in a disaster in disseminating vital information, yet disaster nurses often do not know how to deal with the multitude of media that may be covering an incident. Public information officers, or any other specially designated disaster responder, should follow some simple principles when dealing with the media so that disaster reporting is accurate, timely, and responsible (Nacos, 2007). These may include any or all of the following:

1. Crisis or disaster information that is released must be accurate and timely.
2. Agencies need to designate a spokesperson that has experience in public relations or media relations. No other person should speak with the media; instead, they should be directed to the public information officer.
3. Cooperating with the media is better than having a confrontation with them.
4. Emergency responders may restrict access to the crisis or disaster area (Nacos, 2007, pp. 111–114).
5. Facilitate trust building between the media and responding agencies by collaboration and respect for each other's needs.
6. Use simple explanations and help define complex terminologies or information so the media can responsibly and easily disseminate the information to the public.
7. Plan and practice in agency exercises and drills so that clear channels of communication will be known when the media comes to cover the events that are involved with the disaster.
8. Use the Internet to disseminate information, if feasible (Lowrey et al., 2007).

The Internet is an increasing source of information and news for many individuals. There is support for disaster agencies, both governmental and non-governmental, to establish Web sites prior to a disaster. This allows a responding agency to post warnings or information in a timely fashion for victims, both actual and potential, other disaster responders, or family members of disaster victims (Nacos, 2007).

The media is an important link to information dissemination that must be considered in disaster management. One could view them as a help or a hindrance in disaster mitigation or recovery. They often need to be educated about specific science or medical knowledge they report on so that they can distribute information responsibly and effectively. Their expertise in rapidly collecting and dispersing newsworthy information can be an asset for disaster responders to augment disaster recovery efforts. Planning for how to utilize the media in a disaster should be part of every agency's disaster plan (Lowrey et al., 2007; Nacos, 2007).

Establishing Family Communications in Crisis

Victims in a disaster often face insurmountable difficulties throughout a significant event. From the emergency preparations, disruption or loss of lifestyle, loss of life itself, devastation or disease, and recovery from any form of disaster, victims often feel enormous stresses and disassociations from their families, the community, and public at large. For these reasons, communication is vital in this aspect of disaster management. Communication that flows from victims to family members outside a disaster area and the reverse can be a psychological lifeline to those trying to reestablish their connection with the outside world and return to some semblance of normality.

Two key hindrances are often noted when these important communications are disrupted between family members or social groups. The imminent chaos or devastation in a disaster area leads to isolation of the persons affected by the disaster. The severity or nature of the disaster, structural damage, loss of electricity, overloading of existing phone or cellular networks, and response time of disaster responders who can assist communication reestablishment play an important role in the disaster communications continuum.

Public mobility is important to note as well. Public populations are more mobile and in flux than at past points in history. Families and loved ones are often located in many different and far apart geographical locations. There is often an urgent need for reconnection after a disaster, particularly after the event to assure outside relatives or friends the safety or well-being of a victim. Tracking the movements of individuals being moved from disaster shelters, hospitals, or temporary residences after a disaster can be a major challenge for families (Veenema, 2007).

The best means of facilitating family communications after a disaster is family preparedness before a disaster (Marks & Borden, 2004; Missouri Department of Public Health, 2006). Many governmental and nongovernmental agencies encourage and educate the public about the importance of having a family disaster plan. The Internet hosts numerous sites with practical advice to the public on how to construct, and what should be included in, a family plan. Contact information, evacuation plans, and meeting locations are vital components of this plan as much as the gathering of necessary supplies and sundries for a disaster (FEMA, 2007b; Marks & Borden, 2004).

Conclusion

Disasters are chaotic and random events that disrupt and devastate lives across communities and regions of the world. Communicating within a disaster is often fraught with difficulties both internally and externally. Augmenting communications in any disaster involves preparedness. From individual family disaster planning to the National Incident Management Systems, communications is an integral facet of disaster management.

Nurses are qualified, knowledgeable, and trusted within communities (Willshire et al., n.d). The profession can actively and responsibly engage in the enhancing of all facets of disaster preparations and management, including the facilitation of communications during a disastrous event. Volunteering with disaster relief agencies, maintaining mandated competencies in disaster preparedness, and participating in public health education are few of the many ways nurses can help in emergencies or disaster readiness. They can also develop and teach disaster nursing seminars or continuing education offerings to healthcare professionals to broaden the scope of disaster preparation and response within a given community.

References

After Rita's damage, millions told to stay away. (2005). *USA Today.* Retrieved February 4, 2008, from http://www.usatoday.com/weather/stormcenter/2005-09-24-ritalands_x.htm

Cable News Network. (2003). *Major power outages hit New York, other large cities.* Retrieved February 9, 2008, from http://www.cnn.com/2003/US/08/14/power.outage/

Cable News Network. (2005). *Louisiana, Texas bail out from Rita: Local officials criticize pace of recovery efforts.* Retrieved February 4, 2008, from http://www.cnn.com/2005/WEATHER/09/26/rita

Federal Emergency Management Agency. (2007a). *FEMA: Frequently asked questions.* Retrieved February 7, 2008, from http://www.fema.gov/emergency/nims/faq/compliance.shtm

Federal Emergency Management Agency. (2007b). *Make a disaster kit and a family plan.* Retrieved February 10, 2008, from http://www.fema.gov/news/newsrelease.fema?id=36880.

Goolsby, C., Kulkarni, R., & Mothershead, J. L. (2006). *Disaster planning.* Retrieved January 19, 2008, from http://www.emedicine.com/emerg/topic718.htm

Gunn, S. W. A. (2003). The language of disasters: A brief terminology of disaster management and humanitarian action. In K. M. Cahill (Ed.), *Basics of international humanitarian missions.* New York: Forham University Press.

Lenfant, B., & Soder, M. (n.d.). Disaster communications. *Military Information Technology.* [Electronic version]. Retrieved January 19, 2008, from http://www.military-information-technology.com/print_article.cfm?DocID=1244

Lowrey, W., Evans, W., Gower, K. K., Robinson, J. A., Ginter, P. M., et al. (2007). Effective media communications of disasters: Pressing problems and recommendations. *BMC Public Health* [Electronic version]. Retrieved February 8, 2008, from http://www.pubmedcentral.nih.gov/articlerender.fcgi?artid=1894967

Marks, S., & Borden, L. M. (2004). Encouraging family communication after a disaster: Promoting the health and well-being of families during difficult times. *University of Arizona Cooperative Extension.* Retrieved January 17, 2008, from http://www.cals.arizona.edu/pubs/family/az1341/az1341f.pdf

Matthews, T. J. (2006). *Disaster communications networks: A case study of the Thai Red Cross and their disaster communications.* Retrieved January 17, 2008, from http://contentdm.byu.edu/cdm4/item_viewer.php?CISOROOT=/ETD&CISOPTR=876&CISOBOX=1&REC=7

Merriam-Webster's online dictionary. (2007). Retrieved February 23, 2008, from http://www.merriam-webster.com/

Missouri Department of Mental Health. (2006). *Disaster communications guidebook, preparedness and public education: Promoting emotional well being when preparing for disasters.* Retrieved January 17, 2008, from http://www.dmh.mo.gov/diroffice/disaster/documents/FINALGUIDEBOOKwCov.pdf

Nacos, B. L. (2007). Communication: The role of the media. In T. G. Veenema (Ed.), *Disaster nursing and emergency preparedness for chemical, biological, and radiological terrorism and other hazards* (2nd ed.). New York: Springer.

National Incident Management System. (2004). Lesson 2: Command and management under NIMS. *IS-700 National Incident Management System (NIMS): An Introduction.* Retrieved February 4, 2008, from http://www.training.fema.gov/EMIWeb/IS/is700.asp

Shover, H. (2007). Understanding the chain of command during a disaster. *Perspectives in Psychiatric Care.* Retrieved February 8, 2008, from http://findarticles.com/p/articles/mi_qa3804/is_200702/ai_n18622103/pg_3

Slepski, L. A. (2005). Emergency preparedness: Concept development for nursing practice. *Nursing Clinics of North America: Disaster Management and Response, 40*(3), 419–429.

Smith, P. C., & Simpson, D. M. (2005). The role of mobile emergency tactical communications for disaster response. *University of Louisville, Center for Hazards Research and Policy Development.* Retrieved February 8, 2008, from http://hazardcenter.louisville.edu/pdfs/wp0605.pdf

Sorkin, A. R., & Richtel, M. (2003). The blackout: Communications; cell phone failures cause many to question systems. *New York Times.* Retrieved February 9, 2008, from http://query.nytimes.com/gst/fullpage.html?res=9C0CE2D61430F935A2575BC0A9659C8B63

Twigg, J. (2004). Disaster risk reduction: Mitigation and preparedness in development and emergency programming. Retrieved January 19, 2008, from http://www.odihpn.org/report.asp?id=2893

United Nations. (2006). *International strategy for disaster reduction: Library on disaster risk reduction.* Retrieved February 5, 2008, from http://www.unisdr.org/eng/library/lib-glossaries.htm

Veenema, T. G. (2006). Expanding educational opportunities in disaster response and emergency preparedness for nurses. *Nursing Education Perspectives, 27*(2), 93–99.

Veenema, T. G. (2007). *Disaster nursing and emergency preparedness for chemical, biological, and radiological terrorism and other hazards* (2nd ed.). New York: Springer.

Weiner, E. (2006). Preparing nurses internationally for emergency planning response. *Online Journal of Issues in Nursing.* Retrieved February 10, 2008, from http://nursingworld.org/MainMenuCategories/ANAMarketplace/ANAPeriodicals/OJIN/TableofContents/Volume112006/Number3/PreparingNurses.aspx

Willshire, L., Hassmiller, S. B., & Wodicka, K. A. (n.d.). Disaster preparedness and response for nurses. Retrieved January 3, 2008, from http://www2.nursingsociety.org/education/case_studies/cases/SP0004.html

Wray, R. J., Kreuter, M. W., Jacobsen, H., Clements, B., & Evans, G. (2004). Theoretical perspectives on public communications preparedness for terrorist attacks. *Family Community Health, 27*(3), 232–241.

chapter 10

Legal and Ethical Considerations in a Disaster

Deborah A. DeLuca and Rebecca F. Cady

GOAL

The goal of this chapter is to provide an overview of legal and ethical considerations relevant to disaster situations and disaster nursing.

OBJECTIVES

At the completion of this chapter, the reader will:

1. Describe the differences between federal law and state law as applicable to disaster nursing.
2. Analyze how Good Samaritan laws and immunity from liability provisions in the law affect the disaster nurse in time of disasters and while working in states where the disaster nurse has no license.
3. Define *disaster-specific immunity* and how it impacts the nurse in times of disaster.
4. Evaluate ethical issues that arise in a disaster and how ethical decision making is affected by the legal framework surrounding disaster medical decision making.

Key Terms

- Federal and state laws impacting disaster nursing
- State-based disaster organizations
- Licensure
- Good Samaritan laws
- Disaster-specific immunity
- Professional liability insurance
- Employment issues
- Workers' compensation
- Medical ethics and professional responsibility
- Emergency Medical Treatment and Active Labor Act (EMTALA)

Introduction

Legal issues present an area of concern for all nurses practicing disaster nursing care. As with many areas of the law, the legal framework affecting disaster nursing is complex and constantly evolving. It is therefore imperative that the nurse intending to practice in a disaster situation be well aware ahead of time of the potential legal issues that can affect practice and that the nurse stay up to date on changes in the laws affecting this practice. Disaster nursing practice is affected by both state and federal laws and regulations. These laws address licensure, liability, employment rights, and workers' compensation benefits. Ethical issues also arise when caring for victims of disaster. These issues are related to, guide, and are guided by law. This chapter will explore legal and ethical effects on disaster nursing and will discuss pitfalls for the nurse practicing in this specialty to avoid.

Legal Issues

Federal Laws Affecting Disaster Nursing

> Mr. Vice President, Mr. Speaker, Members of the Senate, and of the House of Representatives: Yesterday, December 7th, 1941—a date which will live in infamy—the United States of America was suddenly and deliberately attacked by naval and air forces of the Empire of Japan. . . . It will be recorded that the distance of Hawaii from Japan makes it obvious that the attack was deliberately planned many days or even weeks ago. (Eidenmuller, 2008)

These words were spoken by then-President Franklin Delano Roosevelt to a shocked nation—a nation provoked to enter World War II by what was, essentially, a terrorist attack on the United States. This is now just another historical fact learned by Americans during their school years. But why are such things like this still taught in school? Because . . . it is 60 years later: September 11, 2001, another date that will live in infamy. Where were you? As Santayana (1905) wrote, "those who cannot remember the past are condemned to repeat it" (p. 284).

On September 11, 2001, a beautifully sunny and clear morning, the peace and tranquility of the nation was interrupted over the course of 20 minutes, during which time airborne terrorists sequentially crashed two hijacked Boeing 767 commercial airliners into the North and South World Trade Towers (WTC) in New York City (Cushman, Pachter, & Beaton, 2003). In moments, this single event created a demoralized, shaken, stunned, and grief-stricken city and nation, with repercussions almost indescribable, and is the "event" that now defines our nation and this generation, just as the Japanese attack on Pearl Harbor did 60 years ago. The nation's sense of security was challenged and, consequently, led to a coordinated in-depth reevaluation of national security and defense reorganization, medical disaster preparedness, economic fall-out strategies, and what the nation might improve to respond more effectively and efficiently, should another such cataclysmic event befall our shores again (McCarthy, Larkin, Greenberg, Ahmad, & Kapp, 2001).

What is most interesting about this event is not the destruction, death, despair, grief, and emotional damage following the collapse of the towers, but how many people selflessly rose to the occasion and went to aid those in distress. The community response was amazing if somewhat chaotic. City planners instituted a disaster plan and, within minutes, lower Manhattan trauma centers did the same (Cushman, Pachter, & Beaton, 2003). Chelsea Piers became one of the primary triage centers, and others were set in local area restaurants, hotel lobbies, or on the street by first responders. Ferries were coordinated to evacuate people to New Jersey and Staten Island and, although overwhelmed, evacuations proceeded for awhile. During the first 24 hours postattack, physicians, nurses, and medical students formed small teams to move to the WTC site to render aid.

Although attempts were made to keep these groups organized and out of harm's way, the reality is that most of the healthcare providers were untrained in providing field medical care to either victims or rescuers, and actually placed themselves in unnecessary risk positions (Cushman, Pachter, & Beaton, 2003). New York City metropolitan area hospitals began preparing to receive large numbers of polytrauma victims; patients were moved by any means possible throughout the city for aid (Yurt et al., 2005). Quickly, it became evident that usual emergency medical response processes were overwhelmed, and it was anticipated that tens of thousands of victims would need acute medical care on this Monday morning. As city planners activated responses, paramedics services dispatched ambulances to the WTC site, upon request of the New York Fire Department, who were put in control. The Fire Department was to remain in contact with the base station and police. Emergency centers, trauma centers, and intensive care units in lower Manhattan all prepared for a large influx of victims, initiating plans to try to assess, resuscitate, stabilize, and triage patients with major injuries (Yurt et al.).

As time progressed it became clear that competition among responders began. A triage team at the site learned that a fireman had traumatic amputations but was rescued. Emergency medicine physicians planned to evaluate, stabilize, and move him by ambulance to a trauma center uptown. A medical officer from the fire department arrived on scene and asserted authority, initiating an intense verbal confrontation while the injured fireman waited, without any basic care, to be transported. Entrepreneurs anxious to get to the site had to be stopped. Undisciplined medical personnel put everyone at risk at the site, including themselves, claiming that undisciplined care without a plan in place is better than no care at all. Impulsiveness and usefulness overrode logic and reason with uncertainty overtaking communication and action. Continued confusion created theories and hierarchies about who was expendable and who was not. Openness, flexible leadership, and goodwill begin to disintegrate while responders wished all would return to normal (Yurt et al., 2005).

It is easy to look retrospectively and criticize what happened in the hours and days surrounding the WTC attack. Mass casualty management principles were applied as well as could be expected under the traumatic, unpredictable circumstances (Cushman, Pachter, & Beaton, 2003). That said, two major errors clearly occurred that forced our nation to rethink how mass casualty disaster preparedness and action must be handled regarding emergency medical volunteerism. The first tragic mistake was that the classic *second hit* phenomenon was not anticipated, where a second event follows directly from the first, though second hits are common occurrences in terrorist activities and well known by the FBI and CIA. The towers' collapse resulted in the needless death and injury of over 400 firemen and police first responders who were dispatched when they probably should have been held back, at least for awhile, until the circumstances could be assessed and the immediate risks settled. Equally tragic was the immediate and inexplicable breakdown of essential communication between police and fire departments, resulting in confused messages to first responders who responded and became victims of unnecessary risk (Cushman, Pachter, & Beaton).

Public Health Security and Bioterrorism Preparedness and Response Act of 2002

In view of the WTC events, the United States Congress authorized federal agencies to help the states develop a system to enroll and organize emergency volunteers ahead of a disaster. On June 12, 2002, President George W. Bush signed into law the Public Health Security and Bioterrorism Preparedness and Response Act of 2002, 42 U.S.C. 201 et seq., 116 Stat. 594, Pub. L. No. 107-188, 107th Congress, June 12, 2002 (Public Health Security, 2002). Under this act, the Secretary of the Department of Health and Human Services (DHHS) is authorized to develop and implement a coordinated strategy according to prior capabilities established under Sec. 319A to "carry(ing) out health-related activities to prepare for and respond effectively to bioterrorism and other public health emergencies, including the preparation of a plan under this section" (Public Health Security, p. 597). For this to occur, the secretary was empowered to collaborate with state and local governments to ensure that all activities regarding bioterrorism and other public health emergencies are coordinated with the activities of the states and local governments.

In Subtitle B, sec. 2811, Emergency Preparedness and Response, 116 Stat 599, the secretary is responsible to coordinate several key activities to ensure proper coordination of the state and federal responses by (a) coordinating interagency interfaces between the DHHS and local entities responsible for emergency preparedness, (b) establishing and coordinating the operations of the National Disaster Medical System (NDMS), (c) coordinating DHHS efforts to bolster state and local emergency preparedness for a bioterrorist attack or other public health emergency and evaluate the progress thereof, and (d) appointing individuals as needed to serve as intermittent personnel of the NDMS in accordance with applicable civil service laws and regulations, with such individuals becoming employees of the Public

Health Service performing medical, surgical, dental, or related functions (Public Health Security, 2002, pp. 599–600).

Emergency System for the Advanced Registration of Health Professions Volunteers (2002)

As part of these requirements, the secretary is empowered to create an Emergency System for the Advanced Registration of Health Professions Volunteers, under Part B, Title III, 319I, of the Public Health Services Act, *as amended* by sec. 106, 42 U.S.C. 247d-7b, 116 Stat. 597 at 608. Part B, Title III empowered the secretary to:

> establish and maintain a system for the advance registration of health professionals for the purpose of verifying the credentials, licenses, accreditations, and hospital privileges of such professionals when, during public health emergencies, the professionals volunteer to provide health services (referred to in this section as the 'verification system'). In carrying out the preceding sentence, the Secretary shall provide an electronic database for the verification system. (Public Health Security, 116 Stat. 597, 2002, at pg. 608)

Uniform Emergency Volunteer Health Practitioners Act (2007)

Although the above act provided for the electronic registry to be prepared expeditiously and had over $2 million appropriated for each of the fiscal years 2002 through 2006 to achieve this database development goal, little development occurred until late 2005 (Public Health Security, 116 Stat. 597, 2002). The Uniform Emergency Volunteer Health Practitioners Act (UEVHPA) and its accompanying database (entitled the Emergency System for Advance Registration of Volunteer Health Professionals [ESAR-VH Programs]) was expeditiously developed and drafted by the National Conference of Commissioners on Uniform State Laws (NCCUSL; last amended November 1, 2007) in 2005 immediately following Hurricanes Katrina and Rita, which struck the nation's Gulf Coast within weeks of each other and completely devastated the coastlines of Texas, Florida, Louisiana, Mississippi, and Alabama. The UEVHPA was drafted with the express purpose of "remedy(ing) significant deficiencies in interstate and intrastate procedures used to authorize and regulate the deployment of public and private sector health practitioners to supplement the resources provided by state and local government employees and other first-responders" (UEVHPA Prefatory Note, 2007, p. 1). The act was approved in its entirety in 2006 excepting Sections 11 and 12 (addressing civil liberties and workers' compensation protections), which were approved in November 2007. The UEVHPA, although adopted, seemed to raise several unanswered questions, such as: (a) what constitutes an emergency, (b) when are volunteers liable for their actions, (c) what about licensure, and (d) should volunteers be compensated for harm to themselves (Hodge, Gable, & Cálves, 2005b)?

When hurricanes Katrina and Rita hit, the UEVHPA did not yet exist. To address concerns about responders licensed in different states than where they were needed and to allow these healthcare professionals to come to areas where assistance was urgently required, affected states would enact emergency management laws to allow modifications or waivers of licensing statutes specifically to allow licensed healthcare practitioners from different states to come to render emergency assistance. Within the public sector, many states had ratified the Emergency Management Assistance Compact (EMAC; see Chapter 2 for more on the EMAC), which formalized the ability of a given state or jurisdiction to accept emergency assistance from licensed health practitioners employed by different state and local governments. All states have ratified the EMAC (UEVHPA Prefatory Note, 2007). Even with ratifying the EMAC, concerns remained regarding the nonlicensure (in the emergency-affected states) of healthcare practitioners responding to different states' calls for assistance. Therefore, UEVHPA addresses this particular concern.

The hurricanes of 2005 brought focus to several deficiencies in federal and state programs used to facilitate interstate use of healthcare practitioners volunteering for emergency service who were not otherwise employed by state or federal agencies. The problem was that interstate licensure reciprocity did not exist, which was necessary to fully utilize volunteer licensed health practitioners (UEVHPA Prefatory Note, 2007). Therefore, since this system of reciprocity did not exist, there was no simple way to link various private and public sector programs. Additionally, there was no uniformly accessible system available to facilitate contact with many healthcare providers and the wide range of nongovernmental organizations vital to all disaster relief organizations. This became problematic because, although states would issue proclamations and executive orders to allow health practitioners from other states to enter and work within their assistance-required boundaries, each state would function independently and differently when coordinating and implementing the programs. Therefore, most responses unfortunately became uncoordinated and ineffective (UEVHPA Prefatory Note, p. 2).

This problem was particularly evident in the immediate days and weeks after Hurricanes Katrina and Rita. These hurricanes added a dimension of difficulty to the already cumbersome process since routine communication was vastly impaired, resulting in a significant breakdown and ineffective, uncoordinated response. Confusion ensued, causing significant delays in deploying many voluntary healthcare practitioners due to the absence of simple communication routes (UEVHPA Prefatory Note, 2007). Physicians and nurses were particularly negatively affected as concerns about availability of workers' compensation and civil liability protections abounded, delaying and limiting the range and scope of services these individuals could provide to individuals located at emergency shelter locations.

As evidenced in the Department of Homeland Security's post-Katrina Medical Response System's Web site report:

> Volunteer practitioners are pouring in to care for the sick, but red tape is keeping hundreds of others from caring for Hurricane Katrina survivors. The North Carolina mobile hospital waiting to help . . . offered impressive state-of-the-art medical care . . . developed with millions of tax dollars through the Office of Homeland Security after 9-11. With capacity for 113 beds, the kit is designed

> to handle disasters and mass casualties. It travels in a convoy that includes two 53-foot trailers, which on Sunday afternoon was parked on a gravel lot 70 miles north of New Orleans because Louisiana officials for several days would not let them deploy to the flooded city. "We have tried so hard to do the right thing . . . it has taken us 30 hours to get here," said one frustrated surgeon. That government officials can't straighten out the mess and get them assigned to a relief effort now that they're just a few miles away "is just mind-boggling," he said. (UEVHPA Prefatory Note, 2007, p. 2)

The sentiment was reiterated by a group of volunteer medical personnel whose resources could not be deployed for several days due to uncertainties in licensure recognition. As the Director of Emergency Services in New Orleans stated, "we need doctors . . . [and] it was pandemonium in the area" (Nevius, 2006, p. A2).

The end result was that practitioners did not treat the sick and injured. Rather, they (a) waited in long lines in futile attempts to navigate through a barely functioning bureaucracy; (b) provided alternative forms of assistance, such as general labor, instead of tending to the sick and injured; (c) reneged on volunteering due to liability concerns, especially regarding noncoverage under their medical malpractice insurance policies since they were practicing, essentially, out of state without a license; or (d) risked facing criminal or administrative penalties or civil liability by consciously violating existing state statutes, all of which are unacceptable options during a public health emergency of disaster magnitude (UEVHPA Prefatory Note, 2007, p. 3).

In response to the ineffective systems and problems created after Hurricanes Katrina and Rita, several organizations developed and implemented systems to promote efficient interstate deployment of volunteer healthcare practitioners. Some of the organizations predominantly involved in this effort were the Federation of State Medical Licensing Boards, the National Council of State Boards of Nursing, the Association of State and Provincial Psychology Licensing Boards, the American Nurses Association, the American Medical Association, the American Psychology Association, the National Association of Chain Drug Stores, and the American Veterinary Medicine Association, which had equally as many problems with their licensees rendering services to animal victims of the hurricanes. Despite these actions, the status of volunteer healthcare practitioners still remained unclear, complicated by concerns about professional licensing sanctions and civil liability, which made these organizations feel compelled to still limit the scope of services available from these volunteers (UEVHPA Prefatory Note, 2007).

In response, the American Red Cross and the NCCUSL decided to address these issues, forming a committee in 2006 to determine if developing a uniform state law could remedy the problems experienced (UEVHPA Prefatory Note, 2007). As previously stated, the end result was the formation and acceptance of the UEVHPA in November 2007, in accordance with the Public Health Services Act. Essentially, the UEVHPA is a federally based supplement to state law that allows health practitioners who are licensed and work for the federal government to respond to disasters and emergencies without compliance with any given state's licensing requirements where their services are being used (UEVHPA Prefatory Note, 2001). In conjunction with the Public Health Services Act, licensed private sector health practitioners are also allowed to practice in different locations than their licensing state during disasters and emergencies.

In general, the UEVHPA accomplishes five goals through the redundant yet robust system for facilitating volunteer medical practitioners' deployment in declared emergencies: (a) establishing a system for using volunteer health practitioners capable of practicing autonomously when routine methods of communication are disrupted; (b) providing reasonable safeguards to assure that volunteer health practitioners are appropriately licensed and regulated to protect the public's health; (c) allowing states to regulate, direct and restrict the scope and extent of services provided by voluntary health practitioners to promote disaster recovery operations; (d) providing limits on the exposure of volunteer health practitioners to civil liability to create a legal environment conducive to volunteerism; and (e) allowing volunteer health practitioners who suffer injury or death while providing services pursuant to this act the option to use workers' compensation benefits from the host state if such coverage is not otherwise available (UEVHPA Prefatory Note, 2007). One circumstance is particularly relevant under the Public Health Services Act: that Medical Reserve Corps in locations throughout the United States are able to recruit, train, and promote deployment of healthcare practitioners in response to emergencies, according to 42 U.S.C. sec. 300hh (UEVHPA Prefatory Note, p. 1). Therefore, the purpose of the act is to remedy defects in state laws to allow states dealing with issues of surge capacity and having to protect the public's health, to utilize effectively private sector volunteers to meet those needs.

Remembering that the UEVHPA does not supplant state emergency management laws nor establish a new emergency response system nationally, the act does require that any health practitioner volunteers first must be registered with either a private or public system that has the capability to determine that the volunteers are in good standing and are properly licensed in their primary practice jurisdiction. The state, if utilizing the UEVHPA, must also be able to communicate this information to the host state's government and entities using the volunteer(s). These primary provisions prevent the likelihood of spontaneous volunteers, especially untrained volunteers, independently traveling to the disaster location without any support from public or private emergency response agencies (UEVHPA Prefatory Note, 2007).

Additionally, and perhaps somewhat cumbersomely, the act allows for volunteers to register with systems located throughout the nation, rather than at the host state's location, which means that any systems utilized by any private or public emergency response agency must work cohesively together, which can be challenging from an electronic perspective (UEVHPA Prefatory Note, 2007). However, considering that registration systems can be developed and implemented only by governmental agencies or private organizations that operate regionally or nationally in accordance with disaster relief of healthcare organizations that have previously demonstrated their capability to recruit, train, and deploy volunteers responsibly, the likelihood of significant difficulty in accounting for registered healthcare volunteers should be minimal.

One benefit to the act is that healthcare practitioner volunteers are restricted to practicing only in their areas of practice in which they are properly licensed, trained, and qualified to perform (UEVHPA Prefatory Note, 2007). This does not mean that the host state cannot make exceptions for qualified practitioners to work outside of their licensed areas of practice under emergent situations. This does, however, justify concerns raised when Sections 11 and 12 of the act were being created.

Sections 11 and 12 of the UEVHPA address specifically concerns in two areas: (a) when and to what extent volunteer healthcare practitioners and entities involved in registering, deploying, and using these individuals are responsible for civil claims arising from a practitioner's act or omission in providing health or veterinary services; and (b) when and to what extent workers' compensation benefits should be provided to these volunteer healthcare practitioners, should they become injured, disabled, or die while providing emergency services (UEVHPA Prefatory Note, 2007). These issues are discussed more thoroughly later in this chapter.

Disaster Relief Act of 2000: Delineating Between a Public Health Emergency/Disaster and Presidentially Declared Emergencies/Major Disasters

An assumption underlies discussions on the UEVHPA that there is clear understanding of the difference between federal and state disaster or emergency responses and the role of volunteer registration in these two categories; this is not necessarily the case. There is a point of delineation that is necessary regarding the meaning of a declared emergency or disaster versus a presidentially declared emergency or disaster. This distinction becomes important regarding the registering of volunteer nurse healthcare professionals under the NDMS of the Federal Response Plan (FRP): The reason that registering under the FRP is important is because it is the single most effective way for healthcare professional volunteers to respond effectively to mass casualties caused by all disasters. Joining a group sponsored at the national level enables these volunteers to respond nationally as well as regionally or locally, provided disaster nurses are also registered at the state/local level or with private organizations at both the state and local levels, such as the American Red Cross, MRC, CERT, or other organization (Schwarz & Kennedy, 2003).

According to the Disaster Mitigation Act of 2000, 42 U.S.C. sec. 5121-5206, implemented in 44 C.F.R., secs. 206.31-206.48, Pub. L. No. 106-390 (Oct. 1, 2006) (Disaster Mitigation Act), an amendment to the Robert T. Stafford Disaster Relief and Emergency Assistance Act, as amended, 42 U.S.C. sec. 5121 et seq, Pub. L. No. 100-707, title 1, Nov. 23, 1988 (Stafford Act), a presidentially declared emergency or disaster must be enacted for the Department of Health and Human Services, through its action agent in the Office of Emergency Response, to reply to all public health and medical needs resulting during a mass casualty event, natural or man-made (Disaster Mitigation Act, 2006; Schwarz & Kennedy, 2003). The only exception is when the emergency is clearly in a subject area that is exclusively or preeminently in the federal purview, under which a federal emergency or disaster is automatically declared (Bazan, 2005). For those healthcare providers interested in volunteering and joining teams that respond to such events, the teams must be sponsored at the national level. This means that healthcare practitioners so registered can respond to any event occurring nationally, as well as regionally or locally.

Under the Disaster Mitigation Act of 2006, the federal government is provided a means by which to supplement state and local resources in major disasters or emergencies where those state and local resources have been or will be overwhelmed, as well as providing similar mechanisms for declaring a major disaster or emergency (Bazan, 2005). Unless the event involves primarily federal interests, both declarations of major disaster (44 C.F.R. 206.36 [10-1-06 Edition], 2006) and declarations of emergency (44 C.F.R. 206.35 [10-1-06 Edition], 2006) are triggered by request to the president from the governor of the affected state (Bazan; Disaster Mitigation Act, 2006).

As defined, when a catastrophe occurs in a state, an *emergency declaration* may be made (sometimes called a "state of emergency"). This is an official pronouncement made by state or local officials authorized to declare the existence of an emergency pursuant to established laws that authorizes the deployment, use, and protection of volunteer healthcare practitioners who comply with provisions (UEVHPA Section 2 Comment, 2007, pg. 14). There is an underlying assumption that the state or local government is well positioned to handle such emergency occurrence.

A *major disaster declaration* (presidential declaration) is made when a catastrophe occurs in a state, and the governor or, in his or her absence, the acting governor, requests the president ensure prompt acknowledgement and processing of the request under the following circumstances: (a) the situation is of such severity and magnitude that effective response is beyond the state's and local governments' capabilities and (b) federal assistance under the Disaster Mitigation Act of 2006 is needed to supplement the efforts and available resources of the state, local governments, disaster relief organizations, and compensation by insurance for disaster-related losses (44 C.F.R. sec. 206.36 [10-1-06 Edition], 2006). Similarly when an incident occurs or threatens to occur in a state, which would normally not qualify under the definition of a major disaster, the governor of that state or, in his or her absence the acting governor, requests the president *declare an emergency* (presidential emergency). In this situation, the following conditions must exist: (a) the situation is of such magnitude and severity that effective response is beyond the normal capability of the state and local government(s); and (b) requires supplementary assistance to save lives, protect property, public health or safety, or to lessen or avert the threat of a disaster (44 C.F.R. 206.35 [10-1-06 Edition], 2006).

Tying these concepts back to the discussion of the UEVHPA, understanding the terminology regarding disasters and emergencies declarations allows one to understand that the UEVHPA defers to other laws currently in effect in all states including those pertaining to declaring public health emergencies (UEVHPA Section 2 Comment, 2007). However, states are allowed to limit or restrict the application of the UEVHPA when issuing an emergency declaration, provided that the state includes within its definitions of emergency and disaster declarations all potentially applicable laws to accomplish the broad objectives of the UEVHPA provisions. This means that no matter how a state decides to define emergency, its declaration of emergency should be the trigger through which the protections of the UEVHPA become effective (UEVHPA Prefatory Note, 2007).

National Response Plan Under the NDMS and Stafford Act

Applying these concepts to the volunteer disaster nurse, government authorities now emphasize the importance of providers volunteering via a structured system versus appearing *ad hoc* at the scene of a disaster, both for the sake of the provider and the patient. In terms of organized participation in the FRP, the disaster nurse has three options: (a) join one of three categories of the NDMS, either the Disaster Medical Assistance Teams (DMAT), Burn Specialty Teams (BSTs), or National Medical Response Teams (NMRTs); (b) join National Nurse Response Teams (NNRTs); or (c) join the Commissioned Corps of the United States Public Health Service (USPHS) (Schwarz & Kennedy, 2003). Each of these options is discussed herein.

The first option is to join one of three categories of the NDMS teams: DMAT, which represents the majority of federal medical assets during a hurricane, flood, earthquake, or other disaster response; Burn Specialty Teams, which are staffed almost entirely by nurses or physicians having substantial education and experience in treating severely burned patients (see Chapters 12 through 15); or National Medical Response Teams, which specialize in responding to chemical and biological agents weapons of mass destruction (Schwarz & Kennedy, 2003). Generally, members of these teams who are activated or called to serve are paid, reimbursed for travel and per diem expenses, and provided liability coverage outside the state of licensure (Schwarz & Kennedy, 2003).

The second option is to join a National Nurse Response Team. This team utilizes the NDMS as part of the Department of Health and Human Services, Office of Preparedness and Response, and is a specialty team that assists with either chemoprophylaxis, vaccination of the public, or in any other scenario that overwhelms the nation's supply of nurses when responding to a weapons of mass destruction event (which has not yet occurred) (U.S. Department of Health and Human Services [DHHS], n.d.; Schwarz & Kennedy, 2003). The NNRT teams are directed by the NDMS in conjunction with a regional team leader in each of 10 established federal regions, and are composed of approximately 200 civilian nurses (DHHS, n.d.). Additionally, the NNRTs are sponsored by the American Nurses Association and are compensated similarly to the DMAT teams in that nurse volunteers are paid upon activation while serving as part-time federal employees, reimbursed for per diem and travel expenses, and are provided liability coverage outside of their licensing state (Schwarz & Kennedy). Additionally, the NNRT requires volunteer members to maintain appropriate certifications and licensure within their discipline; complete Web-based training in disaster response, bioterrorism, humanitarian relief, and other training as relevant; remain current with treatment recommendations for biological weapons; participate in annual training exercises; and be able to deploy if needed (DHHS, n.d.; Schwarz & Kennedy, 2003).

National Response Plan and the Commissioned Corps of the United States Public Health Service

The third option for a volunteer disaster nurse is to become a member of the Commissioned Corps of the USPHS. The USPHS places their volunteers in full-time working positions within a federal agency, particularly the FDA, NIH, CDC, Indian Health Service, or the Federal Bureau of Prisons. When a presidentially declared disaster is called, disaster nurse volunteers are deployed from their assigned agency to assist with the federal response (Schwarz & Kennedy, 2003).

In 2005, the National Response Plan (NRP) was introduced to standardize a national approach for responding to emergency events under the National Incident Management System (NIMS), which updates the USPHS program. The NIMS establishes standardized training, communications, and organization procedures that are usable by multiple jurisdictions to interact in a disaster. The NRP clearly defines authority and leadership responsibilities. Essentially, 15 emergency support functions (ESF) are organized under the NRP, with ESF #8 pertaining specifically to the public health and medical services. The Commissioned Corps (CC) is one of the seven uniformed services within the USPHS, and their officers can be deployed as needed to assist with public health needs when traditional mechanisms and resources are inadequate (Couig, Martinelli, & Lavin, 2005).

The NRP's purpose is to "establish a comprehensive, national, all-hazards approach to domestic incident management across a spectrum of activities including prevention, preparedness, response and recovery . . . using the NIMS . . . which establishes standardized training, organization, and communications procedures for multijurisdictional interaction and clearly identifies authority and leadership responsibilities" (Couig et al., 2005, p. 34). Therefore, the NRP serves as a national framework for coordinating emergency management response and providing standardized protocols. Assuming a national domestic incident occurs, the federal government would use the NRP to coordinate a massive response through its 15 ESFs (Couig et al.).

For nurse volunteers, ESF #8 is of interest as it is the means by which public health and medical services are provided. ESF #8 provides supplemental medical and public health care to local, state, and tribal resources during an incident of national significance. ESF #8 defines five key functional areas: assessing public health and medical needs, determining medical personnel needs, public health surveillance, assessing and securing medical supplies and equipment, and coordinating federal health and medical assistance. Once required to respond to an incident, the Department of Health and Human Services (DHHS) coordinates the ESF #8 through the Secretary's Operations Center (SOC). The DHHS-SOC coordinated focus is on achieving the five ESF #8 functions (Couig et al., 2005).

In summary, the USPHS-CC is the primary recommended volunteer registration system for nurses interested in participating in national disaster response incidents (Schwarz & Kennedy, 2003). Through the NRP, participating in the USPHS-CC lays the foundation for the federal government's comprehensive, systematic, and coordinated response to mass casualty events. Registering with the USPHS-CC fulfills the regulations enhanced through the UEVHPA and enables licensed nurse healthcare practitioners to practice anywhere nationally that they are needed in the event of a mass casualty incident occurring.

UEVHPA Sections 11 and 12: Liability and Workers' Compensation Concerns

Assuming that healthcare professionals appropriately register for service in the event of a mass casualty disaster or emergency occurring, the UEVHPA remains the primary means of coordinating registered information of volunteer health practitioners so that they may respond anywhere needed, regardless of where they are licensed. As explained above, volunteer health practitioners registered with a recognized state disaster response system may practice in a different state experiencing a disaster as though they were licensed in that state, although the laws of the host state will still govern the provision of services (UEVHPA Section 6 and Comment, 2007, p. 28). Also as stated, the act does not impact a health facility's credentialing or privileging standards, nor does it prevent the facility from waiving or modifying these standards during a declared emergency. Rather, the act provides that practitioners must follow the scope of practice for their license as applicable in the disaster state; providers may be subject to licensure discipline if they willfully engage in unauthorized practice (UEVHPA Section 4 Comment, 2007, p. 21).

Because of the suboptimal conditions under which the volunteer healthcare practitioners work during an emergency, many worry about exposure to malpractice liability and the availability of workers' compensation benefits. During emergencies, practitioners are often providing services without access to the resources to which they are usually accustomed. However, they are still responsible for acting appropriately according to professional standards of care, even if they are practicing outside their fields of expertise or have fewer than normal resources available. Complicating the scenario is the higher risk of psychological and physical injury or death while providing services in the emergency care setting. Without appropriate standards in place to alleviate legitimate concerns of these volunteer providers, qualified practitioners may otherwise become reluctant to serve (UEVHPA Prefatory Note, 2007). To address these concerns, the NCCUSL Drafting Committee of the UEVHPA established a process to recognize licensing issues, extend liability protection, and extend workers' compensation protection to volunteer healthcare practitioners (Brewer, 2005). The UEVHPA addresses these issues by building upon the EMAC (see Chapter 2).

The EMAC is a federal law that allows for deployed health practitioners employed by state or local governments to work in host states where they are not normally licensed to practice (Brewer, 2005). The EMAC is a mutual recognition by the states that emergencies require immediate access and present procedures to apply outside resources to make a prompt, effective response to such emergencies (EMAC Legislation, 2007). All 50 states have entered into the EMAC, thereby providing immunity from negligence-based claims to state and certain local government employees deployed from one state to another in reply to disasters and emergencies (UEVHPA Prefatory Note, 2007).

Although the EMAC provides for compensation and death benefits to injured members of emergency forces replying in emergency situations (Article VIII) and reimbursement for loss, damage, or expense incurred in the operation of any equipment or provision of service (Article IX), concerns exist concerning the practical applicability of the EMAC's compensation and asset management procedures between member states during emergency or disaster situations (EMAC Legislation, 2007). For example, although EMAC clearly outlines procedures for assets sharing between states providing mutual assistance, outlines protections for those assets, and provides a reimbursement scheme for the use of these assets, the EMAC does not address utilizing resources beyond the state government as a component of the state's EMAC response. Therefore, incorporating local assets into a state's EMAC response is governed by state law provisions. Although some states have attempted to address this concern by formulating memoranda of understanding (MOUs) for using specific local employees in the response, this is still problematic (Brewer, 2005; Hodge, Gable, & Cálves, 2005b).

Good Samaritan statutes have been enacted by several states to protect volunteers at disaster sites, also. Immunities to other individuals engaged in disaster relief efforts have been extended to groups and organizations providing charitable, disaster, or emergency relief services by several states as well (UEVHPA Prefatory Note, 2007). Unfortunately, the UEVHPA does not clearly delineate the applicability of these laws to volunteer health practitioners, creating a confusing maze of legal protections in very limited settings (Hodge et al., 2005a).

In drafting the UEVHPA, the NCCUSL attempted to clarify the extent to which volunteer health practitioners and the entities engaged in deploying, registering, and using them will be exposed to civil liability. The NCCUSL determined that decisions regarding levels of protection provided belong to the states, but also concluded that failing to include provisions that clearly define the scope of liability exposure creates a significant risk that could deter volunteers from participating. Therefore, the resultant provisions of the UEVHPA provide some level of liability protections under two alternative rule sets in Section 11, entitled Alternative A and Alternative B (UEVHPA Prefatory Note, 2007).

Alternative A, the first alternative, indicates that volunteers are not liable for actions or omissions while giving services during an emergency (UEVHPA Section 11, Alternative A, 2007). This does not absolve the volunteer from willful, wanton, or grossly negligent conduct nor from criminal conduct, other intentional torts, breach of contract, or negligence in the operation of a vehicle. Additionally, volunteer practitioners providing emergency services under this provision are entitled to all other rights, privileges, and immunities otherwise provided by the host state's law and their home state laws. When the volunteer is protected from liability under this alternative, no other individual or entity employing or using these volunteers can be held liable for the actions or omissions of that volunteer under a theory of vicarious liability. This essentially means that when a state adopts Alternative A, it is striking down Good Samaritan and other state volunteer protection acts, illustrating that such legislative determinations satisfy constitutional requirements (UEVHPA Section 11, Alternative A Comment, 2007).

Alternative B, the second alternative, only extends through the UEVHPA the protection described above to uncompensated volunteers under the federal Volunteer Protection Act of 1997, 42 U.S.C. sec. 14501 et seq, 111 Stat. 218, Pub. L. No. 105-19 (VPA), who receive compensation of $500 or less each year for providing services under the UEVHPA (Volunteer Protection Act, 1997). This provision, unlike Alternative A, does not address the issue of vicarious liability (discussed on p. 177), rather leaving it to existing state law to reconcile (UEVHPA Section 11, 2007). Reimbursement for reasonable expenses and continuation of salary while on leave are not counted toward the $500 limit; however, even the question of compensation under the VPA is not a clear, bright line test to determine when the $500 limit is reached. The same types of excluded conduct listed above apply to this alternative as well.

It is important to clarify a few key issues surrounding the Volunteer Protection Act of 1997, since it plays such an important role in the UEVHPA Section 11, Alternative B. As stated, the VPA provides that a volunteer who meets certain criteria will have a complete defense to an action and has no liability. Unfortunately, the VPA does not prohibit lawsuits against volunteers, although it does attempt to provide the volunteer a defense to use should he or she be sued (Runquist & Zybach, 2007). The problem is that any statutory scheme such as the VPA, which merely tailors liability, does not cause a decrease in lawsuits filed against volunteers. For this to occur, it would be necessary for a statute to include two clear provisions: (a) prohibit the filing of lawsuits against volunteers and (b) transfer all liability for the volunteer's conduct to the organization they are affiliated with for the disaster. Logically, this is unrealistic.

The next assumption is that the VPA is still beneficial for volunteers' protection since it is a federal law, thereby preempting the laws of any state. However, state law may provide additional liability protections for the volunteers or may remove protections of the VPA when all parties to the suit are citizens of the same state (Runquist & Zybach, 2007). Therefore, the VPA only applies when the state law does not provide more protection to volunteers than the VPA; it will not apply if the state specifically eliminates the applicability of the VPA to its citizens or provides more protections than the VPA.

Now, assuming that the VPA is used by a state in its adoption of UEVHPA Section 11, Alternative B, a volunteer *acting within the scope of the volunteer's responsibility* is not liable for harm if all of the following criteria are met. Here, acting within the scope of the volunteer's responsibility the act includes all of the following: (a) the volunteer is acting within the scope of the volunteer's responsibilities in the organization at the time of the act or omission (referring to a harm, usually negligence or liability); (b) the volunteer is properly licensed, certified, or authorized by the appropriate authorities of the state for the activities taken, if such is appropriate or required; (c) the volunteer is not guilty of willful or criminal misconduct, gross negligence, reckless misconduct, or a *conscious, flagrant indifference* to the rights or safety of the individual harmed; and (d) the harm was not caused by the operation of a vehicle, vessel, or aircraft where the state requires an operator's license and insurance (Hodge, Gable, & Cálves, 2005b; Runquist & Zybach, 2007; VPA, 1997).

These four rigorous criteria basically assume that the volunteer becomes a full employee of the organization in order to gain protection. It is only under this restrictive provision, where the volunteer becomes a full employee of the organization, that the VPA applies; otherwise, the VPA does not apply to an action brought against the volunteer by the organization nor does it limit the liability exposure of the organization to the extent it would otherwise be responsible for the volunteer's actions (Runquist & Zybach, 2007). (The concepts of vicarious liability, federal protections granted to organizations, and charitable immunity are part of the ethics discussion in this chapter beginning on page 177.) Assuming that a volunteer is acting within the scope of the volunteer's responsibilities to the organization but does not otherwise meet the aforementioned four criteria specified in the VPA, the volunteer's liability is limited under the VPA to the following extent: (a) punitive damages; here unless the injured party bringing suit can establish by clear and convincing evidence that the harm was caused by the volunteer's action and that the action constitutes criminal or willful misconduct or a conscious and flagrant disregard for the rights and safety of the individual, punitive damages may not be awarded; (b) noneconomic damages; here losses such as for pain and suffering or mental anguish will only be assumed by the volunteer to the extent of his or her percentage of the harm actually suffered, which is determined by the court in a separate proceeding; and (c) economic damages; here defendants are jointly and severally liable for economic losses, where joint and several liability means parties are responsible together and individually, and recovery can be sought from either or both wrongdoers, but the injured party cannot receive double compensation (*Black's Law Dictionary,* 1990a).

Therefore, simply put, Alternative B, instead of providing an expanded scope of immunity generally to all jurisdictions under current law as does Alternative A, removes potential impediments to applying existing immunities provisions to volunteer healthcare practitioners providing services under the UEVHPA (UEVHPA, Section 11, Alternative B, Comment). The NCCUSL did not recommend which alternative on liability, A or B, is preferred. However, the NCCUSL included within its Section 11 commentary that each state adopting the UEVHPA must clearly articulate which protections it provides to allow volunteer health practitioners to make informed decisions concerning volunteering (UEVHPA Section 11, Comment, 2007).

Because of obvious concerns that volunteer providers have about serious injury, disability, and death due to entering potentially dangerous working conditions common to emergency or disaster incidents, workers' compensation is another area anticipated and addressed by the NCCUSL and in the UEVHPA Section 12. Before examining how the UEVHPA provides workers' compensation benefits to healthcare volunteers, it is important to understand what workers' compensation benefits are: Workers' compensation is a system administered by each state government and by the federal government to provide limited benefits to employees who suffer work-related injury or death, without regard to fault. These injuries must be reported and compensated according to specific laws. The laws that apply in a particular situation depend on the state in which the injury occurs. These laws cover only employees, and thus usually would not cover unpaid volunteers. Hence, this is the obvious reason for the concern among volunteer healthcare practitioners and the interest by the NCCUSL in addressing effectively the worker's compensation issues for volunteers, who are not employees under the standard worker's compensation definitions existing on the state and federal levels.

The UEVHPA Section 12 is designed to provide redress for injuries, disability, or death directly related to the healthcare provided by the volunteer healthcare practitioners at the time of emergency or disaster (UEVHPA Section 12, Comment, 2007). To invoke this protection, Section 12(a) defines injury as "includ[ing] physical or mental injuries or diseases for which employees of the state, who is injured or contracts the disease in the course of the employee's employment would be entitled to benefits under the workers' compensation [or occupational disease] law of this state" (UEVHPA Section 12(a), 2007, p. 48). This provision simply means that volunteer health practitioners in a host state are entitled to workers' compensation benefits if a state employee of the host state would be entitled under the same circumstances (UEVHPA Section 12, Comment, 2007). The provision regarding occupational disease law pertains only to those states that have occupational disease laws; if a state adopts the UEVHPA and does not have such occupational disease laws in place, they do not have to be concerned with that provision and only regard information on workers' compensation benefits.

Most states value the services provided by volunteer healthcare providers during emergencies and disasters and the concomitant idea that state and local governments should provide workers' compensation benefits to individuals voluntarily providing such valuable services is well settled legally. For example, almost all states extend workers' compensation benefits to their police auxiliary and volunteer fire department members (UEVHPA, Section 12, Comment, 2007). The problem is encountered when state laws are developed *ad hoc* without a base of underlying unifying principles, which usually serves to confound reliance upon the laws when trying to integrate a unified, nationwide volunteer disaster response system.

The problem is further confounded when a licensee's state does not provide workers' compensation benefits to volunteer healthcare providers, if the host state's benefits are more or less expansive than the licensee's state, or the volunteer's licensing state's benefits are more or less expansive than the host state's benefits. Interestingly, the NCCUSL, in drafting Section 12, provided for these possibilities. Consequently, the UEVHPA provides that volunteers can choose to be deemed an employee of the state in which services are being provided for the purposes of receiving workers' compensation benefits. In this situation, injury will be defined according to the law in the disaster state (National Conference of Commissioners on Uniform State Laws, 2008b).

By allowing this provision, the UEVHPA treats all volunteers equally, thereby eliminating the problem of determining whether and to what extent host states' workers' compensation benefits apply. Therefore, Section 12 generally and Section 12(b) specifically are based on the laws of all states that provide workers' compensation benefits to all volunteers who are appropriately registered or provide services pursuant to the direction and control or at the request of emergency management officials. It is important to note however that Section 12 is different from existing state law in that it expressly provides coverage for volunteer healthcare practitioners and accounts for the specialized registration systems and practice requirements imposed by this act upon the states (UEVHPA, Section 12 Comment, Annotated, 2007).

Reading the UEVHPA carefully, the aforementioned provisions may seem to be in contravention with Section 3, that states the UEVHPA applies only to volunteer healthcare practitioners "who provide health or veterinary services in this state for the host entity while an emergency declaration is in effect" (UEVHPA, Section 12, Comment, Annotated, 2007, p. 50). The "emergency declaration in effect" restriction may be problematic for volunteers participating in emergency training and drills who sustain injury, disability, or death and attempt to claim workers' compensation benefits. Again, anticipating this possible conflict in terms, the NCCUSL provides in Section 12 for states to add any provisions regarding benefits during emergency drills or training sessions for volunteers freely as needed, without conflicting with the terms in Section 12. Further, absence of such provisions do not reduce any benefits provided to healthcare volunteer practitioners who qualify directly for those benefits under such laws, unless the laws are designated for repeal under Section 14 of the UEVHPA, as provided for in Section 9(a), stating that the UEVHPA does not limit rights, privileges, or immunities provided to volunteer healthcare practitioners by laws other than this act (UEVHPA Section 9(a), 2007, p. 37; UEVHPA Section 12 Comment, Annotated, p. 50–51). This type of coordinated effort to provide benefits to volunteer healthcare practitioners substantiates the intent of Section 13, which provides that the UEVHPA recognizes the uniformity of interstate recognition of licensure and the granting of particular privileges and protections to these individuals during emergencies or disasters (UEVHPA Section 13, 2007). Therefore, it becomes clear that the intent of the NCCUSL in creating the UEVHPA was to treat equivalently licensed, competent volunteer healthcare practitioners justly so that their vital skills and services would not be lost in an emergency or disaster incident due to concerns for their own safety and well-being.

Some states have passed laws addressing workers' compensation protection to volunteers who are injured during the course of providing assistance during a disaster. An example of a state actively involved in ensuring workers' compensation benefits for its volunteer healthcare practitioners is Minnesota. Minnesota law indicates that individuals who volunteer to assist a local political subdivision of the state during an emergency or disaster, who register with that subdivision, and who are under its direction and control are considered to be the subdivision's employee for purposes of workers' compensation as well as tort claim defense (defense to malpractice or negligence) and indemnity (one party agrees to secure another against an anticipated loss or damage); in a very broad sense insurance is a type of indemnity contract. Individuals in Minnesota who volunteer to assist the state during an emergency or disaster, who register with a state agency, and are under its direction and control are considered a state employee for purposes of workers' compensation, tort claim defense, and indemnity (Minn. Stat. Ann. 12.22 Subd. 2A.).

Finally, the UEVHPA is being adopted by many states since its final adoption in November 2007 by the NCCUSL. Table 10-1 illustrates the status of adoption of this act as of March 10, 2008. This table represents the status of adoption of the UEVHPA in different states in the 2007–2008 year. While only 13 states are in the active phase of adopting UEVHPA currently, the NCCUSL has stated their intention to actively pursue adoption among all the states in the 2008 year (UEVHPA Annotated, 2007, Prefatory Comments).

State-Based Organizations for Volunteer Healthcare Practitioners' Registrations

Medical Reserve Corps

One of the most efficient ways for nurses to volunteer to register to provide services nationwide in the event of emergency or disaster incidents is through the USPHS-CC. To provide volunteer healthcare practitioner services on the state, regional, or local level, volunteers must also be registered within their own licensing state. The MRC (see Chapter 2) provides this option to volunteer healthcare practitioners within the state, and is also registered through to the national level for coordination of teams as needed. The MRC was founded after President G. W. Bush's 2002 State

TABLE 10-1 STATUS OF ADOPTION OF UEVHPA AS OF MARCH 2008

State	Status
Hawaii	Introduced 2007-08 as HB 2424
Pennsylvania	Introduced in 2007-08 as SB 1060
Indiana	Introduced in 2007-08 as SB 363; passed senate
New Mexico	Introduced in 2007-08 as HB 348; passed both houses
Oklahoma	Introduced in 2007-08 as SB 2032
Maryland	Introduced in 2007-08 as HB 666/SB 857
Mississippi	Introduced in 2007-08 as HB 1027; died in committee
Illinois	Introduced in 2007-08 as SB 2285
Minnesota	Introduced in 2007-08 as SB 2932
Utah	Introduced in 2008
Colorado	Adopted
Kentucky	Adopted
Tennessee	Adopted

Source: The National Conference of Commissioners on Uniform State Laws, 2006, 2008a.

of the Union Address, when he asked all Americans to volunteer in support of the nation. MRC teams are sponsored by the Office of the U.S. Surgeon General, but are organized at the state, county, and local level (MRC, 2008). These teams, while under the auspices of the Citizen Corps, are organized according to the needs of each local governmental body and function to locally organize and utilize volunteers wanting to donate time and expertise to prepare for and respond to emergencies among other tasks; they supplement existing emergency and public health resources.

MRC teams are composed of medical and public health specialists, such as nurses, physicians, pharmacists, dentists, epidemiologists, and veterinarians, along with other skilled community members such as chaplains, interpreters, office workers, legal advisors, and others as needed. These healthcare professionals are trained according to Citizen Corps online and on-ground requirements and respond as determined by the local government agency sponsoring the MRC. Most often, MRC units are given specific areas where strengthening of the public health infrastructure is needed. These locations are outlined priorities for the health of individuals and, the nation as a whole, which serve to guide the MRC teams. Health literacy improvement is the overarching goal of the MRC, which is achieved by the MRC developing and implementing programs that increase disease prevention education, eliminate health disparities, and improve public health preparedness generally (MRC, 2008).

Many states have developed other ways to coordinate volunteers in a disaster. For example, New York has developed a Public Health Preparedness Volunteer Practitioner Database. Registered nurses can join this database through the New York State Nurses Association at www.nysna.org.

Licensure

As stated previously, according to the Uniform Law Commission, all 50 states have adopted the EMAC, which provides for the interstate recognition of licenses held by professionals responding to disasters and emergencies. However, this Compact only benefits providers who go through a complicated process of entering into agreements with their home state to be deployed to other states pursuant to mutual aid agreements (National Conference of Commissioners on Uniform State Laws, 2008b).

Some states have passed additional laws that allow reciprocity in disaster situations. New Hampshire law (New Hampshire Revised Statutes Section 21-P:41, 2002) provides for such reciprocity in the form of immunity and exemption from that state's licensure requirements in the provision of care during an emergency. Minnesota law provides for direct reciprocity, in that a professional license from any other state will have the same force and effect during an emergency or disaster as though it were issued by Minnesota (Minnesota Statutes Section 12.42, 2005). Illinois provides that persons licensed elsewhere, who are members of a mobile support team or unit of another state rendering aid in Illinois under the order of the governor of the provider's home state or as requested by the Illinois governor, may practice during the disaster without being licensed in Illinois (20 Illinois Comp. Stat 3305/16, 2005). Utah's Emergency Management Assistance Act (Emergency Management Assistance Act, SB0118, 2001, Utah) was passed to enact the EMAC. This act provides that licensure will be recognized by the state receiving the assistance if the licensure is valid in the healthcare provider's home state, but is subject to any limitations or conditions determined by the governor of the state requesting assistance.

Other Legal Issues

Professional Liability Insurance

It is important for the disaster nurse intending to participate in disaster response to maintain a personal professional liability policy of insurance. The disaster nurse needs to make sure that the policy does not exclude the activities sought to be insured. If the disaster nurse is participating as part of an organized disaster response team, then liability coverage may be provided by way of that team membership.

It should be noted that volunteers are typically not covered by the Federal Tort Claims Act (1946), a federal law providing coverage for employees of the federal government and some federal health centers. MRC teams typically provide liability coverage for their members, but this varies by locality and needs to be confirmed by the disaster nurse member. Members of the New York Public Health Preparedness Volunteer Practitioner Database who are activated and deployed by the New York State Department of Health are considered state employees and are thus provided both defense and indemnity under Public Officers Law Section 17; if the volunteer also has an individual policy, a claim must be filed with the individual policy as well (New York Public Officers Law Section 17, 1909).

There is no harm in having an individual liability policy on top of what may be provided by way of team membership, and it is strongly advised all disaster nurses have one. In assessing an insurance policy, the disaster nurse needs to determine whether the policy is an occurrence policy or a claims made policy. An occurrence policy covers any incident that occurs while the disaster nurse is insured; claims made policies only cover claims made when the policy is active regardless of when the incident occurred. Other aspects of an individual liability policy that need to be evaluated include declarations, coverage agreement, supplementary payments, limitations, and conditions.

In selecting a policy, the disaster nurse should discuss any other potential coverage (i.e., through the federal government or other organization) and get a copy of that policy. The disaster nurse should evaluate the available options in the commercial market, compare premiums, identify the risk of exposure, insure for the biggest exposure with the broadest coverage, check the insurer's rating, ask whether the insurer gives a premium reduction for educational attendance, and investigate the availability of additional services such as state board of nursing disciplinary defense coverage.

Employment Issues

The last thing a disaster nurse volunteer wants to deal with on returning home is the loss of a regular job. The American Nurses Association has published two position statements regarding issues arising with nurses volunteering in disasters, one geared toward the nurse and one toward the employer. According to the ANA (ANA, 2002a, b), at the time the disaster nurse is employed, he or she should inform the employer in writing of any disaster/emergency preparedness education or related certification and time commitment required to maintain proficiency, as well as notice of enlistment on any state or federal medical response team. The disaster nurse should keep the employer up to date regarding his or her competency in disaster/emergency preparedness and should inform the state or federal team of which he or she is a member in writing if the employer refuses to consent or withdraws consent for the disaster nurse to participate in emergency deployment.

The employer should provide a written mechanism of approval for the nurse to participate as a member of such a team and should keep a current list of all of its employee nurses who are educated in disaster/emergency preparedness as well as those who are members of state or federal medical response teams. The employer should also keep a current list of those employee nurses who have been approved for state or federal medical response team service. These position statements emphasize that reemployment should be guaranteed by the employer, with continued pay and benefits while the disaster nurse is deployed for up to 2 months unless the disaster nurse is being paid for his or her disaster work by the government or other entity (ANA, 2002b).

Providers who respond under one of the designated federal response systems or through the EMAC have a protected right to reemployment upon returning home after responding to a disaster. This includes job, seniority, and wage protection. Volunteers who are reserve members of the uniformed services and are called up for active duty receive the same protections under the Uniformed Services Employment and Reemployment Rights Act (Centers for Law and The Public's Health, 2008b).

Volunteers need to be aware that, aside from these federal level protections, they may be vulnerable to adverse effects on their regular employment. Factors that can impact this effect include (a) the amount of time the volunteer is absent, (b) whether the absence causes undue hardship on the employer, and (c) whether the employer's circumstances have changed during the volunteer's absence such that reemployment is unreasonable or impossible (Centers for Law and the Public's Health, 2008a). Some states have laws that address employment issues. For example, Illinois provides for employment protection for employees of a state agency under certain conditions when that employee provides services requiring leave from work in a disaster (5 Ill. Comp. Stat. 335.3, West 2005).

Ethical Considerations in Disaster Response

The law and ethics are inextricably tied. Theoretically, if this statement is true, then to act ethically is to act legally, yet if an action is ethical does that automatically mean it is legal as well? This is the question that often confounds medical practitioners. To understand this conundrum, it is first necessary to understand how the law accommodates ethics and how ethics influences the law. The focus of this section is not on the basic ethical principles of autonomy, beneficence, nonmalfeasance, distributive justice, and veracity, as these are assumed known by licensed medical practitioners. Rather, this discussion begins from a conceptual model of the interplay between law and medical ethics, and continues into the application of that model to legal and ethical concerns underlying decisions to volunteer in disaster emergencies (Olick, 2001).

This section's discussion focuses on two major areas of interest affecting volunteer health practitioners involved in a disaster management situation: the legal implications of particular actions of volunteers (i.e., sovereign immunity, vicarious liability, and the Federal Tort Claims Act [FTCA]), and ethical concerns under the Emergency Medical Treatment and Active Labor Act (EMTALA). The reason these discussions are couched in ethical theory is because it is the fundamental question of the *right action* (ethics) to do in a disaster situation that brings these legal issues into play.

Before engaging in the legal and ethical discussions surrounding disaster nurses volunteering in a disaster, it is important for volunteer responders to understand the law and ethics behind a disaster response that directly affects them and, more disturbingly, may not provide protections legally necessary for an informed volunteer service decision to be made. The concern begins with the conditions under which a disaster responder works: usually an altered medical environment, in a state usually different from where they normally practice, under laws and provisions different from that to which they are normally accustomed, without any guarantees of safety, available resources, or right to reemployment upon their return (ANA, 2008). Without a good base of understanding upon which to make a volunteering decision, a disaster nurse, upon returning home, could be unpleasantly surprised.

Ethically, nurse volunteers must understand that federal and state law does not usually provide the anticipated legal protections considered necessary by the profession (ANA, 2008). The ANA clearly articulates through its nursing *Code of Ethics* and *Nursing Scope and Standards* the level of practice expected by its practitioners. As will be explained, such codes are not legally binding authority. However, state and regulatory issues are often affected by these formalized codes. Therefore, when deciding whether to volunteer or not during a disaster situation, the disaster nurse is responsible for knowing and understanding the expectations of responders and being comfortable acting within those expectation levels (ANA, 2008).

From a legal perspective, disaster nurse volunteers must recognize two primary issues. First, as indicated briefly under the UEVHPA Section 12 on worker's compensation, responding either through EMAC or under designated federal response systems gives volunteer practitioners a minimal level of assurance that they will retain their employment following disaster deployment (ANA, 2008; EMAC, 2007; UEVHPA Section 12, 2007). However, individuals choosing to serve as spontaneous volunteers are not guaranteed a right to reemployment without having clear agreement with their employer in place prior to deploying. Again, this focuses on the quasi-legal and ethical conundrum surrounding the *right actions* for a practitioner balanced against the legal constraints imposed by employment law.

Additionally, as a final prelude to the entire legal and ethical discussion, licensing is probably the single most concerning aspect to volunteering during a disaster. Although several procedures are in place to allow for licensing reciprocity recognition for volunteer health practitioners during disasters (Public Health Services Act, 42 U.S.C. sec. 247(d)-7b [2005]), the problem arises when state regulatory boards are unable to function during the disaster due to circumstances arising such as power outages affecting computer registrations, so that minimal procedures are impossible to execute (ANA, 2008). This type of simple problem could expose the volunteer practitioner to both civil and criminal charges for practicing without a license or worse.

Overview of the Law and Medical Ethics Interplay

Social values, medical practice, and the law are not static creatures. In the course of normal medical practice, several issues arise requiring consultations from lawyers, risk managers, or ethicists. Risk managers usually function at the institutional level and often are attorneys who possess a clear clinical medicine background. Although it may seem awkward to discuss the issue of risk management in the context of a mass disaster situation, the reality is that many decisions made when individuals arrive simultaneously at an institution for acute stabilization and care present the possibility of difficult decision making by healthcare practitioners that automatically call the risk manager into play. Interestingly, it is often the risk manager who bridges the gap between the law and ethics by developing, instituting, and interpreting institutional policies, procedures, and practices that are founded on societal norms and social values regarding care and the ethics behind that care, while reducing risk of liability to both the institution and the licensed medical practitioners within it. When institutional standards of practice extend beyond the minimal standards required by law, law and ethics are called into play to resolve the conflict.

The law is the established societal rules for appropriate conduct, the violation of which may create civil or criminal liability (Vincier, 1998). Often, when ethical questions arise during medical practice, legal concerns also often arise. Therefore, the study of medical ethics in context involves understanding the discipline and methodology involved when considering the implications of any medical practice against what *ought to be* or what the *right action* is (ethics). Thus, the overlap between law and ethics occurs.

Conceptually, the distinction is clear. Law regulates behavior to protect society (Ogloff & Olley, 1998). It is expressed through four major vehicles: (a) federal and state constitutions of the fundamental laws of its character and conformation; (b) federal and state statutes embodying in writing enactments of a legislative body; (c) federal or state regulations, rules, or orders prescribing the behavior of those under its control; and (d) federal and state case law decisions at the appellate level explaining how the law in concept applies in reality, although the case decisions are legally binding only in the jurisdiction where the decision is made. Similarly, yet distinctly, medical ethics is expressed through four similar vehicles: law; institutional policies or practices derived from law and professional standards of practice; policies of professional organizations; and professional standards of care, often defining fiduciary obligations of care in exchange for financial remuneration (Vincier, 1998). Conceptually, a gradual confluence occurs between the law and medical ethics, as seen in Figure 10-1.

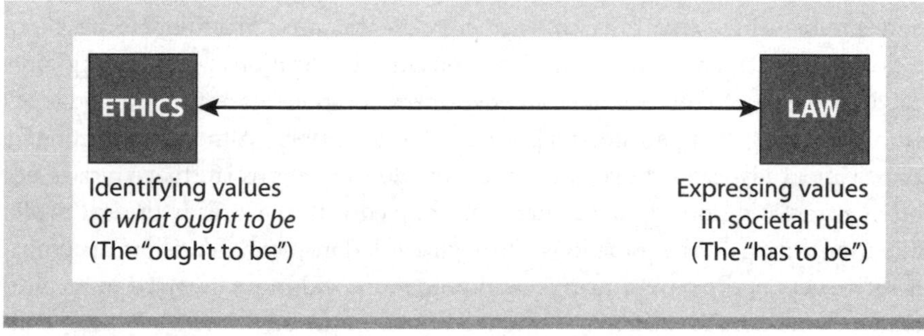

Figure 10-1 The confluence between law and ethics.

The functional role of each is dynamic and in a constant state of change such that new legislation and court decisions occur and medical ethics responds to the challenges created by new technology, law, or other influences (Ogloff & Olley, 1998; Vincier, 1998). However, although the roles of each are distinct, law and ethics have at least seven common points of consideration: (a) access to medical care, particularly in regard to providing care, emergency treatment, stabilization, and patient transfer; (b) confidentiality of protected healthcare information balanced against mandatory reporting requirements defined by law; (c) informed consent; (d) advanced care directives and healthcare proxies; (e) privileged communications and privacy; (f) physician-assisted suicide concerns (applicable only in Oregon and Washington states as of 2008); and (g) abortion. As similar and broad as these seven considerations are, the law and ethics are equally distinct in their respective function, power, and philosophy.

The law does not establish positive duties, defined as that which one should do, to the same extent that professional ethics or medical ethics does (Peabody, 1998). Rather, the law is based on court order and binding decisions that determine the outcome of a particular controversy (Vincier, 1998). Standards of conduct are prescribed through statute or administrative law code, which must be adhered to, or criminal and or civil penalties attach for breaching the code or statute. Conversely, medical ethics is the understanding of principles from which positive duties emerge and begins when good law ends (Peabody; Vincier). Moral conscience precedes legal rule development for social order. Therefore, medical ethics and law share a common goal: creating and maintaining social welfare through a symbiotic relationship. Law and professional ethics both attempt to articulate, interpret, operationalize, and resolve conflicts between ethical principles and values that have evolved throughout the history of man and are operationalized in a variety of ways both within societies and communities. The law frequently turns to policy statements of professional organizations when creating or interpreting laws affecting that profession, thereby reinforcing the connection between the law and ethics. The law shapes ethics and ethics shapes the law such that over time, law and ethics become increasingly consistent through this gradual process (Ogloff & Olley, 1998).

So what does this mean to a disaster nurse volunteer thinking about leaving home and employment to serve in a disaster emergency? Volunteer practitioners must keep a clear line of demarcation between legal and ethical obligations when making clinical decisions, based on current knowledge of key components of the laws and regulations affecting their patients and practice (Peabody, 1998). Although practitioners act as patient advocates, the volunteer practitioners must appreciate that ethical issues often attract widespread public attention, coupled with the already present media attention during disaster situations. Through legislation, judicial decision, or administrative action, the government is becoming more and more involved in medical ethics. Combining the heightened emotional environment that attends disasters with scientific advances, public education, consumer and civil rights movements, law and economic effects on medical practice, and the heterogeneity of the nation's society, practitioners must be well settled on the ethical principles governing their behavior (Peabody).

The problem begins with the core constitutional value that influences all aspects of disaster management, namely federalism. Although federalism has been a fundamental underpinning of the entire chapter and book discussions, it has not been formally exposed for what it is and the impact it has on the legal and ethical questions arising in disaster response. Federalism enures from the U.S. Constitution's Tenth Amendment that states "the powers not delegated to the United States by the Constitution, nor prohibited by it to the States, are reserved to the States respectively, or to the people" (U.S. Constitutional amend. X). This means that the Constitution basically requires a coordinated response to encompass and pass through all levels of the government, from federal to state to local to private actors, during a disaster emergency response. Although it seems simple, this is an extremely complex requirement to meet. Although federal and state governments share the responsibility for appropriate disaster response, the lines of authority are not clearly delineated (Weeks, 2007).

The lines become muddier when states and the federal government each may justifiably claim authority for the response in an attempt to meet the challenge of federalism. When this occurs, finger pointing and blame assigning follow, creating a state of chaos as evidenced in the moments and days following both the WTC attacks and Hurricane Katrina, stymieing attempts by responders to reach victims. As if it could get no worse, federalism also demands complete coordination among separate state governments. Should a disaster impact more than one state, each state has its own separate sovereign authority and discretion to enact different, often conflicting, legal requirements and policy priorities for emergency management and response (Weeks, 2007).

Natural disasters and terrorist disasters are differentiated under federalism. Natural disasters, such as Hurricane Katrina in 2005, are categorized as catastrophes that create new, immediate emergency needs and serious exacerbation of existing conditions with lasting and devastating effects for the region's healthcare infrastructure (Weeks, 2007). Terrorist acts, such as the WTC attacks, inflict widespread human injury, with sudden and unprecedented demands for medical care. The point of similarity is in the number of individuals affected directly or indirectly by either event, usually numbering in the thousands. In trying to understand the legal and ethical ramifications created for volunteer responders under these two schemes, it is important to first understand the conceptual difference between healthcare and public health, which is based on three clear ideas: disaster response; collective approach to healthcare; and public health and safety, all which have legal and ethical concerns attached to them. Each concept is explained below.

First, disaster response requires an entirely different mindset to healthcare planning and response. Here, healthcare volunteers are faced with the problem of having to think in terms of populations (Weeks, 2007). The population-based healthcare approach is unfamiliar to most healthcare providers and is absolutely antithetical to traditional medical treatment models. Authorities and caregivers need to focus not on individualized care, but how to best allocate scarce and stretched resources, facilities, funding, and personnel for the collective benefit of the entire population (Weeks, 2007). Often the legal and ethical conundrum arises when the best medical outcome for an individual patient must be compromised for the collective benefit of the entire population.

Second, healthcare must become a collective response. This means volunteer responders must focus more on how to achieve the best overall outcome for the greatest number of affected individuals (Weeks, 2007). This concept directly contravenes traditional medical approaches, creating a legal and ethical conundrum. Here, the patient–caregiver relationship is sacrificed to a centralized approach of providing health care. Health is traditionally seen as a personal, medical matter, a state of freedom from pathology achieved by an individual in conjunction with their healthcare provider who is guided by the standard of care of his or her profession, which seeks the best outcome possible for the individual patient, regardless of who else is waiting (Gostin, 2002). The conundrum is therefore trying to balance this edict with sacrifice for the greater good demanded by a mass casualty environment.

Third is the public health focus, which requires compromise by healthcare providers in order to ensure the welfare and safety of an entire mass casualty population (Gostin, 2002; Weeks, 2007). Here, sacrificing individual health outcomes for the greater good of the community at large is mandated, allocating resources most efficiently, in the best interest of the collective affected population, forcing a tension to develop between individual rights and interests and the communitarian interest at large (Gostin, 2004). The legal and ethical conundrum often occurs when volunteer responders have to face the harsh reality that one person's medical condition may or must be allowed to deteriorate while another victim's more pressing medical requirements are addressed, contrary to the traditional individual patient standard of care, which is to exercise reasonable skill, care, and diligence as would normally be rendered by medical practitioners under the same or similar circumstances (*Keebler v. Winfield Carraway Hospital,* 1988).

The fact that a practitioner may not have sufficient equipment, training, or capability to properly treat a patient does not excuse failure to exercise due care (*New Biloxi Hospital, Inc. v. Frazier,* 1962). This is where the conundrum rears its ugly head, as in a mass casualty event resources are stretched or significantly limited. Therefore, abandonment is sometimes necessary to achieve the greater benefit for the larger number of patients, whereas the professional standards of care have not yet taken into account competing needs of other patients (Public Health Security, 116 Stat. 597, 2002; NCCUSL, last amended November 1, 2007). Therefore, where liability may be concerned, the role of circumstances related to the emergency playing effectively as a factor adjusting the standard of care for medical practitioners rendering care is still unsettled, which directly affects the practitioner's decisions on how, when, and to whom to render care, creating the legal and ethical confusion.

There is no question that a reasonable healthcare practitioner volunteering in good conscience to attend to victims in a mass casualty event is often confused regarding the line between what constitutes right actions professionally in the care of patients and the legal questions surrounding that care and their status as licensed professionals volunteering to practice in a state other than where they are licensed. Understanding the parameters involved behind this legal and ethical conundrum may help elucidate the role of ethics and law in making an informed choice on whether or not to volunteer.

Understanding the Legal Conundrum Ethically: Immunity, Liability, and Treatment

The following issues underlie the legal and ethical conundrum volunteer healthcare practitioners face when deciding to respond to a mass casualty disaster event: sovereign immunity, vicarious liability, the Federal Tort Claims Act (FTCA), and EMTALA. Although all of these precepts have been alluded to throughout this chapter, these issues will now be explained in the context of legal and ethical concerns for volunteer responders.

Volunteer Liability, Immunity, and Indemnification

When a volunteer healthcare practitioner (VHP) responds to an emergency or disaster, the VHP is immediately confronted with the risk of civil liability for negligent conduct (Hodge, Gable, & Cálves, 2005a). Negligence theories rooted in the VHP's failure to adhere to a particular standard of care when providing services are the most common basis for civil liability claims. In addition to direct liability of the VHPs for their own negligent actions, their employers may be held vicariously liable for their actions (Dobbs, 2000). Although the VHP may also be subject to other torts such as civil battery liability (for performing an invasive bodily procedure without informed consent), the discussion herein is limited to risk of liability related to negligent torts only. However, it is important to note that the VHP may also be subject to criminal liability, and liability is determined by assessing the elements of the crime the VHP is alleged to have committed (Dobbs; Hodge, Gable, & Cálves, 2005a). Interestingly, since the VHP's professional negligence is generally governed by state law, the VHP's acts will be assessed under the laws of the jurisdiction where the acts occurred (Hodge, Gable, & Cálves, 2005a).

To prevail in a claim of negligence or liability, the plaintiff must show that the VHP did not adhere to the appropriate standard of care required for someone of their professional standing and training under the circumstances during which care was rendered (Hodge & Anderson, 2006). This means that the plaintiff must show that the VHP: (a) owed a duty to the injured party, (b) breached the duty by failing to adhere to the requisite standard of care, and (c) caused actual harm to the injured party as a direct consequence of the breach. The last element is called proximate causation and means that *but for* the negligent actions of the VHP, the injury would not have otherwise been incurred (Hodge, Gable, & Cálves, 2005a; *Pratho v. Zapata,* 2005). Duty is met once the provider establishes a relationship with the patient and begins to provide the patient with a healthcare evaluation; this provider–patient relationship may be implied and does not have to be explicitly discussed or agreed upon by the parties to be in effect (Hodge & Anderson, 2006).

The law is not entirely clear on the role the mass casualty emergency plays in the liability determination. Currently it appears that the circumstances of the emergency as a whole play a role in establishing the standard of care for all VHPs, but to what specific level remains unclear, until it is officially addressed under EMTALA (DHHS, 2005). Nonetheless, the standard appears to suggest that in order to save the maximum number of lives possible, it may become necessary to ration scarce medical resources rather than do everything possible to save every human life. Again, this standard directly contravenes the normal medical standard of care for an individual patient and is why the ethical conundrum occurs.

Regarding this civil liability, all VHPs are offered a degree of immunity from liability, circumstance specific. For volunteers who are *government employees, uncompensated* for their VHP role or helping during a declared emergency, immunity from civil liability is broadly available through five sources: volunteer protection statutes; governmental immunity provisions, if the VHP is a government employee or agent; Good Samaritan statutes; emergency statutes; and mutual aid compacts. Immunity merely means an affirmative defense prevents a civil liability claim from proceeding. If these alternatives are not available to the VHP, then the VHP may be protected through indemnification provisions that essentially provide for the payment of damages that are reimbursed by the state or another source, if a civil liability claim against the VHP is successful (Dobbs, 2000).

Sovereign Immunity and Good Samaritan Statutes

Employees or agents of state governments enjoy protection from civil liability pursuant to the government's immunity, which is called sovereign immunity, and is held by all state and federal governments as sovereign entities (Hodge & Anderson, 2006). State governmental immunity is grounded in tradition and is reflected in the Eleventh Amendment to the U.S. Constitution (U.S. Constitutional amend. XI). Here, individuals are prevented from bringing private claims against the state. Although sovereign immunity has been held to be absolute in common law, the passage of tort claims acts, such as the Federal Tort Claims Act, 28 U.S.C. secs. 1346 et seq., has eroded some of its breadth and strength on the federal and state levels (Hodge & Anderson, 2006). The reality of this is that for a VHP to receive sovereign immunity protection, the VHP must be considered an employee or agent of the government.

Regardless and contrary to public belief, sovereign immunity does not afford absolute protection; this has been eroded due to tort claims acts.

In most jurisdictions, tort claims acts provide the exclusive remedy for persons harmed by negligent government employees; therefore, true sovereign governmental immunity really applies only to employees, officers, or agents of the government when and if the acts in question were performed within the scope of their employment (Hodge, Gable, & Cálves, 2005a). It should be noted, however, that the structure and scope of applicability of the tort claims acts vary widely by state; for example, some states generally abolish sovereign immunity entirely, only reserving immunity by specific circumstance (Alaska statute sec. 09.50.250, [2004]; Georgia Code Annotated sec. 50-21-23, 2002). Other states retain sovereign immunity generally and only allow exceptions where civil liability may arise (Colorado Revised Statutes sec. 24-10-106, [2004]; Texas Civil Practice & Remedies Code sec. 101-021, [2005]). In the most extreme circumstance, the state of Washington has completely abolished sovereign immunity (Washington Revised Code Annotated sec. 4.92.090 [West, 2005]).

To confuse matters further, statutory volunteer protections at the federal and state levels also limit VHPs' civil liability when certain criteria are met, predominantly through the federal Volunteer Protection Act of 1997 (VPA of 1997, 111 Stat. 218, as amended, 42 U.S.C. sec. 14503(a), 2000). Here, the statutes provide VHPs with liability immunity for acts performed within their volunteer duties, which do not amount to gross negligence or reckless misconduct, as previously reviewed. Of course, these protections again only extend to volunteers who are not compensated and who are volunteering for a nonprofit organization. If a VHP is receiving compensation for services or working for a for-profit organization, they are not entitled to immunity protections (VPA of 1997, 111 Stat. 218, as amended, 42 U.S.C. sec. 14505, 2000).

Good Samaritan statutes provide another route of protection to VHPs responding to immediate medical emergencies outside of the practitioner's normal practice location. Provisions require the VHP to *volunteer in good faith without compensation* at the scene of an emergency to receive protection from civil liability based in ordinary negligence (Hodge, Gable, & Cálves, 2005a). Additionally, Good Samaritan statutes may apply to volunteer emergency services provided in hospital settings when the practitioner is not on duty and does not charge a fee (*Gordin v. William Beaumont Hospital,* 1989; Veilleur, 2005; *Villamil v. Benages,* 1993). Some Good Samaritan statutes do not apply when services are provided in a hospital on a prearranged basis or if the provider receives compensation for those services regardless of the circumstance (Veilleur). Nonetheless, the intent of the Good Samaritan statutes is to preserve avenues of civil liability against health professionals who have a preexisting duty to provide care by exempting them from liability. However, applicable standards of care and standards of negligence vary widely from state to state (Illinois Compensation Statutes Annotated 49/1-120, 2002; Minnesota Statutes

Annotated sec. 604A.01, 2004; Ohio Revised Code Annotated sec. 2305.23, 2005; Texas Civil Practice & Remedies Code Annotated sec. 74.001(a)).

VHPs are also covered under other federal and state emergency statutes. The difference here is that VHPs who are registered with the state are considered employees of the state for the purpose of tort claim defenses and indemnification, so long as the VHP has not undertaken willful misconduct (Minnesota Statutes Annotated sec. R.12.22, Subd. 2a, 2005). Registering through an advanced registration system is beneficial as well, such as through a DMAT or MRC (Connecticut General Statutes Annotated, 2003). Under federal law provisions, intermittent VHPs are considered employees of the federal government, which entitles them to liability protections under the FTCA (Federal Tort Claims Act, 28 U.S.C. sec. 300hh-11(d)(2), 2003), discussed in the next section.

Corporate Negligence Theory and Liability Protections

Hospitals are also granted liability protection under corporate negligence theory. Relevant to the mass casualty situation, hospitals do not have to ensure the safety of their patients against negligent acts of practitioners (*Decker v. St. Mary's Hospital,* 1993). Rather, they merely must provide a degree of reasonable care as the patient's known condition requires. This means the hospital merely needs to continue to act consistently with its status as a known institution that provides lifesaving medical care.

Hospitals (including clinics and other healthcare organizations involved in emergency response) are found to have four duties to avoid liability claims: to use reasonable care while maintaining safe and adequate facilities and equipment; to select and retain only competent healthcare providers; to oversee all individuals involved in the practice of medicine to patients; and to formulate, adopt, and enforce adequate policies and rules to ensure quality care (*Thompson v. Nason Hospital,* 591 A.2d 703-707, 1991). Based on these duties, a prima facie case of corporate negligence is established by showing that the hospital deviated from the standard of care, the hospital had actual or constructive knowledge of flaws in procedures that caused the injury alleged, and there was a causal link between the conduct and the harm.

However, the ethical and legal conundrum arises in the mass casualty situation even at the hospital institution level, due to the large number of disaster victims that may present. Consider the environment: whether a public health emergency, pandemic, bioterrorism, or terrorism attack, healthcare organizations will likely exceed the ordinary capacity by having to accept and process large numbers of patients quickly and effectively (Hoffman, 2007). Appropriately or not, the institution will also likely deviate from the standard procedures for personnel oversight, treatment protocols, facility management, and other matters. Liability claims against the organization arise in face of deficiencies provided in the care provided by the institution.

Ethically, the problem becomes the need to change treatment approaches to accommodate the best results for the largest number of patients, a dictate that flies in the face of the duty of care aforementioned, for liability protection to attach. Healthcare workers in these institutions during and following a mass casualty incident are placed in the position that the law clearly states should not occur, which is to rethink how medical care is provided to the greatest number, even if the care level of an individual patient must be sacrificed (Gostin, 2002, 2004).

The liability protection attaches merely if the institution acts upon its dictate to prescribe a reasonable level of care, even if it is unable to act consistently with the level of care that a given patient requires, and hence where the ethical conundrum becomes most pronounced. Satisfying the ethical conundrum may prevent a liability claim, but the corresponding actions certainly will not meet the required standards of care necessary to achieve the greatest benefit for the greatest number of individuals. The ANA and Agency for Healthcare Research and Policy are currently considering guidelines addressing altered standards of care in health emergencies, which would account for the extreme circumstances present in mass casualty incidents, thereby reducing the ethical concerns in rendering treatment as well as limiting liability claims against institutions and practitioners within those institutions providing care during mass casualty events (Health Systems Research, 2005).

Vicarious Liability: *Respondeat Superior* and Ostensible Agency Theory

The concept of vicarious liability is usually applied in circumstances where a healthcare practitioner is placed, by his or her education and experience, in a position superior to that of the patient, thereby eliminating the patient's ability to effectively negotiate aspects of care or understand that the practitioner is most likely an independent contractor working within the confines of a medical institution. In the view of surge capacity, utilizing VHPs to increase care levels during emergencies, theories of vicarious civil liability or ostensible agency may arise (Hodge, Gable, & Cálves, 2005a).

When an organization is implicated in liability due to the actions of their employees, the doctrine of *respondeat superior* often enters. *Respondeat superior* means let the superior answer, which simply means that the employer is responsible for the acts of its employees in the course of their employment (*Black's Law Dictionary*, 1990b, p. 1331). A related theory to *respondeat superior* is *vicarious liability*. This states that an organization can be held liable for the tortuous actions of its volunteers who are perceived by patients as being employees of the institution, regardless of whether or not the institution engaged in any negligent activities (Hodge, Gable, & Cálves, 2005a; Hoffman, 2007). Vicarious liability reads exactly as *respondeat superior* in terms of the liability protections afforded, as discussed. However, vicarious liability deviates slightly when plaintiffs seek redress for injuries suffered during care. The courts created the concept of ostensible agency to address the patients' concerns.

Under ostensible agency, the hospital may be liable for the physician's actions when two criteria are met: the patient looks to the hospital rather than the individual physician for care and the hospital holds out the physician as its employee (*Burless v. West Virginia University Hospital Inc.*, 2004). The theory of ostensible agency is particularly applicable in the emergency treatment of mass casualties. When patients enter an emergency room, they seek care; the very nature of the emergent need for care places the hospital in the superior position of knowledge and power in the manner in which the care is provided and rationed, as well as in the evaluation and qualifications of the healthcare practitioners rendering care within their facility (Hodge, Gable & Cálves, 2005a). Patients are in no position to either challenge the practitioners' status or negotiate how or when care is given to them in this environment. Therefore, the patient is certainly not expected to understand the nature of the caregiver's relationship to the institution. In the mass casualty environment, the mere presence of healthcare practitioners working in the emergency room exposes the hospital to vicarious liability as applied through ostensible agency theory, since the institution is essentially holding out the practitioner as its agent-employee (Hodge, Gable, & Cálves, 2005a; *Torrence v. Kusminsky,* 1991). It should be noted that within the mass casualty setting and ostensible agency theory, the healthcare practitioner referred to includes any healthcare practitioner working within the institution with the victims, whether physician, nurse, or other healthcare provider.

Therefore, as stated at the outset, using VHPs within the emergency healthcare environment, either at a hospital emergency room or hospital-sponsored outpost or clinic or other healthcare institutional setting, exposes the institutions to vicarious civil liability exposures (Hodge, Gable, & Cálves, 2005a). Depending on the relationship between the host institution and the VHP and the way the VHP is being utilized, the host institution may be exercising a supervisory role sufficient to expose the institution to vicarious liability for the VHP's actions, which may also be grounded in ostensible agency theory. The ethical concerns arise when one considers the environment in which the VHP is placed during a crisis situation involving massive numbers of casualties.

A Comment on the Federal Tort Claims Act of 1946 and Liability Protection

Personal injuries and wrongful deaths caused by *federal employees* usually fall within the scope of the Federal Tort Claims Act, 28 U.S.C. 1346(b), 60 Stat. 842 (1946) and 28 U.S.C. sec. 2401(b), 2671–2680 (August 2, 2000). The FTCA is a statute enacted by Congress in 1946 permitting private parties to sue the United States in federal court for most torts committed by persons acting on behalf of the United States and applies in circumstances where the United States, if a private person, would be liable to a claimant according to the law of the place where the act or omission occurred (Federal Tort Claims Act, 42 U.S.C. sec. 1346(b) [1946] and Federal Tort Claims Act, 42 U.S.C. sec. 1346(b), 2401(b), 2671–2680 [2000]). This means that the FTCA does not apply to conduct that is uniquely governmental, meaning that it cannot be performed by an individual.

This also means that an individual may sue the United States in federal court for money damages, property loss, personal injury, or death provided that the circumstances under which any of these claims occurred fit within the strict limits of the FTCA. Additionally, the FTCA allows for money damages because of negligent, wrongful acts or omissions by the federal government or an employee of the federal government while acting in the scope of his or her employment (Federal Tort Claims Act, 42 U.S.C. sec. 1346(b), 2401(b), 2671–2680, 2000). However, this discretionary function (extension of liability) does not apply, or does not provide liability to a federal government or its employees, if a statute, regulation, or policy specifically prohibits the course of action taken (*Berkovitz v. United States,* 1988).

The legal issues raised regarding immunity generally, and particularly in regard to the FTCA, are clear based on federal cases that cannot be covered in this text. Ethically, however, the issues are more muddled. In the case of general immunity protections for government employees and VHPs working during disaster situations on a state or federal level, many of the concerns arise in the context of the mass casualty emergency treatment responses and the need to ration healthcare to achieve the best results for the largest number of victim/survivors, potentially resulting in sacrificing care of some patients to achieve the greater benefit with the scarce resources available.

In regard to the FTCA specifically, the ethical conundrum arises where policy decisions versus directives are concerned. Some policies, directives, and procedures that are mandated by federal law raise policy concerns on a societal level. Therefore, the employee or VHP is often faced with having to balance his or her own policy concerns against directives with which the person may not agree; if the VHP complies and follows the procedures or directives, he or she is entitled to immunity protections provided under the FTCA; if the VHP does not follow the procedures and directives, giving into policy concerns by making a conscious choice not to follow them, the VHP loses protections otherwise afforded under the FTCA, opening themselves and the employer or organization to potential liability.

There is no clear answer on ethical versus legal conundrums arising in mass casualty events. However, as stated at the outset, the law shapes ethics and ethics shapes the law such that over time, law and ethics become increasingly consistent through this gradual process (Ogloff & Olley, 1998).

The Emergency Medical Treatment and Active Labor Act in Mass Casualty Incidents

There is one remaining legal protection assigned to healthcare practitioners in a public health emergency context, the EMTALA, 42 U.S.C. sec. 1395dd (1986), and the recently promulgated EMTALA regulation at 68 Fed. Reg. 53221–53264 (September 9, 2003). EMTALA was enacted by Congress in 1986 to prohibit the practice of patient dumping, which involves a hospital's refusal to undertake emergency screening and stabilization services for individual patients who sought emergency room care, usually due to insurance status, inability to pay, or other grounds unrelated to the patient's need for services and the hospital's ability to provide those services.

However, EMTALA has a broader purpose, which is related to the protection of the community and public health (Rosenbaum & Kamoie, 2003). EMTALA further imposes upon all Medicare-participating hospitals a singular, legally enforceable duty of care, entitling all individuals who seek care at hospital emergency departments to an appropriate, nondiscriminatory examination and then to either provide stabilizing treatment or conduct a medically appropriate transfer if an emergency medical condition is identified. The duty to screen is virtually absolute (EMTALA, 68 Fed. Reg. 53221–53264, 2003). EMTALA is held in such high regard by the courts that hospitals and physicians are held to a duty of emergency intervention and rescue even when cases are medically futile (*In the Matter of Baby K*, 1994, Rosenbaum & Kamoie, 2003).

From a liability perspective, EMTALA is controversial. Although EMTALA functions as a condition of Medicare participation, the law creates a duty of care applicable to all persons regardless of health insurance status or Medicare eligibility (EMTALA, Fed. Reg. 53221–53264, 2003; Rosenbaum & Kamoie, 2003). By imposing a duty to undertake care in emergency medical circumstances, EMTALA establishes a provider/patient relationship giving rise to the legal duty of professionally reasonable care, thereby creating potential liability for medical negligence in how emergency medical examinations, stabilizing care, and medical transfers occur, where no such liability may have existed in the absence of the provider/patient relationship (Rosenblatt, Law, & Rosenbaum, 1997).

Despite the liability concerns and costs associated with care rendered under EMTALA's provisions, EMTALA represents Congress' effort to address how best to ensure community-wide access to emergency care through its most potent weapon, Medicare hospital conditions of participation (Rosenbaum & Kamoie, 2003). The law imposes two basic requirements on hospitals with emergency departments and a Medicare provider agreement, and the requirements apply regardless of the Medicare or insurance status of an individual coming to seek care. First, any person arriving at a hospital emergency department and requesting care, or care is requested on the person's behalf, is entitled to an appropriate medical screening exam in a nondiscriminatory manner; whether the proper diagnosis is attained or not (to avoid making EMTALA into a federal medical liability statute) (EMTALA, 42 U.S.C. sec. 1395dd(f), 2000). Second, if the person is found to have an emergency medical condition, the hospital must either provide appropriate stabilization treatment or a medically appropriate transfer that meets certain specified criteria in the statute and regulation must be effected (EMTALA, 42 U.S.C. secs. 1395dd(b)(1), 1395dd(3)(3)(A), 1395dd(c), 2003). Administrative penalties and private causes of action for those aggrieved by EMTALA violations attach when EMTALA provisions are not followed (EMTALA 42 U.S.C. sec. 1395dd(d), 2000).

Consider now the application of EMTALA to a mass casualty event. Emergency rooms will likely become flooded with victims seeking emergency medical care, which means that a hospital may not be able to comply with EMTALA's mandates during a catastrophic event. This raises a serious concern: whether or not a hospital has the legal obligation to treat every one of these disaster victims. Recognizing the community interest in accessing medical care generally, and especially during a mass casualty incident, EMTALA operates as an antidiscrimination statute regarding providing emergency medical care, by preventing hospitals from turning patients away based on ability to pay or on the type of care required (Hodge, Gable, & Cálves, 2005a).

EMTALA protections activate when disaster victims arrive at an emergency room for care; practitioners must determine if presenting patients have emergency medical conditions (via screening) and then, if so, are required to provide stabilizing treatment (EMTALA, 42 U.S.C. secs. 1395dd, 1395dd(e)(1)(A), 2000). Here, emergency medical conditions are defined as acute severe symptoms, including pain, which may result in a threat to the patient's health, serious bodily impairment, or death (EMTALA, 42 U.S.C. sec. 1395dd(e)(1)(A), 2000).

Applying this articulated standard to the mass casualty environment, hospitals are required to provide medical treatment to all patients who present during emergencies under EMTALA, because EMTALA establishes a minimum standard of care for every patient who presents at a hospital's emergency department (Hodge, Gable, & Cálves, 2005a). However, EMTALA is not intended to ensure that every patient receives the correct diagnosis, but ensures that every patient is provided the same level of medical treatment provided to all other patients in the same or similar circumstances (*Kilroy v. Star Valley Medical Center,* 2002). So, in the mass casualty setting, EMTALA has now forced a requirement Congress may not have originally intended, which is the need for hospitals to use VHPs to satisfy their statutorily defined duty to provide every patient with quality emergency care.

Although this may not seem concerning, this presents a very different problem than EMTALA compliance in the individual patient context. EMTALA's mandate is not unlimited; the default position is that EMTALA only requires hospitals to screen and stabilize patients within the capability of their emergency department (EMTALA, 42 U.S.C. 1395dd(a), 2000). Courts have not yet decided whether hospitals must increase surge capacity during an emergency to treat and screen all patients who present for care, and a strict statutory interpretation may not impose a legal duty upon hospitals to recruit additional staff to meet the increasing demand for emergency care during a public health emergency (Hodge, Gable, & Cálves, 2005a). However, if a strict statutory interpretation occurs, hospitals would have to recruit additional VHPs to provide services to meet surge capacity. Additionally, doctrines of corporate negligence and liability would impose a duty upon the hospitals to provide quality medical care to the community, giving rise to a broad interpretation of the hospital's statutory duty to provide emergency care (Hodge, Gable, & Cálves, 2005a; Hoffman, 2007).

This scenario again presents the ethical conundrum for health practitioners during mass casualty events. If a mass casualty event causes a hospital to exceed its capacity to provide the legally required standard of care generally, and EMTALA mandates a quality standard of care for every single individual presenting to the emergency room, the ability to care for any seriously injured individual may be compromised merely by trying to comply with the law to avoid liability, but VHPs are under mandate to behave within the confines of their profession as prescribed by their employer in the emergency situation. Therefore, ethically, a decision of how to conduct oneself professionally according to the standards of one's profession versus the legal demands both of emergency care and stabilization under EMTALA and corporate liability statutes while working within the confines of a hospital emergency department must be made.

The choice is not clear, the decision is not easy, and the legal ramifications are uncertain and yet confusingly obvious. Therefore, although the law and ethics are supposed to merge over time, it is clear that this confluence has not yet occurred in the emergency mass casualty care setting today. Hence, VHPs must be completely settled with the ethical and legal ramifications involved in volunteering during mass casualty disaster incidents to ensure that their legal and ethical positions and ramifications related to deployment are understood prior to leaving to avoid unpleasant surprises during their deployment period of service and upon their return.

This conundrum became very clear to one disaster nurse who responded to the 9/11 terrorist attacks. Being one of only 1600 disaster nurse volunteers with the American Red Cross and with 16 other disasters occurring across the United States at the time, she responded, when asked. She tried to use her paid-time-off to go. When her college, where she was an assistant professor, refused to let her go, she examined her ethical obligations to her country, profession, employer, and students. She returned, 3 weeks later, to find herself fired for abandoning her job. Under Illinois law, since she did not leave her job for discrimination or health reasons, her lawsuit seeking reemployment lost, all the way to the Illinois Appellate Court. To this day, she feels she did the right thing in going, but she has to live with the emotional and financial results of her ethics.

Conclusion

Given the legal uncertainties that apply when nurses volunteer *ad hoc* in a disaster, it is clear that the best way to avoid the legal pitfalls involved in disaster nursing is to become a member of a recognized organized team at the state or federal level. The nurse can then be apprised of the legal rights and benefits available at the time of disaster deployment well ahead of time in order to avoid unpleasant and financially disastrous consequences. As always, the information in this chapter is not meant to replace the fact-specific advice of an attorney experienced in health or employment law. The disaster nurse with further questions regarding these issues is encouraged to seek out competent legal advice as to his or her individual situation.

References

5 Illinois Comp. Statutes 335.3 (West 2005).

20 Illinois Comp. Statutes 3305/16(2005).

Alaska Statute, Alaska Stat. sec. 09.50.250 (2004).

American Nurses Association. (2002a). *Position statement on registered nurses' rights and responsibilities related to work release during a disaster.* Silver Spring, MD: Author.

American Nurses Association. (2002b). *Position statement on work release during a disaster: Guidelines for employers.* Silver Spring, MD: Author.

American Nurses Association. (2008). *Know the law/ethics of disaster response.* Retrieved April 8, 2008, from http://nursingworld.org/MainMenuCategories/HealthcareandPolicy Issues/DPR/The LawEthicsofDisasterResponse.aspx

Bazan, E. B. (2005). Robert T. Stafford Disaster Relief and Emergency Assistance Act: Legal Requirements for Federal and State Roles in Declaration of an Emergency or a Major Disaster, The Declaration Process, *CRS Report for Congress,* Sept. 16, 2005. Retrieved April 5, 2008, from http://cipp.gmu.edu/archive/DisasterDeclarations_Legal.pdf

Berkovitz v. United States, 486 U.S. 531, 108 S.Ct. 1954, 100 L.Ed.2d 531, 56 U.S.L.W. 4549 (1988)

Black's Law Dictionary (6th ed.). (1990a). *Liability, joint and several.* St. Paul, MN: West Publishers.

Black's Law Dictionary (6th ed.). (1990b). *Respondeat superior.* St. Paul, MN: West Publishers.

Brewer, K. (2005). New legislation could smooth the way for the volunteer nurses from across the U.S. to respond to natural and man-made disasters. *Advances for Nurses, 10*(1), 22–24.

Burless v. West Virginia University Hospital, Inc., 601 S.E. 2d 85 (W.Va. 2004).

Centers for Law and the Public's Health. (2008a). *Notice of rights and responsibilities of volunteer health professionals under the registration system.* Baltimore, MD: Author.

Centers for Law and the Public's Health. (2008b). *Uniform emergency volunteer health practitioners act (UEVHPA): An overview.* Baltimore, MD: Author.

Colorado Revised Statutes, Colo. Rev. Stats. Sec. 24-10-106 (2004).

Connecticut General Statutes Annotated, Conn. Gen. Stat. Ann. 28-13 (West 2003).

Couig, M. P., Martinelli, A., & Lavin, R. P. (2005). The National Response Plan: Health and Human Services the lead for emergency support function #8. *Disaster Management & Response, 3*(2), 34–40.

Cushman, J. G., Pachter, H. L., & Beaton, H. L. (2003). Two New York City hospitals' surgical response to the September 11, 2001, terrorist attack in New York City. *Journal of Trauma, 54*(1), 147–154.

Decker v. St. Mary's Hospital, 249 Ill. App. 3d 802 (5th Dist. 1993).

Disaster Relief Act of 1974, Pub L. No. 93-288, May 22, 1974, *as amended,* Robert T. Stafford Disaster Relief and Emergency Assistance Act, 42 U.S.C. 5121 *et seq,* Pub. L. No. 100-707, Nov. 3, 1988, *as amended,* Disaster Mitigation Act of 2000, 42 U.S.C. 5121 *et seq,* Pub. L. No. 106-390, Oct 1, 2006, *as codified,* Requests for Emergency Declarations, 44 C.F.R. 206.35 (10-1-06 Edition). Retrieved April 5, 2008, from http://a247.g.akamaitech.net/7/257/2422/13nov20061500/edocket.access.gpo.gov/cfr_2006/octqtr/pdf/44cfr206.35.pdf

Disaster Relief Act of 1974, Pub L. No. 93-288, May 22, 1974, *as amended,* Robert T. Stafford Disaster Relief and Emergency Assistance Act, 42 U.S.C. 5121 *et seq,* Pub. L. No. 100-707, Nov. 3, 1988, *as amended,* Disaster Mitigation Act of 2000, 42 U.S.C. 5121 *et seq,* Pub. L. No. 106-390, Oct 1, 2006, *as codified,* Requests for Major Disaster Declarations, 44 C.F.R. 206.36 (10-1-06 Edition). Retrieved April 5, 2008, from http://a.247.g.akamaitech.net/7/257/2422/13nov20061500/edocket.access.gpo.gov/cfr_2006/octqtr/pdf/44cfr206.36.pdf

Dobbs, D. B. (2000). *The law of torts* (pp. 269–273). St. Paul, MN: West Group.

Eidenmuller, M. E. (1941). *Franklin Delano Roosevelt Pearl Harbor address to the nation, December 8, 1941* (certified transcript, 2008). Retrieved March 30, 2008, from http://www.americanrhetoric.com/speeches/fdrpearlharbor.htm

Emergency Management Assistance Act, SB0118, 2001, Utah.

Emergency Management Assistance Compact, EMAC Articles of Agreement, Article II, General Implementation. (2007). Retrieved April 5, 2008, from http://www.emacweb.org/?13

Emergency Medical Treatment and Active Labor Act, 42 U.S.C. sec. 1395dd (1986).

Emergency Medical Treatment and Active Labor Act, 42 U.S.C. sec. 1395dd (2000).

Emergency Medical Treatment and Active Labor Act, 68 Fed. Reg. 53221–53264 (Sept. 9, 2003).

Federal Tort Claims Act, U.S. Congress, 28 U.S.C. sec. 1346(b), 60 Stat. 842 (1946).

Federal Tort Claims Act, U.S. Congress, 28 U.S.C. 2401(b), 2671-2680 (2000).

Federal Tort Claims Act, U.S. Congress, 28 U.S.C. sec. 300hh-11(d)(2) (West, 2003).

Friday-Spivey v. Collier, 268 Va. 384, 601 S.E. 2d 591 (2004).

Georgia Code Annotated, GA. Code. Ann. Sec. 50-21-23 (2002).

Gordin v. William Beaumont Hospital, 447 N.W. 2d 793 (Mich. Ct. App. 1989).

Gostin, L. O. (2002). *Public Health Law & Ethics: A Reader, 2,* 41–44.

Gostin, L. O. (2004). Health of the people: The highest law? *Journal of Law, Medicine & Ethics, 32,* 509–510.

Health Systems Research, Inc. (2005). *Altered standards of care in mass casualty events.* Retrieved April 12, 2008, from http://www.ahrq.gov/research/altstand/altstand.pdf

Hodge, J. G., & Anderson, E. (2006). Emergency systems for advanced registration of volunteer healthcare practitioners (ESAR-VHP)—legal and regulatory issues (2005), as reported, May, 2006, 10, 1–180.

Hodge, J. G., Gable, L. A., & Cálves, S. H. (2005a). The legal framework for meeting surge capacity through the use of volunteer health professionals during public health emergencies and other disasters. *Journal of Contemporary Health Law and Policy, 22,* 5–71.

Hodge, J. G., Gable, L. A., & Cálves, S. H. (2005b). Volunteer health professionals and emergencies: Assessing and transforming the legal environment. *Biosecurity & Bioterrorism,* 3(3), 216–223.

Hodge, J. G., Gable, L. A., & Cálves, S. H. (2006). *Centers for Law & the Public's Health, memorandum, Hurricane Katrina response: Legal issues regarding the use of volunteer health personnel in response efforts: Frequently asked questions.* Retrieved April 5, 2008, from http://www.publichealthlaw.net/research/PDF/Katrina%20-%20FAQs.pdf

Hoffman, S. (2007). *Responders' responsibility: Liability and immunity in public health emergencies.* Case Western Reserve University, Case Research Paper Series in Legal Studies, Working Paper 07-29, September 2007. Retrieved, April 13, 2008, from http://www.ssrn.com/abstract=1017277

Illinois Compensation Statutes Annotated, Ill. Comp. Stat. Ann. 49/1-120 (West, 2002).

In the Matter of Baby K, 15 F. 3d. 490 (4th Cir.), *cert. denied,* 513 U.S. 825 (1994).

Keebler v. Winfield Carraway Hospital, 531 So. 2d 841 (Ala. 1988).

Kilroy v. Star Valley Medical Center, 237 F. Supp. 2d 1298 (D. Wyo. 2002).

McCarthy, M., Larkin, M., Greenberg, D. S., Ahmad, K., & Kapp, C. (2001). Special report. *Lancet, 358,* 935–944.

McWilliams, Jr., M. C. & Russell, III, H. E. (1996). Hospital liability for torts of independent contractor physicians. *South Carolina Law Review, 47*, 431.

Medical Reserve Corps. (2008). *Home.* Rockville, MD: Author. Retrieved March 9, 2008, from http://www.medicalreservecorps.gov

Michigan Comp. Laws Annotated. Section 30.411(4) (2004).

Minnesota Statutes Annotated, Minn. Stat. Ann., sec. 604A.01 (West. Supp. 2004).

Minnesota Statutes Annotated, Minn. Stat. Ann., sec. 12.42 (West, 2005).

Minnesota Statutes Annotated, Minn. Stat. Ann., sec. 12.22 Subd. 2a (West 2005)

National Conference of Commissioners on Uniform State Laws. (2006). Uniform Emergency Volunteer Health Practitioners Act *as amended.* Hilton Head, SC: Author. Retrieved March 9, 2008, from http://www.uevhpa.org/DesktopDefault.aspx?tabindex=1&tabid=55

National Conference of Commissioners on Uniform State Laws. (2008a). Emergency Volunteer Health Practitioners Act *as amended.* Hilton Head, SC: Author. Retrieved March 9, 2008, from http://www.nccusl.org/Update/ActSearchResults.aspx

National Conference of Commissioners on Uniform State Laws. (2008b). Summary: Uniform Emergency Volunteer Health Practitioners Act. Hilton Head, SC: Author. Retrieved March 9, 2008, from http://www.nccusl.org/Update.uniformact_summaried/uniformacts-s-uevhpa.asp

Nevius, C. W. (2006, September 2). *State laws become roadblock to medical response in crisis.* San Francisco, p. A2. Retrieved April 3, 2008, from http://www.sfgate.com/cgi-bin/article.cgi?file=c/a/2006/09/02/MNGNEKUD7I1.DTL&type=printable

New Biloxi Hospital, Inc. v. Frazier, 146 So. 2d 882 (Miss. 1962).

New Hampshire Revised Statutes, NH Rev. Stat. sec. 21-P:41 (2002).

New York Public Officers Law Section 17, (1909).

Ogloff, J. R., & Olley, M. C. (1998). Interactions between ethics and the law: Ongoing refinement of ethical standards for psychologists in Canada. *Canadian Psychology* August, 1998. Retrieved April 12, 2008, from http://findarticles.com/p/articles/mi_qa3711/is_199811/ai_n8821122

Ohio Revised Code Annotated, Ohio Rev. Code Ann. Sec. 2305.23 (LexisNexis, 2005).

Olick, R. S. (2001). It's ethical but is it legal? Teaching ethics and law in the medical school curriculum. *Anatomical Record, 265*(1), 5–9.

Peabody, F. W. (1998). Ethics manual (4th ed.). *Annals of Internal Medicine, 128*(7), 576–594.

Pratho v. Zapata, 157 S.W. 3d 832 (Tex. App.-Fort Worth, 2005), pg. 836.

Public Health Security and Bioterrorism Preparedness and Response Act of 2002, 42 U.S.C. 201, 116 Stat. 594, Pub. L. No. 107-188, 107th Cong., June 12, 2002.

Public Health Services Act, 42 U.S.C. sec. 247(d)-7b (2005).

Restatement of Torts 2nd, sec. 299A.

Rosenbaum, S., & Kamoie, B. (2003). Finding a way through the hospital door: The role of EMTALA in public health emergencies. *Journal of Law, Medicine and Ethics, 31,* 590–608.

Rosenblatt, R., Law, S., & Rosenbaum, S. (1997). *Law and the American health care system.* New York: Foundation Press.

Runquist, L. A., & Zybach, J. F. (2007). Volunteer Protection Act of 1997—An imperfect solution. Retrieved April 11, 2008, from http://www.runquist.com/article_vol_protect.htm

Santayana, G. (1905). *Life of reason, reason in common sense.* New York: Scribner's.

Schwarz, T., & Kennedy, M. S. (2003). Critical care extra: Disaster volunteer teams: Where to go when you want help. *American Journal of Nursing, 103*(1), 64AA–64DD.

Texas Civil Practice & Remedies Code Annotated, Tex. Civ. Prac. & Rem. Code Ann. sec. 74.001(a) (2005)

Texas Civil Practice & Remedies Code Annotated, Tex. Civ. Prac. & Rem. Code Ann. sec. 74.151 (2005).

Texas Civil Practice & Remedies Code Annotated, Tex. Civ. Prac. & Rem. Code Ann. sec. 101.021 (2005).

Thompson v. Nason Hospital, 591 A.2d 703, 707 (Pa. 1991).

Torrence v. Kusminsky, 408 S.E. 2d 684 (W. Va. 1991).

Uniform Emergency Volunteer Health Practitioners Act. (2007). Retrieved March 21, 2008, from http://www.law.upenn.edu/bll/archives/ulc/uiehsa/2007act_final.pdf

U.S. Constitutional amendment X.

U.S. Constitutional amendment XI.

U.S. Department of Health and Human Services. (2005). *Altered standards of care in mass casualty events, 2.* Retrieved April 12, 2008, from http://www.ahrq.gov/research/altstand/altstand.pdf

U.S. Department of Health and Human Services. (n.d.). *Assistant secretary for preparedness and response: National nurse response team.* Retrieved April 3, 2008, from http://www.hhs.gov/aspr/opeo/ndms/teams/nnrt.html

Veilleur, D. R. (2005). *Construction and application of "Good Samaritan" statutes,* 68 A.L.R. 4th 294 (2005).

Villamil v. Benages, 628 N.E. 2d 568 (Ill. App. 1993).

Vincier, L. (1998). *Law and medicine ethics: Ethical topics in medicine: Law and medical ethics.* Retrieved April 12, 2008, from http://depts.washington.edu/bioethx/topics/law.html

Virginia Code Annotated, Va.Code Ann. sec. 2.2-3605(D) (2005).

Volunteer Protection Act of 1997, 42 U.S.C. sec. 14501, 111 Stat. 218, Pub. L. No. 105-19, 103rd Cong., (June 18, 1997).

Volunteer Protection Act of 1997, 42 U.S.C. sec. 14503, 111 Stat. 218, 219, *codified as amended,* 42 U.S.C. sec. 14501-14505 (2000).

Washington Revised Code Annotated, Wash. Rev. Code Ann. Sec. 4.92.090 (West, 2005).

Weeks, E. A. (2007). Symposium: Shaping a new direction for law and medicine: An international debate on culture, disaster, biotechnology and public health: Lessons from Katrina: Response, recovery and the public health infrastructure. *DePaul Journal of Health CareLaw, 10,* 251–290.

Yurt, R. W., Bessey, P. Q., Bauer, G. J., Dembicki, R., Laznick, H., Aldenz, N., et al. (2005). A regional burn center's response to a disaster: September 11, 2001 and the days beyond. *Journal of Burn Care Rehabilitation, 26*(2), 117–124.

chapter 11

HAZMAT

Dale Simpson

GOAL

The goal of this chapter is to provide an overview of hazardous materials and their role in hazardous materials disasters.

OBJECTIVES

At the completion of this chapter, the reader will:

1. Examine ways in which HAZMAT disasters can occur.
2. Describe the various types of disaster professionals who respond to HAZMAT incidents.
3. Review the ABCs of a HAZMAT disaster.

Key Terms

- HAZMAT
- First responder
- Time
- Distance
- Shielding
- Topography
- Five senses
- Rule of thumb

Everything Was Fine, But Then . . .

A worker approaches a mixing machine used to prepare raw polyvinyl chloride that will soon become plastic water pipe for someone's new house. The worker has been working on a shift that is longer than his normal shift due to personnel issues and is starting to get tired. This is not a physically taxing job, but his mental focus is not what it was 8 hours ago. Approaching the mixer control panel, he opens a valve that allows two chemicals to enter a sealed chamber. The reaction caused by the two chemicals mixing releases toxic and volatile fumes that must be contained for the first couple of hours of the process. The chamber is made of heavy steel, with several valves to control the flow and amount of the chemicals, and sensors which indicate when levels of chemicals, gases, and other items are met or exceeded.

As the worker monitors the transfer of products, alarms begin to sound and red lights start to flash on the panel. At this point, he focuses more closely on the panels and lights and suddenly realizes valves are open to a mixing machine that is opened for cleaning. The worker runs to the stairs that lead to the floor below where the cleaning is taking place. When he is halfway down the stairs he sees a body laying on the bottom steps and the raw chemicals spilling across the floor. A fellow worker has succumbed to the fumes and has fallen at the steps in an attempt to reach the control room.

The worker turns in an attempt to exit the room and the building, but, before he can, the fumes find an ignition source, and the entire building is leveled by the blast, with fire racing around the complex along with deadly toxic fumes being released into the air. The results of this event take several days and hundreds of response personnel from local, state, and government agencies to bring it under control. The investigation begins after 6 months of waiting for the air in the area where the blast originated to be safe for human entry. The environment is damaged for several years, as plants and crops that were downwind or in the runoff area near this farming community will be affected. A small town's water supply also must be rebuilt.

A housekeeper at a nursing home is cleaning the floors and finds a stain that will not mop up as usual. She calls the nursing home's maintenance man who gets a bottle of floor cleaner, using it according to directions. The stain still will not budge, so he uses the cleaner at full strength. Even then the stain is still there. Remembering his mother's advice for cleaning anything, he applies full strength ammonia to the stain. Immediately a small odd-colored smoke comes from the area of the stain: The ammonia is mixing with the residue of the floor cleaner and the reaction is causing a noxious cloud that is being sucked into a nearby HVAC air intake vent.

The fumes spread throughout the building and older persons with fragile respiratory systems begin to have immediate breathing difficulties, several go into respiratory arrest, and the staff is overwhelmed. Emergency responders arrive to assist and, before long, they and the staff are also having trouble breathing. It is several hours later, and a large response from several emergency agencies examines the disaster before the reason is discovered. The entire nursing home has been evacuated, other nursing homes are trying to absorb the overflow; hospitals in the area are overwhelmed with displaced residents, as well as staff and emergency responders all suffering the effects of the fumes.

Both of the above scenarios are loosely based on actual events. The scenarios are not an exact representation of the actual events that led up to these real-life disasters or the findings of any investigating agency's published reports. They are not meant to be a factual representation of any determined cause for the real-life incidents. However, they are meant to represent disasters that occurred in Illinois, disasters that cost several lives, led to the closing of a chemical plant in a small town that relied on the plant for employment and tax revenues, and put many people in the hospital with life-threatening injuries.

Types of HAZMAT Disasters

The second scenario represents how a miniscule amount of the release of hazardous materials (HAZMAT) can lead to devastating results. These types of disasters are reported every day across the United States and the world. Not every release is recognized as such, and it is believed there are many more releases that are never reported. This may be due to not recognizing this type of incident as a HAZMAT release that may require a concentrated response effort for mitigation, clean up, and recovery, or it may be due to the person or persons who caused the release not wanting to admit they were involved.

There are also releases of HAZMAT that occur during "normal" incidents that responders and professionals mitigate everyday. A problem occurs such as a car accident or the usual "person down with unknown reasons" where a HAZMAT release is either the underlying cause of the incident or, after the initial event, a HAZMAT situation occurs. Sometimes information does not accompany the person who ends up in the back of an ambulance or transport vehicle or the ER for treatment. These responders and clinical personnel find out the patient has been contaminated with a toxic chemical only when they experience burning eyes or respiratory issues.

Another area where professionals need to be aware of their safety and the HAZMAT world is when they come upon an incident while not "on the clock": driving down the street and coming upon a car accident, seeing a person lying alongside the curb while jogging, having dinner in a restaurant and "help me" is being yelled from the kitchen. These may be the most dangerous for professionals for several reasons:

- No information was passed along prior to going hands-on with the event or the patient.
- The professional is out of his or her usual element and comfort zone for treatment.
- The usual supplies and equipment are not readily available.
- No team approach takes place, and the responder is on his or her own.
- The responder is part of the event without even knowing it.

What is "HAZMAT"?

HAZMAT is the term used for hazardous materials. Hazardous materials are of several different types and categories, all of which must be familiar to the professional HAZMAT responder, as well as the disaster nurse who may have to deal with victims contaminated by these materials. By definition, a hazardous material is a substance or material capable of posing an unreasonable risk to a person's health, safety, or property when transported or in commerce (U.S. Department of Transportation Pipeline and Hazardous Materials Safety Administration [PHMSA], n.d.). Additional terms of importance to HAZMAT are hazardous substances and hazardous waste. A hazardous substance is a material listed within Appendix A of the Federal Hazardous Materials Regulations, 49 CFR sec. 172.205 (Jun. 13, 2005), the quantity of which in one package equals or exceeds the reportable quantity (RQ). The material may be in solution or mixture state and the definition excepts petroleum, lubricants, and fuel products (PHMSA, 2008; 49 CFR sec. 172.205 (2005)). Additionally, the term hazardous waste is used to define any material that is subject to the Hazardous Waste Manifest requirements of the Environmental Protection Agency (EPA), as contained in 40 CFR Part 262 (PHMSA, 2008; 49 CFR sec. 172.205, *as amended,* June 13, 2005). Finally, a HAZMAT incident is defined as any actual or potential unplanned release of a hazardous material (Emergency Response Guidebook [EHSO], 2006).

Types of Professional Responders

HAZMAT incidents occur under several different conditions: highway transportation, rail and marine transportation, fixed facilities, pipelines, cryogenic tanks, radioactive materials sites, chemical and biological terrorism, and illegal or clandestine drug laboratories. First responders must be familiar with the special considerations and concerns associated with each type of incident (Environmental, Health, and Safety Online [EHSO], 2006) no matter what the role of the first responder. There are several types of responders: first responders (i.e., firefighters, police, and HAZMAT teams), ambulance personnel, and ER staff. The last two, ambulance and ER staff, usually get involved after some type of control has been taken of the event.

Ambulance

Ambulance personal have a portable "office." They ride around in their office, with access to special communications equipment and telemetry, medical supplies, and a partner, all in a somewhat stable working environment. When an injured person enters the back of the rig secured to the stretcher, ambulance personnel are in control of the situation. Communications are set up with the receiving location, vital signs are taken with the proper equipment, and wounds and immediate health concerns are mitigated using supplies that are in various compartments. Telemetry is sent to the receiving location and the entire team reviews, determines, and agrees on the course of action that is best for the patient based on all the information to date. One member of the ambulance team is responsible for transporting the patient to the receiving location, and there is a limited time before the patient will be handed off to the receiving location.

On top of the "normal" health concerns, HAZMAT issues may play a role in how the patient is cared for, what can and cannot be done in caring for the patient, and how the receiving location will respond when the ambulance arrives. If the ambulance team knows the patient has been exposed to HAZMAT, proper steps can be taken to contain the contamination and protect healthcare and disaster responders from further exposure. If the exposure is not known immediately, the potential for spreading the HAZMAT exists, thus creating many more victims through exposure.

Hospital

Imagine the following scenario:

> You follow routines of completing your day: park in the same spot, begin your shift with a cup of coffee, and receive information from the previous shift. Suddenly, a call comes in of an in-bound patient, information is transferred, and a treatment room and supplies are prepared based on what you are told is about to arrive. The patient is transferred to your care and, based on what healthcare issues the patient presents, proper personnel are either waiting or will arrive to mitigate. Most equipment and supplies you will use are in their usual places and you know where to go and get them or have someone retrieve them for your use. Protocols are followed, operating procedures are followed, and most patients leave your area much better than they were when you first got them.

The above scenario presents a picture of everything working as it should in the hospital ER. It assumes there will be no surprises and that the receiving hospital has all of the proper and complete information on the patient. Hospitals must have adequate plans in place to address HAZMAT incidents that are incorporated into their employee training for attending to contaminated patients since attempting to transport such individuals to another facility constitutes a violation of the Emergency Medical Treatment and Active Labor Act (EMTALA) (Cox & Lee, 2006). This occurrence is most likely to arise in a mass casualty situation when individuals are moved to a healthcare facility of their choice not by ambulance or EMT transport, but by private vehicle. However, hospital preparedness for HAZMAT may not always be the case. Even if the receiving hospital and personnel know that a HAZMAT incident has occurred and a contaminated patient is being brought in, the proper supplies for the type of HAZMAT may not be available and personnel may not be trained on how to care for a patient exposed to a particular HAZMAT. If the patient is not known to be exposed, the potential for an even greater disaster is set up, with contamination spreading throughout the ER as well as the rest of the hospital.

Handling a HAZMAT Disaster

How can ambulance personnel and ER staff respond when a HAZMAT incident occurs when there are thousands of possible hazardous materials? How can all disaster responders be prepared for any and all HAZMAT situations? Often, there is no usual support group, equipment, communications capability, or normal items for any and all possible HAZMAT disasters, and local responders cannot "call in the cavalry" (i.e., higher level disaster response agencies) to help out during the first moments of the incident. With that in mind, all those who may respond to a HAZMAT situation need to be aware of basic steps that are necessary for protecting the patient and responders from almost all HAZMAT. At a minimum, however, there should be an emergency response plan (ERP) in place that provides for how persons exposed to hazardous materials will be decontaminated on site and prepared for transport (Cox & Lee, 2006).

The very first scenario above is a perfect example of an unknown HAZMAT situation and contains some of the indicators that may be a sign there is more going on than the disaster responder may know. These signs can alert the responder that he or she may be in the middle of a very hazardous situation.

> You happen to be driving along the road that borders the chemical plant mentioned above when you see a large amount of yellow smoke coming from a building in the center of the complex. People from inside the plant are running out of the gate and continue running once they get to the street. You notice two of the people have obvious injuries, but continue to run even though you have stopped your car and announced you are a nurse. You hear a high-pressure hissing sound coming from somewhere inside the plant and an odor similar to acetone is in the air. You are the first person with any kind of healthcare knowledge to happen on the scene and it is up to you to do something . . . but what?

While this may seem like a situation that could never happen, it does happen in many different scenarios every day to the average citizen. The healthcare professional has a special responsibility to respond, because of the special knowledge he or she has (see Chapter 10). However, the wrong response is worse than no response at all and knowing what clues exist that may point to a HAZMAT situation could be the difference between life and death for the responders as well as the victims.

In the above scenario, indicators to be aware of include:

- The yellow smoke may not be from a fire. This may be a plume coming from a released product. Look for the direction the plume is taking and proceed opposite that direction. The direction the people are running in may be a good place to go as personnel employed in this environment should have, at the least, awareness-level training concerning the chemicals and substances they work with each day. Usually, they are heading to the upwind side of the plume. Dead birds may be lying on the ground on the plume side of the release, or worse, people may be lying on the ground who were downwind when the plume presented itself.
- People are running out of the plant and continue running once they get to the street. Again, these personnel should have awareness training, and they may be attempting to put as much distance as possible between themselves and the

plant. A good question to ask is: Why? It is a good possibility there is an imminent threat of explosion or additional release about to take place, or a good enough likelihood of it happening that even injured personnel are not stopping for help, even if someone is standing at the trunk of his or her car with a first aid kit ready. Getting as far away as their protocols call for is the only thing they are thinking of at the moment and is something the first responder should consider as well.

- A high pressure hissing sound is coming from the plant. Many of these types of plants have containers designed to hold gases under high pressure. The sound may be coming from a safety vent that is responding to an overpressure situation to prevent a rupture of the tank. Or the sound may be caused by a rupture in one of these tanks beginning to occur. Again a good indicator is people running from the site: Those with awareness of their equipment know the difference between a safety valve and a rupture. If they are running from the area, all people in the area should follow heed.
- The acetone-like smell is a clue. If someone drives a road a lot and this is the first time this smell is coming from the plant and people are running for their lives, then a HAZMAT release probably is happening or has happened. There are already fumes in the immediate atmosphere, as evidenced by the plume and smell, and everyone in the area is in danger. Depending on the chemicals that are present at a HAZMAT event, once released from their containers, the properties of these chemicals will factor into the path they will follow into the outside world.

As can be seen, there are many indicators or clues here that should tell anyone on or near the scene of the HAZMAT incident that more help is needed and the area should be evacuated. Sometimes the first few moments make the difference in the number of victims and the victims' and responders' long-term health and capabilities.

When dealing with a HAZMAT situation, there are always indicators present that a person with awareness-level training can recognize. These indicators are usually present in some form or another, though not always. Being able to recognize these indicators are important to the disaster responder's safety and well being. All personnel who deal with emergency response or patient care in both the field and the clinical setting should seek training in HAZMAT awareness.

There are several things the disaster nurse can do to prepare for dealing with a HAZMAT situation. Just like other training taken that may not always be used on a daily basis, an awareness of what is going on around a disaster scene and with disaster victims, especially in a HAZMAT situation, can greatly affect the person's future health and well-being.

The ABCs of a HAZMAT Response

Most of the principles in managing a HAZMAT incident are similar to those involved in any mass casualty event (Stephens & Gossman, 2005). The first role is to secure the area and ascertain the severity and nature of the threat. A safe scene with clearly delineated primary and secondary perimeters should be secured and, if a downwind area is needed, it should be immediately established.

Second, involving support and ancillary services early in the disaster, along with mutual aid agencies and local emergency preparedness and response teams, is crucial. Emphasis in this stage is placed on determining what protective equipment may be needed, with protecting and decontaminating rescuers and victims immediately following. Third, rescuers should wear appropriate protective equipment before entering the affected area, if the contaminant is known, and before beginning rescue efforts (Stephens & Gossman, 2005). For the on-site disaster nurse responder, the first focus will be on supportive care with aggressive airway control if needed and dealing with decontamination issues associated with simultaneous containment, neutralization, and decontamination handled by ancillary personnel if available. Additionally, disaster victims need to be prioritized for care based on their presentation, severity of injury, and resources available on site. Disaster victims are subsequently decontaminated and transported to a facility that is informed regarding the etiology of the event and patients. Finally, appropriate recordkeeping, incident analysis, and investigations conclude the initial response.

While all of these events are occurring, it is important for the responding disaster nurse to remember his or her own security and safety in the event as well. There are some basic ABCs to remember that will help protect the nurse who happens upon a HAZMAT situation. REMEMBER: These are only the basics and, depending on the material release, these may be adequate, but there is always the chance these will not protect the responder and others.

Time, Distance, and Shielding

Time, distance, and shielding are the three basics to remember in responding to any disaster, but especially to a HAZMAT situation. They are taught when dealing with radiological emergencies and apply to chemical HAZMAT situations as well. The disaster nurse plays an important role in minimizing fear in low-risk patients as well as in colleagues (Waselenko & Goans, 2006) and recognize the lack of threat these low-risk disaster victims present. Disaster nurse responders should be cautious and not allow risk of exposure to any contaminant interfere with rapid triage and removal of trauma victims from the field of injury.

Protection is based on the previously mentioned three points of time, distance, and shielding: First, limit the time of exposure to any HAZMAT. The longer one is exposed, the more time there is for the chemical to penetrate the skin or be ingested in some manner. Second, put as much distance between the material and the responder as possible. The further away one is from any HAZMAT, the weaker the concentration. This is best achieved by placing the disaster nurse responder behind a protective barrier or at a safe distance upwind from the hazard and returning to a safe area when the shift is completed. Last, the responder should shield or protect him-

or herself from coming into contact with the HAZMAT. Even the most lightweight clothing can protect the skin from a powder that has fallen on it and limit the time and amount of exposure. Any contaminated clothing or waste should be placed in secured containers and removed from the immediate work areas (Waselenko & Goans, 2006).

One of the key underlying issues in first response at a HAZMAT site is the location and weather conditions under which the incident occurred. Therefore, understanding weather and topography becomes important. As a disaster nurse responder, priority in this regard should be placed on performing a hazard vulnerability analysis (HVA) (Gum & Hoyle, 2007). This analysis involves defining any potential hazards within the local geographic area (topography) and environmental conditions analysis (weather).

Weather

Disaster victims, first responders, and disaster nurses can all be placed at risk due to the weather conditions while present at the incident in question (Gum & Hoyle, 2007). The concern here is that practical solutions should be available when needed to address weather-related concerns, such as cold weather, and disaster victims requiring decontamination, especially if the decontamination location is not well protected from the elements. For example, if large numbers of disaster victims are being triaged and held for treatment, those who are chronically ill, elderly, or very young will be more susceptible to heat and cold; they need to be protected from extremes in temperature. Similarly, response personnel working outside in hot conditions, especially those wearing personal protective equipment (PPE), are at high risk for heat exhaustion and injury. Areas should be identified to protect them from this condition and to allow for appropriate cooling during and after shifts are completed.

Simply stated, be aware of the weather. Notice the way the wind is blowing, so that all responders can stay uphill and upwind of the HAZMAT. Look for flags, smoke, or vapor plumes, paper blowing on the ground, and other such clues and move towards the upwind side. This is usually the uncontaminated side of the incident. Most, not all but most, vapor releases are lighter than air and go up and with the wind. Stay on the clean side.

Topography

Geography also plays a key role in developing and implementing realistic inclusive plans for treating victims of a HAZMAT incident. Regarding first responders, the Occupational Safety and Health Administration (OSHA) is concerned with appropriately coordinated plans and decision making between medical and non-medical personnel in developing an HVA on-site (Gum & Hoyle, 2007). By identifying appropriate staff, specialized teams, appropriate protective clothing, and other specific equipment and materials suitable to the geographic location of the incident, better protection of disaster victims, disaster nurses, and first responders can be assured. Taking time to observe the landscape can allow for a successful, efficient, collaborative effort with effective communication capabilities that can transcend land hindrances to address possible overwhelming numbers of casualties.

So, heed simple advice: Be aware of the "lay of the land." Some vapors or liquid chemicals have properties that make them heavier than the surrounding air. HAZMAT such as these will flow downhill. To avoid this HAZMAT risk, the response should stay out of low-lying areas, ditches, and gullies. Taking the high ground, though still remaining downwind of the HAZMAT, is how to avoid this problem.

The Five Senses

One of the most important tools the disaster responder has to any HAZMAT situation is the five senses. If one can see, hear, taste, smell, or even feel something on or around the person and it is not something that is usual for the area the responder may be too close or have been exposed already. Although it is important to be aware of how the body responds via the five senses, *do not* intentionally taste or smell containers, liquids, or solids to verify what it is. This may seem like simple advice, but there are instances all the time where some "expert" does this very thing.

The Rule of Thumb

One of the simplest "tools" in the disaster responder's arsenal is the thumb. When near an object or an incident where a HAZMAT may be or has been released, the responder should hold out his or her hand at arm's length and make the thumbs up sign. If any part of the incident can be seen around the outside of the thumb, the responder is too close. This is a basic axiom that is taught to citizen responders to keep them out of harm's way. This may be far enough away, but it can also be too close, depending on what the material is that has been released (FEMA, n.d.).

Being Ready

There is no way to prepare adequately for every situation and every type of HAZMAT release that may occur. Even professional responders have to take steps in order to determine what they are dealing with and what type of personal protective equipment is needed to mitigate the problem. HAZMAT response teams are taught to use a minimum of three available resources to identify the product, what protection is needed, and the mitigation steps to take *before* getting involved in dealing with the HAZMAT incident. The old saying "Don't bring a knife to a gun fight" applies to everyone when dealing with HAZMAT.

The question remains, "If I can't prepare for everything, what am I supposed to do?" The best things that the nurse responding to a disaster can do include:

1. Research the "Big 5" in the community where you live: Find out what five of the main chemicals used in the area are and prepare for them to be released. There may be more than five, and it is good to research all the possibilities, but five is in the midrange "span of control" that one person can handle alone as

applied to any incident command situation. This is also a relatively easy amount of information to absorb. HAZMAT releases do not happen every day. It may be months, years, or never between learning the knowledge necessary to deal with the "Big 5" and using it. By learning the basic responses to the "Big 5" in your area, it will be easier to remember, review, and use the knowledge if the time comes. Check with your local emergency planner, fire department, or the agency that will deal with a HAZMAT incident for help in identifying the "Big 5" and learning what supplies the receiving hospital should keep on hand for a HAZMAT response to a spill.

2. Learn where these "Big 5" reside in your community: Farm chemical supply stores, propane facilities, water treatment plants, and industrial processing centers, all may have some, all, or more than the "Big 5" in one place. Take the time to learn the most common locations of these materials, so that, when you are on the late shift and the "person down, unknown cause" type of call comes in, your knowledge of this address is on hand and beneficial for all concerned.
3. Get a copy of the *Emergency Response Guidebook* (ERG) for your agency library. This is a yellow soft-cover book available to emergency responders through the United States Department of Transportation. Contact your local emergency planner, fire department, or other emergency response agency to find out how to get a copy and ask for instructions on using the information inside the book. It is a simple book to use and is designed for first responders to use during the first 30 minutes of a HAZMAT incident, but it can be confusing, especially when in the midst of a HAZMAT incident and hard to figure out under stress. There are far more technical resources that come into play after this 30-minute threshold that this book does not cover, but it has great information to assist during the early stages.
4. Find out if there are any groups that offer disaster preparation training to citizen volunteers in your community. An example of this is the Community Emergency Response Team (CERT) and Medical Reserve Corps (MRC). These organizations train citizen volunteers to assist first responders during large-scale incidents. Most offer training on HAZMAT response. This program is a part of the Citizen Corps Council developed after the World Trade Center disaster on September 11, 2001, because of the large number of citizens who arrived to help without any organization or disaster training, creating another mini-disaster within the incident of what to do with the volunteers, how to utilize, feed, house, protect, register, and protect these people.

Conclusion

HAZMAT releases happen all around us all the time. When a release contains a sufficient amount of a certain chemical or a reaction of several chemicals that cause a problem for life and the environment, we actually notice and must control, stop, and recover from the release. Being as prepared as possible assists us and those we are trying to help to recover from any damages they may suffer from the release and keeps the responder from becoming a victim.

References

Cox, R. D., & Lee, D. C. (2006). Hazmat. *The Medscape Journal.* Retrieved June 15, 2008, from http://www.emedicine.com/emerg/TOPIC228.HTM

Environment, Health, and Safety Online. (2006). *USFA hazardous materials guide for first responders, glossary terms, and abbreviations: HAZMAT incident.* Retrieved June 15, 2008, from http://www.ehso.com/EmergencyResponseGlossary1.htm

Federal Emergency Management Association. (n.d.) *What to do during a hazardous materials incident.* Retrieved June 15, 2008 from http://www.fema.gov/hazard/hazmat/hz_during.shtm

Federal Hazardous Materials Regulations, 49 C.F.R. 100-185, at sec.172.205 (1999), *as amended,* Amdt. 172-58, 45 FR 34698, May 22, 1980, *as amended,* by Amdt. 172-90, 49 FR 10510, Mar. 20, 194; 49 FR 11184, Mar. 26, 1984; Amdt. 172-248, 61 FR 28675, June 5, 1996; 70 FR 34075, June 13, 2005. Retrieved June 15, 2008, from http://www.hazmat/dot/gov/regs/rules.htm

Gum, R. M., & Hoyle, J. D. (2007). CBRNE—Chemical warfare mass casualty management. *The Medscape Journal.* Retrieved June 15, from http://www.emedicine.com/emerg/TOPICS895.HTM

Stephens, E., & Gossman, W. (2005). EMS and terrorism. *The Medscape Journal.* Retrieved June 15, 2008, from http://www.emedicine.com/emerg/TOPIC712.HTM

U.S. Department of Transportation Pipeline and Hazardous Materials Safety Administration. (n.d.). *Regulations.* Retrieved June 16, 2008, from http://www.phmsa.dot.gov/portal/site/PHMSA/menuitem.34c72e46d5e5364f4148451067c27789/?vgnextoid=a45a764e4da7e010VgnVCM1000008055a8c0RCRD&vgnextchannel=a45a764e4da7e010VgnVCM1000008055a8c0RCRD&vgnextfmt=print

Waselenko, J., & Goans, R. (2006). Terrorism & disaster: What clinicians need to know: Radiation attack. *The Medscape Journal.* Retrieved June 15, 2008, from http://www.medscape.com/viewarticle/540572

chapter 12

Burns: Overview of Etiology, Pathophysiology, and Determining When Referral Is Needed

Deborah A. DeLuca and Deborah S. Adelman

GOAL

The goal of this chapter is to provide the reader with an overview of burns, including their etiology and pathophysiology.

OBJECTIVES

At the completion of this chapter, the reader will:

1. Analyze the epidemiology of burns in the United States.
2. Describe the pathophysiologic processes involved in the burn injury at the dermal and epidermal levels.
3. Assess the level of a burn.
4. Prioritize disaster nursing care of the burn victim.

Key Terms

- Dermis
- Epidermis
- Thermal burn
- Nonthermal burn
- Chemical burn
- Electrical burn
- Radiation burn
- Carbon monoxide poisoning
- Minor or major burn

OBJECTIVES *(continued)*

5. Identify different types of burns.
6. Classify burns as major or minor.
7. Discuss the role of the disaster nurse in triage of the burn patient.
8. List differences between thermal, chemical, electrical, and radiation burns.

Overview of Burn Chapters

Chapters 12, 13, 14, and 15 all focus on understanding the basic epidemiology, pathophysiology, categorization, and treatment options available in disaster burn wound care. In the polytrauma or mass burn casualty setting, the same concepts and principles apply and are used to allow for prehospitalization triage and stabilization of burn victims on site to provide appropriate care and support until the patient can be transported safely to the hospital setting for further evaluation, referral, and treatment if warranted.

When reviewing this section on burns, the natural question to ask is, "Why are there so many chapters dedicated to this topic?" There are three answers: First, burn wound management is a very complex pathology, and understanding the parameters involved is essential to appropriate identification, triage, stabilization, and support of burn wound victims generally. Second, without understanding the parameters of successful burn wound management on a small scale, the task becomes nearly impossible in the face of a mass casualty disaster when hundreds or thousands of burn wound victims must be processed simultaneously and effectively. Third, bombs aimed at civilian populations are the most common weapons employed by terrorists globally. Therefore, clinicians and healthcare practitioners can no longer believe that caring for victims of explosions and bombings is only a remote possibility, but rather they must be ready to respond efficiently and effectively to address the massive burden imposed by sudden mass casualty incidents upon trauma, emergency, and critical care systems.

The Mass Burn Casualty Disaster

Complex and challenging, burn wound management, whether for a single burned victim or multiple victims of a mass casualty burn incident, requires a coordinated and cohesive team response by highly skilled and trained healthcare personnel, many of whom have burn care experience, and often several who do not. Nonetheless, favorable patient outcomes are directly related to decisive actions covering the spectrum of care: from successful initial assessment and stabilization on site from the time of injury; to referral and transport to a burn center or hospital facility; to emergent, acute, and secondary resuscitation phases of care; and to final rehabilitation and long-term care, maintenance, and support. Understanding the concepts, procedures, and processes involved in burn wound care is imperative and integral to the facilitation of the team response to burn wounds, thereby reducing morbidity and mortality statistics, and ensuring maximization of function of the burn victim postinjury.

Applied to the mass burn casualty disaster incident, the very same concepts, procedures, and processes involved in successful burn wound management are used, only on a much larger scale, with the added dimension of limited supplies, equipment, and resources, and possible unavoidable delays in transporting victims to the appropriate burn center, hospital, or other clinic facilities. The mass burn casualty disaster environment therefore forces the same highly trained team of healthcare personnel to assess, stabilize, and maintain the victims on site for as long as 72 hours postinjury in the most extreme cases. This adds an entirely new dimension to the burn wound care processes and procedures and highlights the need for specific management approaches to all phases of burn wound care to ensure maximized patient outcomes for each of the multiple victims.

It is important to note that Chapters 12, 13, 14, and 15 are not intended to be the definitive guide to burn wound care and management of single or multiple numbers of burn-injured individuals. Rather, these chapters provide the minimally accepted guidelines and procedures engaged in burn wound management, as developed by the American Burn Association in conjunction with the American College of Surgeons in the United States, with the understanding that each burn wound injury, whether of a single victim or of multiple victims in the mass casualty burn incident environment, is unique and assessed individually. Therefore, these chapters together capture the basic processes and procedures employed with each victim, from on-site triage through final rehabilitation and long-term care, while allowing for the provision of additional approaches to care as determined by the healthcare team leader, who is usually a highly trained and experienced burn wound surgeon. Finally, Chapter 15 shows the application of all the principles and concepts previously discussed to specific mass casualty burn wound disaster incidents, particularly blast, chemical, and radiation exposures.

Burn Epidemiology

In the United States, a tragic event occurred in 1942 that resulted in 491 deaths from smoke inhalation injury and hospitalization of several hundred more individuals (Saffle, 1993). The event was Boston's infamous Cocoanut Grove Nightclub fire and, because of this disaster, the nation's recognition of both the seriousness of sustaining burn injury and the need for specialized burn centers developed, and advances occurred in the management and treatment of burn injuries (LaBorde, 2004; Saffle, 1993). As of 2006, according to FEMA and the U.S. Fire Administration, 3,245 American civilians lost their lives due to fire, with another 16,400 civilians injured.

Fire has killed more Americans than all natural disasters combined (FEMA, 2007). Additionally, direct property loss from fire is estimated at $11.3 billion, and intentionally set structure fires resulted in property damage of approximately $755 million. In 2007, the number of burn injuries requiring treatment in the United States was estimated at 500,000 annually, including fire-related deaths totaling 4,000, indicating that burn injuries are still one of the most expensive catastrophic injuries that occur annually, resulting in suffering, high consumption of expensive healthcare resources, and work-time losses (American Burn Association [ABA], 2007).

Historically, the United Sates has focused on improving burn care resources since the 1950s. In the 1950s, fewer than 10% of all hospitals nationally specialized in burn injury treatment. Growth in this sector was slow until the 1970s, when congressional involvement accelerated development through the initiation of funding initiatives (Dimick, Potts, Shaw, Story, & Reed, 1985). Within the decade, burn centers were established in every metropolitan city. Additionally, Congress approved funding for the National Burn Injury Program, which was implemented to track the incidence of the nation's burn injuries as well as report morbidity, mortality, and treatment outcomes of burns. By 1977, Feller and Tholen (1980) indicated that at least 160 hospitals in the United States were dedicated to providing burn care, with another 440 needed. The problem, however, was that there were insufficient statistics available on actual burn injuries sustained that could be used to secure additional funding for new burn care centers. Consequently, although improvements in burn care continued on a national level, progress was never quite as robust as in the 1970s.

Fortunately, since the late 1970s, the incidence of burn injuries has been declining steadily. In the period between 1957 and 1961, 2 million burn-related injuries were reported (Brigham & McLoughlin, 1996; LaBorde, 2004). In 2001, comparatively, only 1 million were reported. However, when reviewing the annual reports of burn unit admissions, the figures are misleading, as there is actually an increase in burn center admissions since the American Burn Association (ABA) began surveying burn centers in 1976. This data suggests that the number of overall hospital admissions from burn injuries is shifting to burn centers specializing in burn treatment; this additionally suggests a trend toward more efficient treatment of burns in emergency rooms, increased use of outpatient treatment settings, improved technology, education on burns prevention, and changes in financial strategies for burn treatment. This suggests that survival rates will continue to increase through the use of highly specialized burn centers for patients with extensive burn injuries, despite their high cost and labor-intensive care (Brigham & McLoughlin; FEMA, 1999). This also suggests that the nation needs to be prepared to deal with a changing epidemiological demographic that points to polytrauma of mass casualties who are victims of disasters and terrorist acts.

Epidemiologists link injury to characteristics of the environment, such as recreation, travel, and products used in the work environment. Further, demographics such as age, sex, occupation, and economic and geographic factors are often linked to incidence and severity of an injury, with demographics often cited as greatly affecting particular injury-based death rates (LaBorde, 2004). Extending these concepts to burn epidemiology, it becomes possible to correlate specific factors contributing to burn injuries: humans, burn-prone people, the elderly, children, intentional acts (suicide, abuse, assault, and terrorism), seasonality, urbanization of America, natural disaster, and occupation (Brigham & McLoughlin, 1996). Similarly, by using epidemiology studies as the base for monitoring data trends in burn- and fire-related injury, it becomes possible to establish prevention programs by region, as well as to understand the impact upon the care system that burn types, treatment strategies, and outcomes related to the burn injury make (Saffle, Davis, Williams, & ABA Registry Participation Group, 1995). More important, however, epidemiological studies today point to a weakness in the system: the need for facilities capable of efficiently and effectively handling polytrauma burn victims.

In September 2001, the nation suffered another tragedy: the destruction of the World Trade Center Towers in New York City by terrorists. Although burn trauma was not the primary injury suffered by the victims of this terrorist attack, this terrorist activity in the United States is yet another reminder of the need to have available facilities, resources, and healthcare personnel capable of providing care for multiple-trauma victims with extensive burn injuries caused by massive explosions, chemical exposure, and weapons of mass destruction.

Physiologic Considerations of the Burn Wound

Survival after burn injury depends on two factors: effective wound management and complete wound closure (Klein, Heimbach, & Gibran, 2002). To understand burn management in both the single patient and mass casualty environments, it is important to first understand the biology and physiology of human skin in regard to burn wound pathophysiology. This is because burn wounds involve anatomic, physiologic, and immunologic alterations and endocrine effects which, if sufficiently severe, can result in a total systemic response, but at a minimum create a localized response (Garner & Magee, 2005). Localized responses affect surgical decision making and the understanding of short- and long-term outcomes. Systemic responses can result in multiple system organ dysfunction caused by the cascade of cellular alterations that result (Garner & Magee; Monafo, 1996). Advances in burn management have reduced morbidity and mortality and increased the quality of life for burn survivors. Areas including specialized knowledge, acute injury, effectiveness of infection control, quality of initial resuscitation, and surgical assessment and management are directly affecting short- and long-term outcomes (Sheridan, 2003).

In burn centers, a comprehensive team approach is employed to improve survival rates and rehabilitation outcomes for victims of increasingly more complex burn injuries. These teams are often composed of physicians, surgeons, critical care specialists, nursing care specialists, pharmacists, nutritionists, and physical and occupational therapists (Sheridan, 2003). Because of this advanced team approach, predictors of morbidity and mortality in burn wounds have also changed and no longer merely rely on the traditional indicators of patient age, depth of burn wound, and surface area involvement (Garner & Magee, 2005; Sheridan, 2003).

Understanding Skin and the Multifactorial Localized Response to Burns

A complex physiology is involved in burn injury, and understanding all of the components is integral for appropriate care and treatment of the critically injured patient. Burn wounds are indiscriminate and occur across the lifespan, thereby requiring healthcare personnel to use a wide range of clinical skills and competencies from the critical acute phase through rehabilitation of the burn injury. Understanding burn wounds requires a review of basic skin pathophysiology.

The skin is the largest organ of the human body, comprising a total body surface area (TBSA) of approximately 7,620 cm^2 with varying thickness (Supple, 1994). The thickest skin is found on the back, soles of the feet, and palms of the hands; the thinnest skin is found on the face, particularly on the eyelids. Adults have thicker skin than infants and toddlers; geriatric patients have thin skin due to integumentary changes that commonly occur with aging. The skin serves as the body's envelope.

The Epidermis and Dermis

Skin is a laminar structure and is generally divided into two layers: the epidermis and the dermis. These layers are integrated together by a structure called the basement membrane zone (BMZ) (Garner & Magee, 2005; Gomez & Cancio, 2007; Klein, Heimbach, & Gibran, 2002; Supple, 1994). The epidermis serves primarily as a barrier between the body tissues and the body's external environment and functions to protect the body from infection, fluid evaporation, and ultraviolet light, and maintains thermal regulation (Klein, Heimbach, & Gibran). Additionally, the epidermis provides specialized functions in moisture, communication, and vascularity, while remaining strong and flexible (Garner & Magee). Since the epidermis derives from fetal ectoderm, it is capable of regenerating, and wound repair to the epidermis begins from epidermal cells located at both the perimeter of the wound and the adnexal structures of the epidermis, particularly the sweat glands, sebaceous glands, and hair follicles (Klein, Heimbach, & Gibran). Pure injuries to the epidermis heal without scarring.

The epidermis is subdivided into five layers, which are arranged into *strata,* or five progressively differentiated layers, that all derive from the keratinocyte or principal cell of the epidermis (Gomez & Cancio, 2007; Klein, Heimbach, & Gibran, 2002; Supple, 1994). Progressing from outermost to innermost, the strata of the epidermis are the stratum corneum, stratum lucidum, stratum granulosum, stratum spinosum, and stratum basale. The outermost layer, the stratum corneum, is relatively impermeable and serves as the barrier protecting the underlying tissues and is comprised of keratin fibers surrounded by lipids. The next layers, the stratum lucidum and stratum granulosum, are where epithelial cells die and become keratinized or thickened. The stratum lucidum is most easily identified in the thick-skin areas of the palms of the hands, the back, and soles of the feet. Next is the stratum spinosum, which provides the elasticity for the skin. The innermost layer, the stratum basale, contains epidermal cells capable of mitotic division (Supple, 1994).

The cells other than keratinocytes that are found within the epidermis consist of melanocytes and Langerhans cells (Klein, Heimbach, & Gibran, 2002). Melanocytes are derived from fetal neuroectoderm and produce melanosomes, which become colored or pigmented through the action of an enzyme tyrosinase that results in the formation of melanin. The pigmentation that results serves two primary functions: skin coloration and protection from ultraviolet radiation. Langerhans cells are derived from bone marrow cells and provide the immune function of the skin. The Langerhans cells are capable of recognizing, phagocytizing, processing, and presenting foreign antigens and initiate the process of rejection in skin transplantation through their expression of class II antigens (Gomez & Cancio, 2007; Klein, Heimbach, & Gibran, 2002).

The dermis, or dermal layer, lies below the epidermis and comprises the bulk of the skin (Garner & Magee, 2005; Gomez & Cancio, 2007; Klein, Heimbach, & Gibran, 2002; Supple, 1994). The dermis is composed of two primary sublayers, which contain cellular and acellular components: the papillary dermis, which is the superficial layer, and the reticular dermis, or deeper layer. The structure of the dermis is defined by two particular fibers: collagen fibers, the major structural matrix molecule that constitutes 70% of the skin's dry weight, and elastic fibers, which account for approximately 2% of the skin's dry weight and are responsible for maintaining the skin's integrity. Glycosaminoglycans, or GAGs, serve as the third extracellular component of the dermis and are responsible for regulating intracellular and intercellular functions by binding to, releasing, and neutralizing growth factors and cytokines (Klein, Heimbach, & Gibran, 2002). Generally, if conditions are ideal, the dermis can rejuvenate itself, and it is for this reason that essential burn wound care focuses on salvaging the dermis (Supple, 1994).

The primary cell of the dermis is the fibroblast, which is responsible for the generation and destruction of fibrous and elastic dermal proteins (Klein, Heimbach, & Gibran, 2002). The dermis also contains epidermal appendages: particularly nerve endings, blood vessels, and immunocytes, which are derived from bone marrow stem cells, mast cells, and cells associated with nervous, vascular, and lymphatic tissues (Gomez & Cancio, 2007; Supple, 1994).

The integration of the epidermal and dermal layers is achieved with the BMZ. The BMZ simply is an extracellular matrix that connects the basal cells of the epidermis to the papillary dermis (Gomez & Cancio, 2007). The BMZ structure is identifiable under electron microscopy and appears to be trilaminar in form, consisting of a central lamina densa, or electron-dense region, surrounded by regions of lower electron density. The epidermal–dermal junction is characterized by protrusions of the dermal papillae, or dermal connective tissue, which interdigitate with the rete ridges, or epidermal projections (Gomez & Cancio).

The last functional unit of note in the dermis is the hemidesmosomes, or sites of attachment to the basal lamina through the basal cells of the epidermis. Anchoring fibrils reach from the lamina into the connective tissue of the dermis on the dermal side. The significance of the BMZ is its burn wound healing function that occurs when epithelialized wounds blister until the anchoring structures of the BMZ mature sufficiently to provide protection from shearing (Gomez & Cancio, 2007).

Assessment and Resuscitation Levels

There are two classifications and four mechanisms by which burn injury occurs: thermal, caused by heat from flame, scalding liquid, or thermal contact with other substances; and nonthermal, most commonly involving electrical, chemical, or radiation sources. Correspondingly, the local response to burn is multifaceted (Garner & Magee, 2005; Gomez & Cancio, 2007; Mertens, Jenkins, & Warden, 1997; Sicoutris & Holmes, 2006; Supple, 1994). Generally, in burn wounding, some tissue destruction occurs directly in any of these mechanisms, which results in cell rupture and protein denaturing. Necrosis ensues after injury, which is followed by blood vessel thrombosis in the dermal layer. Stasis often occurs subsequently in the surrounding tissue, which is exacerbated when the patient becomes hypovolemic (Garner & Magee, 2005).

Survival postinjury depends on the integrity of the vapor and bacterial barriers afforded by normal skin, as provided by the epidermal layer, and maintenance of flexibility and skin strength, as afforded by the dermis (Sheridan, 2001). When these functions become impaired by burn injury, durable bonding between these two layers can become compromised, as evidenced by development of specific disease processes, particularly toxic epidermal necrolysis and epidermolysis bullosa. These compromises to the skin occur when substantial areas of the skin are burned, which also accounts for the large volume of electrolyte and fluid loss and increased incidence of infection concomitant with the burn disease process (Sheridan). Improving survival for burn victims involves four key stages: (a) assessment of the acute injury, (b) resuscitation or treatment phase approaches, (c) effectiveness of infection control, and (d) surgical decision making for improved short- and long-term outcomes (Garner & Magee, 2005).

General Trauma Priorities and Triage Approaches

When a person receives a burn injury, whether as a single person injury or as part of a group trauma environment, two assessments must be made: first, determination of the type of burn injury (i.e., thermal or nonthermal) and, second, categorization of the burn as minor or major (Gomez & Cancio, 2007). These two initial assessments taken together provide the guidelines for decision making regarding referral of the patient to a burn center, emergency room, or other care facility for treatment as appropriate. Table 12-1 summarizes the American Burn Association guidelines for the determination of burn center referral (Gomez & Cancio, 2007; DeBoer & O'Connor, 2004).

It should be noted that burn center referral does not necessarily imply burn center admission (Gomez & Cancio, 2007). Rather, referral is made because the nature of the burn and its location is classified as major rather than minor and thus requires evaluation by a physician experienced in burn wound care. Referral and admission are not mutually exclusive. However, in several cases referral leads to admission because the burns are sufficiently severe as to require immediate attention in an emergency department setting with probable admission to a burn-focused intensive care unit (BICU) (ACS, 1999; Gomez & Cancio; DeBoer & O'Connor, 2004). Generally, patients with symptomatic inhalation injury or more than a minor burn should be admitted to a hospital. Similarly, if burns cover more than 5% to 10% of the TBSA or are a result of either chemical or high-voltage electrical injury, the patient should be transferred to a designated burn center after being stabilized (Gomez & Cancio; Sicoutris & Holmes, 2006).

Many burn patients suffer concomitant injuries that are nonthermal in nature. These patients should be assessed initially according to the American College of

TABLE 12-1 SUMMARY OF BURN UNIT REFERRAL CRITERIA, BURNS THAT SHOULD BE REFERRED TO A BURN UNIT

Criteria
1. Partial-thickness burns covering more than 10% TBSA
2. Burns involving the face, hands, feet, genitalia, perineum, or major joints
3. Third-degree burns in any age population
4. Electrical burns and or lightning injury
5. Chemical burns
6. Inhalation injury
7. Burn injury in patients with preexisting medical conditions that could exacerbate management of the patient, prolong recovery, or affect mortality
8. Burns and concomitant trauma such as fractures in which the burn injury poses the greatest risk of morbidity or mortality. In these cases, if the trauma poses the greater risk, patients should be stabilized in a trauma center initially before being transferred to a burn unit. Physician judgment is necessary and should be in concert with the regional medical control plan and triage protocols
9. Burns in children who are in hospitals without qualified personnel or equipment for the specific care of children
10. Burn injury in patients who require special emotional, social, or long-term care and or rehabilitation interventions

Source: Adapted from American College of Surgeons Committee on Trauma [ACS], 1999.

Surgeons Advanced Trauma Life Support (ATLS) algorithm for nonthermal injuries (ACS, 2004; Gomez & Cancio, 2007). Recognition that nonthermal injuries may actually take precedence over thermal-based injuries is important; similarly, if patients present without serious nonthermal injuries evident, decisions should be made to submit these patients for burn center referral (Gomez & Cancio).

Determining Whether a Burn Is Thermal or Nonthermal

In this preliminary process, the goal is merely identification of a wound as being thermal or nonthermal. Once a burn is identified as thermal or nonthermal, actual classification of the burn based on depth of injury and size of involvement becomes intelligible. Properly identifying a burn wound as thermal- or nonthermal-based is essential to appropriate decision making concerning burn unit referral for the victim, as well as securing the healthcare provider on site from harm, and properly securing the victim from further injury prior to transport when warranted.

Identifying a Thermal Burn

The majority of burns seen in burn centers are thermal, accounting for 82% of all burn injury admissions in the period between 1974 and 2002, according to the National Burn Repository. Of these, 45% of the burns were caused by fire or flame, 30% by scalding, and 7% by thermal contact. More disturbing are the statistics affecting children: Of the 82% of thermal burn injuries, 69% were sustained by children, most under the age of 2 years; similarly, 29% of scald injuries and 7% of thermal contact injuries were sustained by children (ABA, 2007; Supple, 1994).

Generally, thermal burns occur when excessive temperature causes damage directly to the entire skin, to the epidermis and dermis, and, in the most severe cases, to the underlying subcutaneous tissues (Klein, Heimbach, & Gibran, 2002). The severity of any thermal or flame-based burn is directly related to the depth and size of the actual injury as well as to the area of the body that is burned (Sicoutris & Holmes, 2006; Supple, 1994). Of these criteria, the overall size of the burn in proportion to the TBSA is the primary predictor of need for specialized care and type and likelihood of complications developing and burn-related mortality (Morgan, Bledsoe, & Barker, 2000; Sicoutris & Holmes).

The Jackson classification further delineates thermal injury into three zones: coagulation, stasis, and hyperemia, which are arranged as concentric volumes of tissue damage. These zones are visualized from the core of the injury outward to the area of least involvement. The centermost area, the zone of coagulation, is characterized by cells that have coagulated or necrotized and is considered the most severely injured volume of tissue (Gomez & Cancio, 2007; Klein, Heimbach, & Gibran, 2002; Sicoutris & Holmes, 2006; Supple, 1994). Tissue debridement in this zone is necessary. The zone of coagulation is surrounded by the zone of stasis, which is characterized by potentially viable tissue but vasoconstriction and ischemia are present, which can cause this area to convert to coagulation should edema, decreased perfusion, or infection develop (Klein, Heimbach, & Gibran; Supple). The outermost zone surrounding the zone of stasis is the zone of hyperemia. The zone of hyperemia is characterized by vasodilation resulting from a release of inflammatory mediators from resident cutaneous cells (Gomez & Cancio; Klein, Heimbach, & Gibran; Sicoutris & Holmes; Supple).

Theoretically, permanent damage occurs in the zone of coagulation, possible viability of tissue occurs in the zone of stasis although ischemia is present, and increased blood flow results in the zone of hyperemia making it the most viable of the three regions owing to the cellular inflammatory response occurring there (Gomez & Cancio, 2007; Klein, Heimbach, & Gibran, 2002; Sicoutris & Holmes, 2006; Supple, 1994). Hence, initial proper determination of the type of burn suffered, appropriate fluid resuscitation, and attentive wound care can result in either spontaneous wound healing, keeping the burn superficial, or increasing the depth and extent of the injury to full-thickness (Gomez & Cancio; Supple).

Identifying a Nonthermal or Special Burn Injury

Nonthermal or special burn injuries are usually caused by chemical, electrical, or radiation exposure. Tar burns are a special subclass of nonthermal injuries as it has both thermal and nonthermal components (DeBoer & O'Connor, 2004). Appropriate identification of the causative element ensures safety of the medical personnel attending to the victim on site as well as defining the decision-making parameters and support needed during transport to the burn center. Recognizing that some injuries could be missed during the initial evaluation is also important since they are not usually immediately visually evident, and therefore can become a source of significant mortality later (Sheridan, 2001).

Identifying a Chemical Burn Injury

Chemical burns usually result from exposure to an acid, an alkali, or an organic compound. Injury severity depends on the degree of chemical exposure, the duration of exposure, the chemical concentration, and type of chemical involved (Gomez & Cancio, 2007; Supple, 1994). Mortality from chemical burns often results from the systemic absorption of the chemical as well as the depth and extent of the injured area (Supple). The problem with chemical burns particularly is that the true depth and extent of the chemical burns may not be immediately apparent, because the chemical absorption often takes several hours to days to manifest as tissue injury. Burn center referral is necessary to minimize the risk of significant damage or death (Gomez & Cancio; DeBoer & O'Connor, 2004; Supple). Interestingly, according to the National Burn Repository statistics, only 3% of burn center admissions are due to chemical burns (ABA, 2007; Supple).

The most common types of chemical exposures resulting in injury are classified as either industrial or household. Industrial chemical burns commonly occur when an individual falls into or is splashed with a caustic chemical, resulting in a severe chemical burn. Household chemical burns may be caused by intentionally or accidentally mishandling cleaning substances, such as drain-opening chemicals (Supple, 1994). In both types of exposures, the injury may or may not be immediately apparent, and thus identification of the causative agent becomes important for further assessment and treatment while on site, during transport to, and at the burn center.

Identifying an Electrical Burn Injury

Electrical injuries most commonly occur when a person becomes exposed to either a high-voltage electrical current, which is defined as contact greater than 1,000 volts, or a low-voltage electrical current, which ranges between 500 volts and 1,000 volts, but can be as low as 110 volts or 220 volts, as is common in a home environment (DeBoer & O'Connor, 2004; Gomez & Cancio, 2007; Supple, 1994). Consequently, burn center referral is warranted not only because of the high degree of internal injury that may result, but because the victim often sustains cervical and spinal injury requiring complete immobilization prior to transport (DeBoer & O'Connor; Gomez & Cancio). Furthermore, burn referral is necessary because, although the initial burns may appear minimally concerning, the real concern develops 3 to 5 days postinjury, when delayed hemorrhage from the labial artery can occur (DeBoer & O'Connor).

High-voltage burns are usually occupational in nature. These electrical burns result either when a lineperson climbs electrical transformers and telephone poles, or when other workers interact with high-voltage lines (Supple, 1994). Low-voltage exposures are usually incurred during normal contact with electrical cords and wires, most commonly by children teething on electrical cords, resulting in a mouth injury, or inserting a metal object into an electrical outlet, resulting in a hand, arm, or body injury (DeBoer & O'Connor, 2004; Supple). Although most of these injuries are usually minor, they can be severe should a flame ignite causing an additional flame burn (Supple).

Normally, skin provides a secure, resistant barrier to electrical exposure, but once electrical current breaks through the skin resistance, the electrical current travels along nerves and through fluids (DeBoer & O'Connor, 2004; Supple, 1994). Since nerves are attached to muscles and organs, severe muscle contraction could result when stimulated by high-voltage current. Such forced contractions often result in either musculoskeletal injury of the spine and support structures or direct severe muscle damage, evidenced by gross myoglobinuria, which requires aggressive fluid resuscitation and possible surgical fasciotomy to release the resultant contractures (Cancio et al., 2005; DeBoer & O'Connor; Gomez & Cancio, 2007). Additional concerns warranting burn referral for electrical exposures come from internal injuries that are not immediately apparent, due to thermal damage to deep tissues that occurs as the electricity moves through the body (Cancio et al.; DeBoer & O'Connor; Gomez & Cancio; Supple, 1994).

Lightning: A Subcategory of Electrical Burn Injury

Recognizing that a low-voltage electrical injury can occur from just 110 volts to 220 volts as found in a home environment, the voltage involved in lightning strikes is almost unfathomable. Lightning has been measured to range between 2,000 to 2 billion volts of energy, usually lethal, yet some victims survive (Cancio et al., 2005; DeBoer & O'Connor, 2004; Gomez & Cancio, 2007; Supple, 1994). Although lightning strike victims are usually identified during or immediately following storm conditions, some strikes occur without warning during clement weather conditions. Others, such as during natural disasters, are found either after the storm conditions pass or as soon as conditions allow and identification and separation of their injury from others during triage is essential to their possible survival.

All victims of lightning strikes must be referred to a burn unit for assessment for at least 24 to 36 hours poststrike, for continuous cardiac observation and monitoring (DeBoer & O'Connor, 2004). Initial identification of lightning strike injuries can be tricky, as a direct or indirect strike may result in little identifiable cutaneous damage. Although rare, presentation of lightning injuries can be devastating due to the high risk of associated trauma, extensive deep tissue and internal organ damage, musculoskeletal damage to the spine, and severe muscle contraction, not dissimilar from any high-voltage electrical injury (DeBoer & O'Connor, 2004; Supple, 1994).

Morbidity in lightning injury is most commonly attributed to cardiac arrest caused by a massive countershock to the myocardium and paralysis of the medullary respiratory center (DeBoer & O'Connor, 2004; Supple, 1994). Victims who do not suffer cardiac arrest usually survive a lightning strike injury, but long-term neurologic, ophthalmologic, and cardiac sequelae are common. Myoglobinuria rarely occurs in lightning strike, unlike in high-voltage electrical injury, due to the fact that the lightning strike is usually of very short contact duration, instead causing a flash over the body with resultant deep entrance and exit wounds, and fewer or no deep muscle contractures (DeBoer & O'Connor).

Identifying Radiation Burns

In the non-mass casualty setting, radiation burns account for only 0.4% of burn center admissions according to National Burn Repository statistics (ABA, 2007; Supple, 1994). Factors used for burn center referral decisions are not well documented, but seem to rely on the degree of radiation exposure, type of radiation, duration of exposure, and number of rads of exposure absorbed (Supple).

Identifying victims of radiation exposure is difficult unless the exposure is known; therefore, knowing the circumstances common to radiation exposure becomes vitally important. Exposure to radiation resulting in possible burn injury may result from air transmission, ingestion, inhalation, or by direct cutaneous contact with a radioactive element or substance (Supple, 1994). Radiation burns may range from minor to deadly, and the burns result subsequent to α-, β- or γ-particles or waves exposure. The most common radiation burn injury sustained occurs from prolonged exposure to solar ultraviolet radiation, which is called "sunburn" (Merck Manual, 2008). Other sources of intense radiation exposure include X-rays or other nonsolar radiation sources (Merck; Supple). Radiation burn wound injuries management is more fully developed in Chapter 15.

Identifying Inhalation Injury with or without Carbon Monoxide Poisoning

Burn center referral is recommended for individuals suffering from inhalation injury (Gomez & Cancio, 2007). According to the National Burn Repository, 10% to 20% of inhalation injury patients are admitted to burn centers (ABA, 2007; Gomez & Cancio). Although inhalation injury most commonly occurs concomitantly with thermal injury, patients exhibiting inhalation injury without cutaneous burns can be difficult to identify initially (Heinback & Waeckerle, 1988). Initial indicators of inhalation injury are evidenced by changes in the character of the voice, intraoral mucosal edema, and/or blisters and singed facial, nasal, or scalp hairs.

Occasionally, sputum that is soot tinged may be observed and may be attended by wheezing, coughing, or associated muscle use, or intraoral soot and ulceration (Garner & Magee, 2005). When large cutaneous burns are present, inhalation injury should be suspected, especially if the victim is at either end of extreme age (child or elderly), has facial burns, or was injured in an enclosed area (Gomez & Cancio, 2007). It cannot be overstated that the severity of inhalation injury is not readily identifiable by outward physical findings alone (Park et al., 2003).

Additionally, concerns that laryngeal edema may develop and progress rapidly support the need for burn referral for these victims. This is particularly important for patients having large cutaneous burn injury without any evidence of inhalation effects (Gomez & Cancio, 2007). Further, early prophylactic endotracheal intubation is recommended to prevent the progress of laryngeal edema. Last, in any suspected case of inhalation injury 100% oxygen support is essential until carboxyhemoglobin levels can be tested and brought under 10% (Gomez & Cancio; Sicoutris & Holmes, 2006; Weaver et al., 2000). This is because, although low levels of CO can be well tolerated, levels greater than 40% are correlated to significant neurologic deficits and or death (Garner & Magee, 2006; Sicoutris & Holmes).

Where inhalation mortality is concerned, respiratory tract involvement is the primary identified cause (Garner & Magee, 2005; Sicoutris & Holmes, 2006; Thompson, Herndon, Traber, & Abston, 1986). Three primary components are identified in inhalation injury that can occur either alone or in combination: carbon monoxide (CO) poisoning, upper airway swelling, and lung injury. When CO injury is suspected, pulse oximetry measurement cannot be relied upon to eliminate the possible existence of dangerous levels of carboxyhemoglobinemia. The only confirmatory evidence of CO poisoning is provided by direct observation of the airway passages through laryngoscopy or bronchoscopy (Garner & Magee; Nguyen, Gilpin, & Meyer, 1996; Sicoutris & Holmes). Table 12-2 presents a summary of the signs of inhalation injury along with signs and symptoms of CO poisoning.

TABLE 12-2 SIGNS OF INHALATION INJURY AND CARBON MONOXIDE POISONING

Condition	Symptomology	
Inhalation injury is evidenced by any of the following:	Burn occurred in a closed space Burn occurred in a motor vehicle Carbonaceous sputum or carbonaceous particles in larynx Change in voice characteristics Singed nasal, facial, or scalp hairs New onset hoarseness not previously present Wheezing, coughing, or associated muscle use Oral or mucosal blistering or edema	
Carbon monoxide poisoning is identified as follows:	**Percentage of CO in Hgb**	**Symptomology**
	0–10%	None
	10–20%	Headache, confusion
	20–40%	Disorientation, nausea, visual changes, and or fatigue
	40–60%	Combativeness, hallucination, shock, and or coma
	> 60%	Death likely more than 50% of the time

Source: Adapted from Garner & Magee, 2005; Gomez & Cancio, 2007; Muller & Herndon, 1994; Sicoutris & Holmes, 2006.

Although this chapter deals with burns, it is important to include some comments on carbon monoxide (CO), a tasteless, colorless, odorless gas produced by incomplete combustion in fuel-burning devices such as gas-powered furnaces in buildings, motor vehicles, and portable generators (King & Bailey, 2008). Possible carbon monoxide poisoning is of concern in a disaster because undetected exposure can be fatal, and most people with CO poisoning ignore or overlook the indicators as not poisoning, but something else such as headache, dizziness, nausea, and/or confusion (CDC, 2001; King & Bailey). Approximately 15,000 ER visits and 500 unintentional deaths in the United States occur annually due to unintentional CO exposure (CDC). These statistics suggest that where inhalation of CO is possible, such as in a disaster with or without actual evidence of burn wound or inhalation injury, possible CO poisoning should be assumed and appropriate precautions with 100% oxygen made available.

Classifying a Burn Wound as Minor or Major

As part of the initial assessment to determine if a patient must be transferred for specialized burn wound care, a wound must be initially classified as minor or major. The reason for this is that major burns generally require specialized care whereas minor wounds can usually be managed on an outpatient basis.

Classifying a Burn Wound as Minor

In looking at the Burn Unit Referral Criteria in Table 12-1, burn injuries of less than 10% TBSA are not considered. This is because wounds involving less than 10% TBSA are considered to be minor and, because these patients do not usually require fluid resuscitation for shock, they can be treated on an outpatient basis. Should a burn patient evidence shock, the burn is not categorized as minor, and serious reassessment is required for a missed nonthermal injury or other concomitant problem. Not all patients categorized with a minor burn injury are candidates for outpatient management owing to specialized support services that may be required, such as dressing changes, range of motion exercises, patient transport to outpatient appointments such as physicians, and occupational or physical therapists (Gomez & Cancio, 2007). Table 12-3 presents an adapted summary of care and management considerations for outpatient burn wounds classified as minor.

TABLE 12-3 OUTPATIENT MANAGEMENT OF MINOR (<10% TBSA) BURN WOUNDS: CONSIDERATIONS

Considerations

1. Check status of tetanus immunization and bring up to date if required.
2. Provide adequate analgesia—for outpatient care a nonsteroidal anti-inflammatory drug is usually adequate; orally administered prescribed narcotics can be used during dressing changes.
3. Clean burn wound with a sterile detergent such as chlorhexidine gluconate.
4. Debride dead skin with moistened sterile gauze or sharp scissors and forceps. Blisters greater than 2 cm diameter should be unroofed.
5. Apply dressings.
6. Reevaluate the patient within 24 hours at a burn center, clinic, or other location where reevaluation of the wound can be achieved to check for progression, possible infection, and patient compliance with instructions.
7. Prepare for untoward events developing such as infection that provide for patient access to additional care.
8. Discuss social and medical concerns for patient support during the care phase and, if necessary, make provisions for patient referral to an appropriate care facility.

Source: Adapted from Gomez & Cancio, 2007; Mertens, Jenkins, & Warden, 1977; Rockwell & Erlich, 1990.

Classifying a Burn Wound as Major

Usually, based on the American Burn Association's criteria for burn center referral (Table 12-1), referral is made either because the anatomic location of the burn requires assessment by an experienced burn practitioner or the burn(s) visually appear(s) to be sufficiently severe to require immediate treatment in an emergency room with subsequent admission to a burn intensive care unit (Gomez & Cancio, 2007). Patients often categorized with major burn wounds are those with inhalation injury, thermal burns comprising more than 10–20% TBSA, or extensive chemical injury or burns from high-voltage electrical exposure (Gomez & Cancio; Sicoutris & Holmes, 2006).

Burn patients with concomitant nonthermal injuries are also included in this category (Gomez & Cancio, 2007). These patients are initially assessed as multiple trauma victims, according to the Advanced Trauma Life Support (ATLS) algorithm (Sheridan, 2001). The ATLS algorithm consists of five assessments for severe trauma injury triage for life-threatening injury and resuscitation, designated A-B-C-D-E, where A represents establishing an airway with cervical spine support, B represents breathing and ventilation, C represents circulation with hematological assessment and support, D represents neurologic evaluation for disability, and E represents exposure and environment in which the injury(ies) occurred (Rockwell & Erlich, 1990).

Of these five assessments, the A-B-C portion (i.e., airway, breathing, and circulation) are the most crucial to gain control of for the patient. Under the ATLS assessment, nonthermal injuries could take precedent over burn wounds; likewise, if the thermal injury is more severe than the nonthermal injury, then referral to a burn center is warranted. Table 12-4 summarizes some guidelines from the ABA on whether

TABLE 12-4 SUMMARY GUIDELINES FOR PATIENT RECOMMENDED REFERRAL BASED ON CATEGORIZATION OF BURN SEVERITY

Major Burn	Moderate Burn	Minor Burn
> 20% TBSA adult > 10% TBSA young, old > 5% full thickness burn 3%+ partial thickness burn Covering > 3% TBSA	10–20% TBSA adult 5–10% TBSA young, old 2–5% full thickness burn 3%+ partial thickness burn covering 3% TBSA	< 10% TBSA adult < 5% TBSA young, old < 2% full-thickness burn
High-voltage, electrical Inhalation injury, known	High-voltage, electrical Inhalation injury, suspected	
Eyes, ears, genitalia, face, or joints-significant injury	Circumferential injury	
Polytrauma nonburn injury, e.g., fracture, head wound	Concomitant preexisting medical condition that could exacerbate infection	Can be treated outpatient
Refer to burn center	Refer to hospital/admission	

Source: Adapted from Morgan, Bledsoe, & Barker, 2000.

a patient can be treated on an outpatient basis or requires inpatient care and support. Burn wound depth is discussed in a later chapter.

In summary, once determination of the type of burn injury sustained and classification of the burn as major or minor occurs, actual burn assessment is conducted on site during triage. This assessment progresses from the prehospital, on-site assessment phase to the three stages of burn injury management essential to give any burn victim the best possible opportunity to return to preburn functional activities.

Conclusion

This chapter has presented the epidemiology, pathology, and assessment of burns. In the next chapter, management of the burn victim will be covered. The chapter will cover the initial assessment to the final outcome.

References

American Burn Association. (2007). *Burn incidence and treatment in the US: 2007 Fact Sheet, National Burn Repository 2006 Dataset Report.* Retrieved March 4, 2008, from www.ameriburn.org/2006NBR.pdf

American College of Surgeons, Committee on Trauma. (1999). Guidelines for the operations of burn units. Resources for optimal care of the injured patient. *American College of Surgeons, 55,* 55–62.

American College of Surgeons, Committee on Trauma. (2004). Advanced trauma life support for doctors (7th ed.). Chicago: Author.

Brigham, P. A., & McLoughlin, E. (1996). Burn incidence and medical care use in the United States: Estimates, trends and data sources. *Journal of Burn Care Rehabilitation, 17*(2), 95–107.

Cancio, L. C., Jiminez-Reyna, J. F., Barillo, D. J., Walker, S. C., McManus, A. T., & Vaughn, G. M. (2005). One hundred ninety-five cases of high-voltage electric injury. *Journal of Burn Care Rehabilitation, 26,* 331–340.

Centers for Disease Control and Prevention. (2001). Unintentional non-fire related carbon monoxide exposures in the United States, 2001–2003. *Morbidity and Mortality Weekly Report, 54*(2), 36–39.

DeBoer, S., & O'Connor, A. (2004). Prehospital and emergency department burn care. *Critical Care Nursing Clinics of North America, 16,* 61–73.

Dimick, A. R., Potts, L. H., Shaw, S. S., Story, K., & Reed, I. M. (1985). Ten-year profile of 1271 burn patients. *Journal of Burn Care Rehabilitation, 6*(4), 341–346.

Federal Emergency Management Agency. (1999). *A profile of fire in the United States: 1989–1998* (12th ed.). Emmitsburg, MD: Author.

Federal Emergency Management Agency. (2007). *QuickStats: The overall fire picture—2006.* Retrieved March 6, 2008, from http://www.usfa/djs/gov/statistics/quickstats

Feller, I., & Tholen, D. (1980). Improvements in burn care, 1965–1979. *Journal of the American Medical Association, 7*(244): 2074–2078.

Garner, W., & Magee, W. (2005). Acute burn injury. *Clinics in Plastic Surgery, 32,* 187–193.

Gomez, R., & Cancio, L. (2007). Management of burn wounds in the Emergency Department. *Emergency Medicine Clinics of North America, 25,* 135–146.

Heinbach, D. M., & Waeckerle, J. F. (1988). Inhalation injury. *American Journal of Emergency Medicine, 17,* 316–320.

King, M., & Bailey, C. (2008). From the Centers for Disease Control and Prevention: Carbon monoxide—related deaths—United States, 1999–2004. *Journal of the American Medical Association, 299*(9), 1011–1012.

Klein, M., Heimbach, D., & Gibran, N. (2002). Trauma and thermal injury: Management of the burn wound: Introduction. *ACS Surgery Online 2002.* Retrieved March 5, 2008, from http://www.medscape.com/viewarticle/535520_print

LaBorde, P. (2004). Burn epidemiology: The patient, the nation, the statistics and the data resources [Electronic version]. *Critical Care Nursing Clinics of North America, 16,* 13–25.

Merck Manual Professional Edition. (2008). *Burns, injuries, poisoning.* Retrieved January 31, 2008, from http://www.merck.com/mmpe/sec21/ch315/ch315a.html

Mertens, D. M., Jenkins, M. E., & Warden, G. D. (1997). Outpatient burn management. *Nursing Clinics of North America, 32,* 343–346.

Monafo, W. W. (1996). Initial management of burns. *New England Journal of Medicine, 335,* 1581–1586.

Morgan, E. D., Bledsoe, S. C., & Barker, J. (2000). Ambulatory management of burns. *American Family Physician, 62,* 2015–2032.

Muller, M., & Herndon, D. (1994). The challenge of burns. *Lancet, 343,* 216–220.

Nguyen, T., Gilpin, D., & Meyer, N. (1996). Current treatment of severely burned patient. *American Surgeon, 14,* 14–25.

Park, M. S, Cancio, L. C., Batchinsky, A. I., McCarthy, M. J., Jordan, B. S., & Brinkley, W. W. (2003). Assessment of the severity of ovine smoke inhalation injury by analysis of CT scans. *Journal of Trauma, 55,* 417–427.

Rockwell, W. B., & Erlich, H. P. (1990). Should burn blister fluid be evacuated? *Journal of Burn Care Rehabilitation, 11,* 93–95.

Saffle, J. R. (1993). The 1942 fire at Boston's Cocoanut Grove nightclub. *American Journal of Surgery, 166*(1), 581–591.

Saffle, J. R., Davis, B., Williams, P., & the American Burn Association Registry Participation Group. (1995). Recent outcomes in the treatment of burn injury in the United States: A report from the American Burn Association Patient Registry. *Journal of Burn Care Rehabilitation, 16*(3), 219–232.

Sheridan, R. (2001). Current problems in surgery: Comprehensive treatment of burns. *Current Problems in Surgery, 38,* 641–756.

Sheridan, R. (2003). Burn care: Results of technical and organizational progress. *Journal of the American Medical Association, 290,* 719–722.

Sicoutris, C., & Holmes, J. (2006). Fire and smoke injuries. *Critical Care Nursing Clinics of North America, 18,* 403–417.

Supple, K. G. (1994). Physiologic response to burn injury. *Critical Care Nursing Clinics of North America, 16,* 119–126.

Thompson, P. B., Herndon, D. N., Traber, D. L., & Abston, S. (1986). Effect on mortality of inhalation injury. *Journal of Trauma, 26,* 163–165.

Weaver, L. K., Howe, S., Hopkins, R., & Chan, K. J. (2000). Carboxyhemoglobin half-life in carbon monoxide poisoned patients treated with 100% at atmospheric pressure. *Chest, 117,* 801–808.

chapter 13

Management of the Burned Trauma Patient: From Initial Assessment to Ultimate Outcome

Deborah A. DeLuca and Deborah S. Adelman

GOAL

The goal of this chapter is to instruct the reader on how to manage a burn disaster victim, from the initial assessment through final outcome.

OBJECTIVES

At the completion of this chapter, the reader will:

1. Evaluate the burn disaster victim based on stage of burn.
2. Assess the burn disaster victims' level of injury.
3. List the ABCs of prehospital burn management.
4. Prioritize nursing care needs in the prehospital environment.
5. Provide stage-appropriate disaster nursing care for the burn victim.
6. Examine the stages of resuscitation involved in the burn injury and nursing care needs at each stage.

Key Terms

- Prehospital assessment
- Classification of burns
- Rule of Nines
- Rule of Hands

Introduction

A complex management problem ensues when a major burn injury presents with concomitant polytrauma. No matter the cause, the reality is that burn injuries with concomitant trauma are directly correlated to whether single or multiple organ systems are involved. Triage of the burn injury polytrauma patient is the goal of disaster response and is determined by which injury is more critical (Beaver, 1990; Dougherty & Waxman, 1996). Therefore, effective triage, referral decision making, timely and accurate diagnosis, and assignment precision for surgical intervention is necessary to effect optimal survival and function of the victim (Dougherty & Waxman).

Optimal management of major burn injury with concomitant polytrauma begins with appropriate initial assessment, support, and treatment as needed on site and continues through transporting the referred patient by ambulance to the burn center. Decisions concerning who should be referred to a burn or specialized trauma center and who should be treated locally have a profound effect on the ultimate patient outcome (Dougherty & Waxman, 1996; Sheridan, 2001). Because most burn victims admitted to burn centers suffer from thermal, nonthermal, and other trauma injuries, the patient presents serious healthcare challenges (Dougherty & Waxman; Rosenkranz & Sheridan, 2002). The goal is to reduce the likelihood of morbidity and mortality. Successful achievement of this goal depends on accomplishing three key processes: (a) determining the proper patient destination (i.e., burn center vs. trauma center, inpatient vs. outpatient care) and coordinating safe, efficient transport to the end destination; (b) performing a thorough primary and secondary survey of the patient on site and at the end destination; and (c) appropriately orchestrating care between multiple healthcare specialist providers and multiple injuries (Rosenkranz & Sheridan; Sheridan, 2001).

The three aforementioned processes are performed in a series of treatment protocols, which occur in four distinct stages, each of which is crucial to the survival of the burn victim. These four stages are stage 1: prehospital phase, with on-site assessment; stage 2: emergent phase, immediate resuscitation, within 0 to 48 hours postinjury; stage 3: acute phase, secondary resuscitation, beginning on day 2 postinjury until near wound closure; and stage 4: final rehabilitative phase, outpatient maintenance and support (DeBoer & O'Connor, 2004; Garner & Magee, 2005; Gomez & Cancio, 2007; Klein, Heimbach & Gibran, 2002; Rosenkranz & Sheridan, 2002; Sheridan, 2001; Supple, 1994). Each of these stages is explained thoroughly for complete understanding of the dynamics involved and the interventions necessary to ensure the best chance for patient survival.

Initial Evaluation of Burns: Stage 1: The Prehospital On-Site Assessment

Once the disaster site is secured, since burn injury often involves trauma resulting from explosion or falls, disaster nurses responding in the field need to understand the mechanism of injury involved, as this information allows for assessment of primary and secondary injuries (DeBoer & O'Connor, 2004; Dougherty & Waxman, 1996). This information is usually gleaned by direct questioning of the victim, witnesses, and any on-scene EMS personnel present (DeBoer & O'Connor). Examples of questions used to determine the mechanism of injury and the presence or absence of potential or concomitant injuries include: Where was the victim found? Was explosion involved? Did the victim jump from any height to avoid fire or smoke? Was the victim assaulted? (DeBoer & O'Connor; Dougherty & Waxman). Other than the obvious need to understand the presence or absence of concomitant trauma with the burn, such questioning provides a beginning timeline for assessing the extent of tissue damage and need for treatment of associated traumatic injuries and airway and fluid resuscitation management (DeBoer & O'Connor). Understanding the injury mechanism also provides a base of comparison to the visible injuries (DeBoer & O'Connor; Dougherty & Waxman).

Initial decisions affecting victim survival and outcome lie with the on-site care and transport team who must triage the victim to the appropriate care facility (Rosenkranz & Sheridan, 2002). Although centers having both level 1 trauma and burn capabilities are preferred for the burn-trauma victim, these facilities are not always available or accessible in the initial acute phases of injury management. Therefore, the default approach is to transport the burn-trauma victim to a trauma center for full trauma evaluation, stabilization, and initial burn resuscitation, if possible (Rosenkranz & Sheridan; Sheridan, 2001). Once the life-threatening traumatic injuries are isolated and stabilized, transfer to a burn center for further management and reconstruction can be arranged.

Prehospital Priorities 1 and 2: Stop the Burn and ABCs

There are four priorities in the prehospital, burn-trauma on-site setting: (a) stop the burning process; (b) address the ABCs of the advanced trauma life support (ATLS) algorithm (i.e., airway, breathing, and circulation); (c) provide analgesia; and (d) cover the wound with dressings (DeBoer & O'Connor, 2004; Dougherty & Waxman, 1996; Rosenkranz & Sheridan, 2002). Once these four priorities are addressed, the victim is ready for transport.

Stopping the burning process is the first priority and relies on appropriate determination of the mechanism of injury and type of burn injury sustained (i.e., thermal or nonthermal) (ACS, 2004; DeBoer & O'Connor, 2004; Dougherty & Waxman, 1996; Sheridan, 2001). The second priority, addressing the ABCs of the ATLS algorithm actually takes priority over care of the actual burn injury (ACS; Brown & Muller, 2004; Dougherty & Waxman; Sheridan). This is important because the most immediate threat to life is asphyxia from airway obstruction, which is usually due to edema, foreign body invasion, or unconsciousness. However, if the burn, especially in thermal burns, is continuing, the disaster responder is also in danger, so stopping the burn may come first. Secondary concerns indicating prioritizing airway stabilization before burn wound care include neurologic injury, circumferential chest burn, circulatory collapse from exsanguinations, and or acute hypovolemia due to the burn or sucking chest wound, and tamponade or tension pneumothorax must be corrected prior to any burn wound care (Dougherty & Waxman, 1996; Rosenkranz & Sheridan, 2002; Sheridan, 2001).

It All Starts with the Letter A

A starts all trauma management in the ABCs of ATLS. Airway control is pursued first to prevent asphyxia and ensure oxygenation levels are adequate (Sheridan, 2001). Securing and maintaining an airway involves specific evaluation of the nasopharynx and oropharynx for indications of inhalation injury. In-line cervical spine stabilization is necessary next. If further injury is imminent or the level of consciousness may interfere with protection of the airway, medical paralysis and intubation are warranted. When probable inhalation injury is suspected, one additional step in airway maintenance is required. Since supraglottal edema rarely presents initially but progresses slowly over 24 to 36 hours postexposure, intubation should be performed to prevent against deleterious outcome in the event surgical intervention is needed, when severe pharyngeal edema may develop. Once an airway is established or maintained, sufficient oxygenation and ventilation must be provided (Dougherty & Waxman, 1996; Rosenkranz & Sheridan, 2002).

B *is for Breathing Support*

The *B* in the ABCs of ATLS refers to breathing support. The goal is oxygenation at the 100% level, administered by mask or endotracheal tube, either at the scene or upon arrival at the triage center, until carboxyhemoglobin levels can be assessed and reduced to under the 10% level (Dougherty & Waxman, 2002; Gomez & Cancio, 2007; Sicoutris & Holmes, 2006; Weaver, Howe, Hopkins & Chan, 2000). Breathing assessment is determined by oxygenation measurement, which looks at O_2 saturation and or gas exchange adequacy evidenced by absence of cyanosis or pallor (Dougherty & Waxman; Weaver et al., 2000). Additional signs of adequate gas exchange are noted by breath sounds and chest wall motion.

For smoke inhalation injuries, blood gas analysis must occur, checking for carboxyhemoglobin, methemoglobin, and oxygen saturation (Dougherty & Waxman, 1996). Pulse oximetry is unable to differentiate between hemoglobin bound to CO and hemoglobin bound to O_2; therefore, pulse oximetry often reveals normal oxygen saturation when profound hypoxia due to CO is present and is often misleading in the presence of carboxyhemoglobinemia. Thus, using pulse oximetry in the acute care setting on site or in transit is misplaced and should be replaced with arterial carboxyhemoglobin assessment. Because patients suffering smoke inhalation or CO poisoning often do not show signs of peripheral cyanosis, 100% oxygen saturation is the mainstay treatment and should be commenced immediately after airway stabilization (Dougherty & Waxman; Ramzy, Barret, & Herndon, 1999).

Deciding to intubate on site depends on EMS protocols and burn victim assessments (DeBoer & O'Connor, 2004). Paramedics usually intubate on site when a victim is either unconscious or in an arrest state. Unconscious victims possessing a gag reflex or patients with severe facial burns who are conscious should be intubated using rapid sequence intubation (RSI). When RSI cannot be performed, 100% oxygen perfusion by face mask should be administered until the airway is secured in the ER or burn center (DeBoer & O'Connor, 2004).

C *Stands for Circulation and Resuscitation*

Once breathing is controlled, the *C* of the ATLS algorithm is employed: circulation and resuscitation. Following trauma, hypotension from hemorrhage and or hypovolemia should be automatically assumed until proven otherwise (Dougherty & Waxman, 1996). Normally, if transport will take less than 1 hour, venous access for fluid administration is not required. However, where transport may be delayed for several hours, obtaining venous access should be pursued (Ramzy, Barrett, & Herndon, 1999; Sheridan, 2001). Fluid administration is usually aimed to begin within the first 24 to 48 hours postinjury, when the possible development of hypovolemia remains greatest. Knowing that total body water remains constant despite massive shifts between fluid compartments, with intracellular and interstitial volumes increasing at the expense of intravascular volume, is key to understanding the process of fluid resuscitation (Sicoutris & Holmes, 2006).

Assuming on-site resuscitation is required, fluid requirements for the thermal trauma are usually set by the parameters of the initial injury, particularly the surface area and depth of burn and the absence or presence of inhalation injury. However, as a rule, the Brooke (2 mL/kg/dL with albumin) and Parkland (4 mL/kg/dL with no albumin) protocols are used to estimate the patient's initial 24-hour fluid consumption based on the percentage of body surface area affected by second- and third-degree burns, in conjunction with the patient's weight (Dougherty & Waxman, 1996).

Considering any resuscitation formula employed as a general resuscitation guideline to prevent or resuscitate burn shock is essential (Sicoutris & Holmes, 2006). Most practitioners use 2 to 3 liters of warmed lactated Ringer's solution (crystalloid) for resuscitation as the initial diagnostic and therapeutic maneuver in a field situation with a hypovolemic trauma victim while isolation and identification of the cause of hypovolemia is ascertained. The fluids are infused according to the Parkland protocol (Dougherty & Waxman, 1996; Garner & Magee, 2005; Ramzy, Barret, & Herndon, 1999). Normal saline is avoided since the volume required for resuscitation often leads to developing a complicating hyperchloremic metabolic acidosis (Ramzy, Barret, & Herndon; Sicoutris & Holmes).

Colloid infusion under the Brooke protocol is usually reserved for the second 24-hour postinjury period. However, in massive burn injuries, burns complicated by inhalation injury, or young children, a combination of crystalloid lactated Ringer's and colloid using the Brooke protocol can be used to minimize the formation of edema while achieving the desired goal of end-organ perfusion (Ramzy, Barret, &

Herndon, 1999; Sicoutris & Holmes, 2006). Failure to respond to on-site fluid resuscitation indicates either hemorrhage or ongoing massive fluid loss (Dougherty & Waxman, 1996). In this case, an infusion of type O blood may be required until the victim can be relocated to an ICU for continued critical evaluation, management of failing organ systems, and nutritional support (Dougherty & Waxman; Garner & Magee, 2005).

Successful resuscitation is achieved when predetermined end points have been met, no further edema results, and the infused fluid volume required to maintain adequate urine output approximates the victim's maintenance fluid volume (Sicoutris & Holmes, 2006). The maintenance fluid volume is calculated as the normal maintenance volume plus evaporative water loss. For adults suffering major thermal injury, required urine output ranging between 1000–1500 mL/24 hours is required; in pediatric patients, a required urine output of 3 mL/kg/h to 4 mL/kg/h is expected (Garner & Magee, 2005; Sicoutris & Holmes). In victims having less than 50% total body surface area (TBSA) involvement, two large-bore intravenous catheters inserted percutaneously should be used to facilitate fluid resuscitation (Dougherty & Waxman, 1996; Garner & Magee; Sicoutris & Holmes). Upper extremity insertion is preferable, even if the lines must pass through eschar or burned skin (Garner & Magee; Sicoutris & Holmes). If the only veins available are those within the burn area, they should be used. Additionally, venous cutdown, if needed, should be placed as far distal on the extremity as possible to allow for line changes to occur more proximally on the same vein (Dougherty & Waxman; Garner & Magee). For patients with more than 50% TBSA involvement, central venous access should be additionally established with invasive hemodynamic monitoring (Sicoutris & Holmes). If peripheral venous access is impossible in an adult, the femoral site should be used first, followed by the subclavian vein, and the internal jugular veins last (Dougherty & Waxman). Additionally, a Foley catheter should be inserted to monitor hourly urine output (Sicoutris & Holmes, 2006).

Once successful resuscitation is achieved, monitor intravascular volume status using cardiac efficiency parameters, laboratory measurements of lactate and base deficit (if such are available), skin temperature and color, and hemodynamics and mentation status. Again, transporting the victim to an appropriate burn unit or ICU is needed for continued fluid maintenance and assessment (Dougherty & Waxman, 1996; Garner & Magee, 2005; Ramzy, Barret, & Herndon, 1999; Sicoutris & Holmes, 2006).

As mentioned previously, the prehospital, on-site burn victim evaluation requires understanding the concepts of burn depth, burn size or TBSA measurement, and burn classification, as mastery of these concepts significantly facilitates the fluid resuscitation effort (Garner & Magee, 2005; Ramzy, Barret, & Herndon, 1999; Sicoutris & Holmes, 2006). Further, subsequent nutritional requirements are related directly to burn size (Klein, Heimbach, & Gibran, 2002; Sicoutris & Holmes).

Understanding Burn Size, Burn Depth, and Burn Wound Classification

When a burn wound exceeds 20% TBSA, which is classified as a major burn, the ensuing systemic response is extensive and is stimulated by tissue cellular mediators and loss of the physical barrier (Garner & Magee, 2005). Qualification and quantification of burn wounds aids resuscitation efforts. Therefore, by recording essential burn wound information such as surface area involvement, depth of penetration, and location of the wound(s), calculations used in resuscitation will be more accurate and likely to aid survival (Garner & Magee; Gomez & Cancio, 2007; Ramzy, Barret, & Herndon, 1999; Sicoutris & Holmes, 2006; Supple, 1994).

There are three ways to record an estimation of TBSA involvement. One of the simplest is either the Lund-Browder or Berkow charts or the Rule of Hands. The Lund-Browder or Berkow charts correlate the percentage of TBSA of different areas of the body as a function of developmental age (Garner & Magee, 2005; Gomez & Cancio, 2007; Rossiter, Chapman & Haywood, 1996; Sicoutris & Holmes, 2006). The Rule of Hands, a less accurate measure, assumes that a normal person's hand, particularly the palm and fingers, equates to approximately 1% of TBSA (Gomez & Cancio; DeBoer & O'Connor, 2004; Rossiter, Chapman & Haywood; Sicoutris & Holmes). Recent studies show that the palm, excluding the fingers, comprises only 0.4% to 0.5% TBSA; when the fingers are included, the TBSA estimates increase, ranging from 0.7% to 0.8% TBSA, which is rounded to the simpler 1% rule (DeBoer & O'Connor; Morgan, Bledsoe & Barker, 2000; Rossiter, Chapman & Haywood).

Because careful estimation of TBSA is important to the early management of burn victims, overestimation or underestimation can be devastating. Therefore, the third and probably best known and accepted tool for quantification of burn size on the body is the Rule of Nines (Brown & Muller, 2004; Garner & Magee, 2005; Gomez & Cancio, 2007; Sicoutris & Holmes, 2006). The Rule of Nines is a division of the human body into regions: the arms, hands, neck, legs, anterior trunk, posterior trunk, and genitalia. The regions are assigned a percentage value that is a multiple of 9, indicating that each regionalized area of the body constitutes 9% of the body's total surface area.

It should be noted that children have a disproportionately larger head than the body, and this anatomical variant directly affects calculating burn wound percentages (DeBoer & O'Connor, 2004; Sicoutris & Holmes, 2006). Therefore, in this adjustment model, the head and neck comprise 18% TBSA in a child versus the 9% TBSA allocated to an adult. To prevent against possible overestimation where children are concerned, the Lund-Browder chart provides a possibly more accurate assessment of TBSA involvement for children (DeBoer & O'Connor; Garner & Magee, 2005; Sicoutris & Holmes; Supple, 1994).

Finally, a simple comparison allows visualization of the Rule of Nines estimate and the Rule of Hands estimate: generally, the whole hand may be used to assess small burns; the Rule of Nines is used to estimate extensive burns (DeBoer & O'Connor, 2004). A burn to an entire arm approximates 9% TBSA; likewise, a burn to the elbow only is approximately the same size as an adult's palm and fingers or only 1% TBSA. This example illustrates how easily over- or underestimation of a burn wound can occur due to the generalization by percentage of the anatomy used for the corresponding estimations. Once the percentage of TBSA involved is estimated, the burn depth must be determined, as burn depth and burn size, taken together, is a primary predictor of a victim's long-term appearance and functional outcome, as well as of mortality (Sicoutris & Holmes, 2006).

Several factors affect the depth of any burn wound. Burn depth injury depends on duration of exposure, skin thickness, temperature, heat capacity of the causative agent, location of the wound, heat dissipation potential of the skin due to blood flow, and initial treatment rendered (Gomez & Cancio, 2007; Sicoutris & Holmes, 2006; Supple, 1994). Age of the victim is also important (Supple): Children under age 2 years who are exposed to 130°F water will sustain a burn in 10 seconds; an adult exposed to the same water requires 30 seconds to sustain the same burn. Similarly, only 5 seconds is needed to burn a child in 140° F water (Gomez & Cancio). Since age and skin thickness are related, age can predict the depth and severity of a burn wound. This corollary holds true in reverse as well; as age increases, starting at 50 years, skin loses its elasticity, thickness, and suppleness and becomes atrophic. The aging process causes the characteristic fragile, translucent skin often seen in the elderly to develop, which increases their risk for a deeper, or full-thickness burn (Gomez & Cancio; Supple).

Skin thickness varies across the body, in both adults and children. Because of this, burn wound location becomes an important predictor to the depth and severity of the wound sustained (Gomez & Cancio, 2007; Sicoutris & Holmes, 2006; Supple, 1994). Mechanism of injury and duration of exposure of the causative substance to the skin also serves as predictors of burn depth (Sicoutris & Holmes; Supple). Duration of exposure is related to the type of substance causing the burn wound. For example, gasoline flames burn at very high temperature; although exposure is short, the heat is intense causing a deep, severe wound (Gomez & Cancio). Similarly, cooking grease spilled or splattered on skin will continue to keep heat in the skin because grease bonds easily to the skin's cellular lipid bilayer. Duration of exposure is also affected by the treatment rendered initially; agents applied to soothe a wound that are greasy in nature, such as an antibiotic ointment or butter, should never be applied, because they will hold heat in the skin, whereas a cooling water-based gel reduces skin temperature (Supple).

Although burn depth as a predictor of burn wound severity is important, its real function is as a determinant for wound healing. Unfortunately, determining the depth of burns during on-site initial assessment may prove challenging for the most experienced burn specialists, because burns may appear to be of one type initially, but may be of another depending on the mechanism of burn injury

(DeBoer & O'Connor, 2004; Garner & Magee, 2005; Morgan, Bledsoe, & Barker, 2000). Therefore, knowing as much information as possible about how the burn occurred can assist the disaster nurse with proper burn wound identification. Additionally, burn depth estimations should be reviewed and revised as needed in the first 24 to 72 hours postinjury, and frequently during the ensuing 2 to 3 weeks (Morgan, Bledsoe, & Barker).

Burns are classified generally as first, second, third, fourth, and fifth degree (DeBoer & O'Connor, 2004; Garner & Magee, 2005; Gomez & Cancio, 2007; Merck, 2008; Morgan, Bledsoe, & Barker, 2000; Supple, 1994). More recently, depth of burn is referred to either as a partial-thickness or full-thickness burn, which relates to the increasing depth of epidermal damage (DeBoer & O'Connor; Merck, 2008; Klein, Heimbach, & Gibran, 2002; Morgan, Bledsoe, & Barker; Sicoutris & Holmes, 2006). The result is a four-part grading system: first-degree burns are epidermal burns; second-degree burns are either superficial or deep partial-thickness burns; third-degree burns are full-thickness burns; fourth-degree burns are deep full-thickness burns and usually categorized as extending to the muscle, although some disagreement exists about just how deep this particular burn extends (DeBoer & O'Connor; Sicoutris & Holmes). Fifth-degree burns are those burns that reach the muscle and bone, though not all sources further classify fourth-degree burns into fifth-degree burns. Some sources do subdivide fourth-degree burns not only into fifth, but also into sixth degree. For the purposes of this chapter, all fourth-, fifth-, and sixth-degree burns should be considered under caring for fourth-degree burns (Walker & Morgan, LLC, 2007). Most burns have a mixture of clinical characteristics, which serves to complicate the classification process, making designating the burn as one type difficult (Sicoutris & Holmes).

First-degree or epidermal burns are often called superficial. These burns are caused by brief heat exposure, flash burns of very short duration, solar energy (i.e., sunburn), or ultraviolet radiation (e.g., tanning beds) (DeBoer & O'Connor, 2004; Gomez & Cancio, 2007; Morgan, Bledsoe, & Barker, 2000; Sicoutris & Holmes, 2006). Superficial burns remain confined to the epidermis, and the epidermis remains intact. Such burns are often dry to the touch, erythematous, and hypersensitive (DeBoer & O'Connor; Garner & Magee, 2005; Gomez & Cancio; Sicoutris & Holmes). Patient care for first-degree burns involves cooling the area with moist towels, providing mild analgesia and mild fluid resuscitation, usually administered orally, and applying a topical antimicrobial (DeBoer & O'Connor, 2004; Garner & Magee). Applying a topical moisturizer containing aloe vera may provide cooling comfort as well as increase the reepithelialization rate (Klein, Heimbach, & Gibran, 2002). First-degree or superficial burns are not included in burn size estimations for fluid resuscitation, a fact which is often legally significant in litigation. Excepting first-degree burn wounds, from this point forward, the following rule applies: The deeper the dermal injury, the greater the challenge to the healing process (Garner & Magee).

There are two types of second-degree or partial-thickness burns, both of which are characterized by extending into the dermal layer: superficial partial thickness and deep partial thickness (DeBoer & O'Connor, 2004; Garner & Magee, 2005; Gomez & Cancio, 2007; Klein, Heimbach, & Gibran, 2002; Merck, 2008; Morgan, Bledsoe & Barker, 2000). In both of these burns, the epidermal layer is completely destroyed, and the burn extends into the layers of the dermis, creating partial dermal loss (Garner & Magee). The degree of dermal destruction differentiates superficial partial-thickness burns from deep partial-thickness burns.

Partial-thickness burns are categorized as second degree, superficial partial thickness, when they involve only the superficial layer of the dermis, without extending into the reticular layers (DeBoer & O'Connor, 2004; Klein, Heimbach, & Gibran, 2002; Merck, 2008; Sicoutris & Holmes, 2006). Fluid-filled blisters are the hallmark of superficial partial-thickness burns. Blistering is usually seen either on initial presentation or several hours later and is accompanied by severe pain. Breaking the blister, which can occur naturally or by intentional removal, reveals moist, pink, wet, and painful skin, which blanches under pressure (DeBoer & O'Connor; Sicoutris & Holmes). Treatment is focused on preventing wound progression.

Deep partial-thickness burns extend through the epidermis into the dermal reticular layers (Garner & Magee, 2005; Klein, Heimbach, & Gibran, 2002; Merck, 2008; Sicoutris & Holmes, 2006). Similar to superficial partial-thickness burn wounds, these deep partial-thickness wounds are dry to the touch yet also blister, but here the wound surface is uneven in color, often taking on a mottled pink-white appearance (Gomez & Cancio, 2007; Klein, Heimbach, & Gibran; Sicoutris & Holmes). Because nerve injury is usually present and capillary refill is slow to absent, the wound is usually less sensitive and the victim will usually express discomfort rather than pain, one of the key differences between a deep partial-thickness burn and a superficial partial-thickness burn (Sicoutris & Holmes).

The next level of burn wound is called full thickness. All full-thickness burns extend through the dermis into the subcutaneous layers of skin located below the dermis (DeBoer & O'Connor, 2004; Garner & Magee, 2005; Gomez & Cancio, 2007; Klein, Heimbach, & Gibran, 2002; Merck, 2008; Morgan, Bledsoe, & Barker, 2000; Sicoutris & Holmes, 2006). There are three types of full-thickness burn wounds: third-degree full-thickness, fourth-degree full-thickness, and fifth-degree full-thickness. Full-thickness (third-degree) wounds are those that affect only the subcutaneous fat layer located under the dermis. Third-degree full-thickness burns are characterized by their coloration: they are usually pale white, cherry red, or charred brown or black; blistering may or may not be present. When touched, full-thickness burns feel firm, leathery, and depressed or contracted (DeBoer & O'Connor; Garner & Magee; Klein, Heimbach & Gibran; Sicoutris & Holmes).

Fourth-degree full-thickness wounds are differentiated from third-degree full-thickness wounds because these burns extend into the muscle layer, extending through all the skin layers, from the epidermis through the dermis into the subcutaneous layer and muscle (DeBoer & O'Connor, 2004; Sicoutris & Holmes, 2006). Charring is always present, giving the wound a brown or black appearance although some pink or red areas may also be apparent; the wound is characterized as dry and insensate. Coagulated blood vessels may also be observed (Sicoutris & Holmes). Fourth-degree burns, due to their severity, usually occur from substantial exposure to the material that has caused the burn. The difference between the fourth- and fifth-degree wounding depends on the depth of the wound. Most references categorize fourth- and fifth-degree burns as one and the same (DeBoer & O'Connor, 2004; Garner & Magee, 2005; Gomez & Cancio, 2007; Klein, Heimbach, & Gibran, 2002; Merck, 2008; Morgan, Bledsoe, & Barker, 2000). When separation is made between fourth- and fifth-degree wounds, the fourth-degree wound is defined as extending through to the muscle layer, whereas the fifth-degree wound extends through the muscle layer to the bone. All other wound characteristics common to fourth-degree full-thickness burns apply to the fifth-degree designation (Supple, 1994).

Once the ABCs of ATLS algorithm have been met, the next goal of prehospital, on-site burn wound care is pain management until the victim can be released for outpatient care or transported to the hospital or burn center for more intensive acute assessment and care. The next section addresses this issue.

Prehospital Priority 3: Pain Management

Excepting the simplest superficial burns, in the initial phases of burn care, pain medications are administered intravenously (DeBoer & O'Connor, 2004; Sicoutris & Holmes, 2006). Due to the intense pain caused by burns, higher than normal dosages of analgesia are necessary: In the acute stage of burn care, pain is best managed with intravenous doses of an opiate, usually either morphine or fentanyl, until analgesia is adequate, while not inducing hypotension (DeBoer & O'Connor; Merck, 2008; Sicoutris & Holmes). If expeditious transport is not immediately possible and more severe burn is involved, the disaster nurse should follow the guidance of medical staff at the identified receiving hospital or burn center regarding analgesia management on site (DeBoer & O'Connor).

It should be noted that, the deeper the burn, the less the pain, since nerve endings are often destroyed in these burns. However, almost all burns have varying levels of burns with the deepest in the center, progressing outwards to the burn's edges, which are often first- or second-degree burns. As anyone who has ever had a sunburn can attest, the more superficial the burn, the more painful the burn tends to be.

For minor superficial burn wounds, applying topical anesthetics or administering oral medications, such as acetaminophen or ibuprofen, can provide adequate pain relief (DeBoer & O'Connor, 2004; Merck, 2008). When topically applied anesthetic is appropriate, care must be taken, particularly in children with larger body surface area involvement, so that absorption of the anesthetic through the wound surface does not induce seizures (DeBoer & O'Connor). Once pain management is addressed on site, the last priority in the prehospital management of a burn wound is dressing application prior to transport.

Prehospital Priority 4: Applying Dressings for Transport or Release

Once all of the initial assessments have been made and completed, attention to the burn wound itself is necessary. Few studies have been conducted to allow any dogmatic recommendations to be proffered. However, covering burn wounds serves several purposes: anesthetic relief, infection barrier, fluid absorption, and drying (Sheridan, 2001). Dressing decisions are made based on the location and depth of the burn.

First, superficial wounds generally are not covered (Merck, 2008). After gently cleaning and drying the burned area(s), a simple skin lubricant or moisturizer, usually containing aloe vera, is sufficient, and no further treatment is medically necessitated unless blistering develops (Morgan, Bledsoe, & Barker, 2000).

At a minimum, all partial-thickness and full-thickness burns are covered with sterile dressings. Generally, dressing with either dry, sterile gauze or Water Jel, if preferred by the burn center, is indicated for patients who will be transferred within 24 hours of the initial injury (DeBoer & O'Connor, 2004; Merck, 2008; Sicoutris & Holmes, 2006). Applying topicals should be undertaken with caution as the burn center will have to clean and dress the wound with agents of their choice upon arrival (DeBoer & O'Connor, 2004), and if deep cleaning is needed to remove the topical, the victim will undergo a pain process to clean the burn wound.

All full-thickness and partial-thickness burns must be covered with a sterile dressing (Morgan, Bledsoe, & Barker, 2000). When transport cannot be accomplished within 24 hours postinjury, such as in a mass casualty setting, using a nonadherent fine mesh covering after applying a topical antimicrobial is recommended to prevent infection and to maintain tissue hydration until the wound can be further assessed and treated (Garner & Magee, 2002; Gomez & Cancio, 2007; Morgan, Bledsoe, & Barker). Applying the mesh covering in successive strips rather than wrapping it around the wound avoids circulatory impairment. Nonadherent tubular gauze is used to hold the mesh in place. For children, tubular gauze can be used on the trunk to hold bandaging in place (Morgan, Bledsoe, & Barker). However, if transport is possible within 24 hours postinjury, there is no reason to apply topical antimicrobials before transfer to the burn center (Gomez & Cancio).

When transport is not possible immediately, bandage maintenance on site is needed. Changing bandages when they become filled with exudates, other fluid, or dirt is essential. Whenever a bandage is changed in the field, prior applications of topical antimicrobial should be gently removed with gentle washing and a sterile dressing reapplied. Sharp debridement and scrubbing should be avoided (Morgan, Bledsoe, & Barker, 2000).

Blister management ranges from leaving them alone to full debridement. Small blisters are usually left intact to maintain the biologic barrier to infection afforded by the top layer (DeBoer & O'Connor, 2004; Morgan, Bledsoe, & Barker, 2000). Managing large, intact blisters remains somewhat controversial. Previously, larger blisters were aspirated with a fine needle to withdraw the fluid that may impair leukocyte activity, without disrupting the top layer so exposure of the burn and pain from dressing contact to the burn wound was avoided (DeBoer & O'Connor; Merck, 2008). More recently, however, fine-needle aspiration is eschewed due to the increased risk of infection; additionally, the presence of blisters for several weeks showing no signs of resorption indicates the possible presence of either partial deep thickness or full-thickness burn (Morgan, Bledsoe, & Barker, 2000).

Removing ruptured blisters and debriding intact blisters is occasionally undertaken to avoid impairing wound healing (DeBoer & O'Connor, 2004; Merck, 2008; Morgan, Bledsoe, & Barker, 2000). Blisters are debrided when they evidence either cloudy fluid or are likely to rupture imminently on their own (Morgan, Bledsoe, & Barker). Regardless of the approach taken with blister management, all blisters should be covered with a topical antimicrobial, such as bacitracin, for victims who will not be transferred; for victims being transported, the blisters should be covered with a dry sterile gauze dressing (DeBoer & O'Connor; Morgan, Bledsoe, & Barker).

If prehospital, on-site triage and management occurs and recommended transfer commences, transporting the victim begins the second phase of critical burn care. This phase, Stage 2, is termed the *emergent phase, immediate resuscitation,* and extends from 0 to 48 hours postinjury. The next section discusses this stage.

Stage 2: Emergent Phase, Immediate Resuscitation

Stage 2, colloquially known as the *critical care phase,* involves several aggressive treatment strategies essential to patient survival: maintaining breathing and airway, aggressive fluid resuscitation, depth and extent of wound determinations, pain control, and initial wound debridement or surgical intervention (Supple, 1994). Treatment strategy in the emergent phase involves ongoing resuscitation efforts focusing on hemodynamic, physiologic, and volume support; surgical planning and intervention; and nutritional support and wound care; continuing the on-site trauma team's initial interventions (Ramzy, Barret, & Herndon, 1999; Sheridan, 2001; Sicoutris & Holmes, 2006; Supple, 1994). Treatment is divided into two survey periods: the primary survey, which focuses on the ABCs of the ATLS algorithm, and the secondary survey, which involves a thorough patient history and examination of the burn victim (DeBoer & O'Connor, 2004; Love & Nguyen, 1999; Ramzy, Barret, & Herndon, 1999).

As stated above, the primary survey in the emergent phase of care commences with the ABCs of the ATLS algorithm. The risk of upper airway constriction, due to the rapid onset of edema from suspected inhalation of noxious fumes or superheated air, is of concern, and, although security of the airway is paramount, it should be approached in a careful and controlled manner (DeBoer & O'Connor, 2004; Ramzy,

Barret, & Herndon, 1999; Sheridan, 2001). Victim assessment for possible intubation occurs first, if intubation has not been done in the field (DeBoer & O'Connor). Treatment for airway injury is supportive, and urgent intubation is reserved for adult or pediatric victims who exhibit airway edema (Ramzy, Barret, & Herndon, 1999). Other intubation candidates are all victims evidencing impending upper airway obstruction indicated by retractions or hoarseness or are otherwise physically compromised due to shock or drugs or alcohol ingestion (Sheridan). It is best to secure an airway as soon as possible to avoid possible airway compromise that can develop in the several hours postinjury (DeBoer & O'Connor).

Invasively creating an airway by either surgical cricothyroidotomy or needle is a viable option; however, the complexity of the techniques involved usually precludes their use (DeBoer & O'Connor, 2004). More commonly, in both the ER and operating room arenas, airways are secured using rapid sequence intubation (RSI) under adequate sedation and analgesia in conjunction with a short-acting neuromuscular blocking agent (SA-NMBA); this is rarely practical in the disaster situation. Upon securing airway control, the next concern in emergent care is inadequate fluid resuscitation causing hypovolemia (Love & Nguyen, 1999; Sheridan, 2001).

Burn shock results from a combination of local tissue and hemodynamic alterations occurring in the body of the burn victim (Love & Nguyen, 1999; Sheridan, 2001). These changes result in decreased circulating and extracellular plasma fluid volumes and decreased cardiac output. Therefore, as is common with hypovolemia treatments generally, the goal in burn wound treatment initially is to stabilize circulatory fluid volumes, which return tissue perfusion to normal levels (DeBoer & O'Connor, 2004; Love & Nguyen; Sheridan). However, care must be taken in assessing fluid resuscitation requirements because of present edema in both the burned and unburned tissues that will increase during the next 24-hour period (Love & Nguyen).

There is always concern about establishing peripheral vascular access in burned areas to support fluid resuscitation measures. If a peripheral vascular line was started during the prehospital stage, these lines can be sutured into place once the victim arrives in the triage unit, ER, or burn unit. If a line was not placed, there are two attendant concerns for consideration: having to place a peripheral vascular line into burned areas and the attendant risk of infection.

First, regarding the placement of a peripheral vascular line in burned areas: Under the best of conditions, in a disaster, vascular access is difficult to attain under hypovolemic conditions. Here, whether the victim is an adult or child, an intraosseous line will be useful (DeBoer & O'Connor, 2004; Sheridan, 2001). In adults, intraosseous cannulation is appropriate in the arm, tibia, or sternum (DeBoer & O'Connor), though tibial access is generally preferred and easier to obtain. In children, the intraosseous cannulation is properly placed below the tibial tuberosity, with the needle distally directed away from the epiphysis, using a commercially available heavy spinal needle or catheter (Sheridan, 2001).

Second, regarding infection risk, burned areas should not be used for intravenous lines unless there are no other viable veins available due to the ever-present risk of infection in exposed skin areas. However, resuscitating fluid levels always takes priority over infection risk (DeBoer & O'Connor, 2004). As mentioned previously, the Parkland formula is the most commonly used formula for estimating initial fluid resuscitation. The preferred solutions at this stage are either lactated Ringers (non-colloid) or normal saline (0.9%), both isotonic fluids that reestablish perfusion and allow maximum fluid to remain in the intravascular space. Finally, evaluating urine output, acid–base balance, and hemodynamic status is necessary to ensure proper fluid resuscitation is achieved, if at all possible (DeBoer & O'Connor; Gomez & Cancio, 2007). Once stabilization of the airway and fluid levels occurs, the secondary survey stage in emergent care begins.

Priorities in the Primary Survey in Emergent Care

Complementing the primary survey, the burn specific second survey focuses on nine specific parameters: (a) otolaryngologic, (b) chest, (c) cardiac, (d) genitourinary, (e) abdominal and (f) neurologic points, (g) extremity issues, and (h) radiography with (i) laboratory studies. (Gang, Sanyal, LalBang, Modkaddas, & Lari, 2000; Supple, 1994). Thorough examination of the victim from head to toe occurs along with identifying the mechanism of burn injury (Supple). Identifying the mechanism of injury allows proper efficient examination and extent of injury determinations to occur.

The first assessment made in the secondary survey is the otolaryngologic assessment. Otolaryngologic assessments include appropriate treatment of corneal epithelial and external ear wounds, particularly focusing on the burned auricle and preventing auricular chondritis from developing, especially since blood supply to the ear is poor at best (DeBoer & O'Connor, 2004; Sheridan, 2001). Fluorescein staining is usually undertaken to assess both subtle corneal epithelial and deep corneal stromal burn wounds. Daily treatment after debridement of the external ear with mafenide acetate, a synthetic sulfonamide antimicrobial and potent carbonic anhydrase inhibitor, reduces the development of infection (Klein, Heimbach & Gibran, 2002; Sheridan, 2001).

The second assessment performed in the secondary survey is the chest assessment. Ensuring sufficient ventilation of the hemithoraces is the focus of chest examination in burn injury (Sheridan, 2001). Two concerns are present: The presence of circumferential deep eschar often causes decreased chest wall compliance, and bronchospasm due to inhalation injury often complicates ventilation. Escharotomy resolves chest wall compliance inhibition (Love & Nguyen, 1999; Sheridan), though it is rarely performed in the disaster setting and rarely develops to an extent that respirations are compromised in the immediate disaster. Electrocautery may be used to minimize blood loss. Incisions are made along the flanks until separation is attained, at which point they are connected midline. This restores chest motions to ensure adequate ventilation levels (Love & Nguyen).

Bronchospasm is addressed with aerosolized bronchodilators and ventilation strategies as needed to reduce the occurrence of dynamic hyperinflation and breath stacking that often attends increased small airway resistance. Identifying structural fire as the burn injury mechanism warrants an additional assessment for CO poisoning or serious CO exposure (Sheridan, 2001). Administering 100% oxygen by mask generally clears the blood of carboxyhemoglobin, which has a half-life of 2.5 hours and elimination half-life of 4 hours on ambient air and 45 to 60 minutes on 100% oxygen (Dougherty & Waxman, 1996).

The third assessment performed in the secondary survey is cardiac. Dramatic effects on the cardiovascular system are evidenced during the progression of burn injury. Initially, during the first 24 to 72 hours postinjury, decreased cardiac output and plasma volume and increased capillary permeability occur (Supple, 1994). These effects result in burn shock, which initially resembles generalized hypovolemic shock as previously indicated, since additional decreased cardiac output, pulmonary artery pressures, central venous pressure, and urine output, along with hypotension and tachycardia, result. Interestingly, however, these are not hypovolemic occurrences; rather they are due to humoral and neurogenic influence (Sicoutris & Holmes, 2006; Supple). For example, decreased cardiac output is a result of cellular myocyte shock, resulting from impaired signaling dysregulation, which comes from impaired calcium homeostasis (White, Maass, Sanders, & Horton, 2002). Burn shock resolution and capillary integrity reestablishment occur during the flow phase that follows the ebb phase by approximately 24 hours, during which diuresis and fluid mobilization result (Sicoutris & Holmes, 2006; Supple; White et al.).

Vascular changes postburn involve several concomitant processes, three of which are noteworthy: The first, impaired cellular membrane function, results from an intravascular water shift into the nonburned tissue by hypoproteinemia and cellular swelling secondary to an extracellular to intracellular water shift (Demling & LaLonde, 1989; Supple). The second, burn edema, increases due to osmotic pressure increases, further complicating circulating volume. Third, intravascular loss occurs due to edema in burned and nonburned tissue and evaporative loss. Additionally, microcirculation experiences marked changes due to direct thermal injury (Supple). Electrolyte alterations occur rapidly and must be monitored and treated accordingly to avoid further degradation of the cardiovascular system (Demling & LaLonde; Supple). Potassium release from damaged cells causes hyperkalemia in the initial resuscitative phase, which can be corrected by addressing the attendant acidosis and hypovolemia. Altered levels of phosphorus, magnesium, calcium, and sodium occur regularly due to fluid loss by evaporation through the open wounds, which can result in arrhythmias developing (Sheridan, 2001; Supple). Cardiovascular response to burn injury varies among individuals, and the general rule is careful monitoring and recovery of subtle changes in electrolyte balances to avoid abrupt or extreme cardiovascular response (Supple).

The fourth assessment performed in the secondary survey is genitourinary. Genitourinary considerations in the emergent phase are limited. In males, foreskin reduction after catheterization to prevent the development of paraphimosis as soft tissue edema ensues is indicated (Sheridan, 2001). In both adults and children, renal impairment is a primary concern, as urine output is the first indicator of kidney function (Supple, 1994). Here, renal impairment usually occurs due to hypoperfusion, hemoglobinuria, or myoglobinuria. Renal failure frequently attends electrical burn injury as it results in the depositing of myoglobin or hemoglobin in the urine. For low output levels, fluid resuscitation is indicated and should be adjusted to achieve a urine output of 75 mL to 100 mL per hour if pigment clearance is desired; adding sodium bicarbonate ($NaHCO_3^-$) facilitates the process (Supple).

Acute renal failure often attends burn injury. In acute burn injury, acute renal failure is usually due to decreased blood flow; fluid resuscitation can reverse this effect. If infection is present, immediate adjustments in fluid resuscitation, infection control, and wound excision will facilitate reversal of renal compromise. Optimizing fluid resuscitation, infection control, and wound closure decreases renal compromise in all injured patients (Supple, 1994).

The fifth assessment performed in the secondary survey is the abdominal assessment. Abdominal evaluations in burn injuries are performed to exclude injuries, reduce the chance of gastroduodenal ulceration or gastric dilation development and to ensure torso compliance (Sheridan, 2001). Injuries occur most commonly during escape from buildings, electrical voltage falls, and motor vehicle accidents. There are several events that can be indicators of abdominal injury in thermal burns. One of the first events suggestive of abdominal injury is a paradoxically falling hematocrit level or need for excessive fluid in the early resuscitation phase (Sheridan). Compartment syndrome, where significant accumulation of intraperitoneal fluid or bowel edema occurs, is also of concern with abdominal injury, potentially causing difficult breathing and reduced urine output. Circumferential torso eschar can cause the same problem, but it is usually corrected with escharotomy.

When significant visceral edema results in the abdominal cavity, abdominal decompression is usually warranted (Sheridan, 2001). Abdominal decompression is also performed to avoid abdominal distension due to swallowing air or peristaltic immobility due to narcotic medications (Love & Nguyen, 1999). Splanchnic blood flow, often compromised in severe thermal injury, causes gastroduodenal ulceration; administering histaminic receptor antagonist drugs during emergent resuscitation often resolves the problem (Czaja, McAlhany, & Pruitt, 1974; McAlhany, Czaja, Villarreal, & Pruitt, 1974; Sheridan, 2001).

Neurological assessment follows next in the emergent secondary phase. Performing a neurological assessment in the emergent phase of burn wound care is important as sensory and motor functions can be impaired by administering medications or by fluid instability occurring immediately postinjury. Assessing intracranial trauma early in the emergent care cycle is also important when victims, in the ensuing hours and days, become obtunded due to pain management, fluid shifts, exhaustion, and sleep deprivation and may not be able to respond appropriately (Sheridan, 2001). CO poisoning, anxiety, and pain management control are also important considerations in the neurological workup. In the disaster setting, the disaster nurse should assess for level of consciousness, grip strengths, and ability to move extremities on command, as appropriate, and as discussed further below.

The last assessment performed in the emergent secondary survey phase is extremity assessment and radiography, which cannot usually be done in the acute disaster setting. Radiographic studies, if possible, and physical examination eliminate other remaining injuries. Knowing the mechanism of injury is important in this phase, as it provides the basis upon which selecting radiographic studies relies.

Extremity perfusion is concerning; initial extremity examination focuses on locating any circumferential eschar on the limbs and identifying any progressive soft tissue edema accompanied by rigid compartments. However, continual extremity examination throughout the resuscitative period is necessary to avoid the development of further burn-related systemic stresses, and the extremities must be dressed to facilitate frequent reexamination. Reexaminations focus on assessing all of the following functions: pliability, active and passive ROM, pain with motion, temperature differences, named vessel pulsations, and evaluating capillary refill. Assessing capillary refill requires extremity elevation to avoid identifying a false-positive venous refill from mottled, nonperfused extremities as elevating the extremity avoids dependence (Sheridan, 2001).

Radiographic studies, where possible, are usually selected based on the mechanism of injury or to eliminate head, extremity, or truncal injury; to eliminate gastric dilation; and to identify the position of resuscitative cannulas. High-voltage injuries usually require radiographic studies to eliminate spinal fracture or tetanic contractures of the paravertebral musculature. Last, laboratory studies, where possible, are performed to assess organ function, carboxyhemoglobin levels, urine myoglobin levels, and hematocrit levels (Sheridan, 2001).

Stage 3: Acute Phase, Secondary Resuscitation

Determining that inpatient care is needed at this point begins stage 3: acute phase, secondary resuscitation, for the burn victim. However, it should be noted that stage 3 also applies to patients who are released after stage 2 stabilization for continued outpatient-based care. It should also be noted that, depending on the duration of the disaster and postdisaster situation, the disaster nurse may have to care for the burn victim longer than "usually" expected in a disaster. This section will briefly address those areas of concern that the disaster nurse might face.

Stage 3, acute phase, secondary resuscitation (successful postresuscitation phase) follows stage 2, beginning approximately 72 hours postinjury. Infection control, surgical intervention, wound care, nutritional support, adequate analgesia, psychosocial support, and occupational and physical therapy become the focus of care. This acute phase continues through the duration of the burn victim's hospitalization and usually extends through discharge to home (Supple, 1994). Successful, high-quality critical care is essential to the survival of burn victims having serious injury (Sheridan, 2001). Surgeons usually direct and provide the majority of this care in the United States, with the support and expertise of critical care nursing within the specialized burn intensive care unit setting.

Stage 3: Acute Phase Resuscitation: Infection Control

Understanding infection control in burn wound management requires acknowledging the complexity of the immunologic response to burn injury in the body (Supple, 1994). Infection development requires three conditions to exist concomitantly: (a) organism source, (b) transmission modality, and (c) body susceptibility (Weber & McManus, 2004). Because burn wounds substantially negatively impact the body's immune system response, infection risk due to burn injury is different than infection risk in other patients. Understanding each condition is essential to understanding how to minimize infection risk to burn victims.

Pathogens ensue from the burn victim's own skin, the environment, and the healthcare environment. Predominant pathogens particularly concerning to burn victims are antibiotic-susceptible gram-negative organisms, gram-positive organisms, yeasts, and fungi. Specific antibiotics should be used for each type of organism when possible in the disaster setting. Burn patients possess a unique susceptibility to colonization from environmentally present organisms. Additionally, burn victims essentially self-infect as well by dispensing organisms from the wounds into the surrounding environment. Interestingly, despite these unique features common to burn-injured victims, the most common infection routes are through droplet, airborne, or direct contact modes (Weber & McManus, 2004). This usually occurs through contact with improperly decontaminated equipment or direct or indirect healthcare provider contact.

The human body is unique in its ability to defend itself against infection unless it suffers a burn injury. Once burn injury results, the body's physical defense system, the skin, and the body's nonspecific and specific immune responses are negatively altered, raising the body's level of susceptibility. Five major organ systems frequently exposed to invasive devices lose their defense to organism invasion: the skin, gastrointestinal tract, urogenital tract, respiratory tract, and external ear and conjunctiva (Weber & McManus, 2004).

Burn injury causes exposure of extensive areas and devastation of tissues (Bang, Gang, Sanyal, Modkaddas, & Ebrahim, 1998). Serous exudate at a temperature of 37°C or above occurs, causing the wound(s) to remain moist. Burned eschar and serous moisture invite proliferation and colonization of a variety of microorganisms. Host immune responses are compromised by severe burns; bacteria such as MRSA, MRSE, group A beta hemolytic streptococci, and VRE colonize rapidly (Gang et al., 2000). Coupled with the depression of the immune response resulting from the burn injury, sepsis is a likely outcome because of the severe catabolism that develops proportionally to the extent of the burn wound injury (Bang et al., 1998; Ninneman, 1987). These conditions exacerbate developing sepsis by encouraging bacterial endotoxin release, which creates another immunologic response by another inflammatory mediator release (Ninneman; Supple, 1994). Therefore, burn victim mortality is directly related to the immunological status of the victim. Immunologic response is dependent on the host response to thermal injury, which activates cell-mediated immunity through the arachidonic and cytokine cascades, each releasing inflammatory mediators (Goodwin, 1990).

Unless there is clear evidence of infection, prophylactic antibiotic therapy is not usually instituted due to the high risk of developing resistant bacterial strains (Merck, 2008). Diagnosing infection is difficult in burn victims as elevated temperature and white blood cell counts attend the injury as well as indicate infection (Dougherty & Waxman, 1996). The symptoms that are confusing are grouped together and are termed SIRS, or systemic inflammatory response syndrome. SIRS refers to a general inflammatory process regardless of cause in the absence of any underlying cause. Localized inflammatory responses are normal and beneficial in combating infection and promoting healing; however, an excessive response predisposes the body to sepsis development and further tissue damage (O'Sullivan & O'Connor, 1997).

Generally, parenteral antibiotic therapy in burn wound management is not started until two signs of systemic and generic infection are present, such as ileus and confusion, leukopenia and glucose intolerance, or confusion with high fever (Dougherty & Waxman, 1996). Where the very young and elderly are involved, parenteral antibiotics are started before a second sign of sepsis evidences.

Multiple organ dysfunction occurs due to prolonged shock, tissue hypoxia, and uncontrolled systemic inflammation, gut translocation, or exposure to severe or repeated infections, all of which are common to severe burn injuries (Sheridan, 2001). Multiple organ dysfunction develops in a progressive manner: from increasing obtundation to progressive hypoxia and intrapulmonary shunting, ileus, non-oliguric renal failure, rising cholestatic chemistries, thrombocytopenia, anuria, vasomotor failure, and death (Goodwin, 1990; Sheridan, 2001). Treatment becomes a two-fold approach: first, to support the failing organs and, second, to identify the occult infection. Usually, identifying wound sepsis as the primary cause for multiple organ dysfunction is uncommon unless deep wounds are not promptly excised and closed (Sheridan, 2001). Death becomes the inevitable outcome unless the infectious underlying focus is identified and addressed. However, prevention is the best treatment to total organ collapse and is accomplished by avoiding infection exposure and carefully managing hemodynamic support.

Clearly, several factors possibly affect the pathogenesis of postburn immunosuppression. Unfortunately, there is no clear indication of which factor exactly affects the immunosuppressive cascade. Identifying the possible factors will provide the means for healthcare providers to restore normal immune function sooner in severely injured burn victims, thereby preventing infection overload and reducing mortality attendant to major burn trauma.

Stage 3: Acute Phase Resuscitation: Hypermetabolism and Hyperglycemia

Another phenomenon that requires attention in the acute resuscitative phase is the hypermetabolic response to burn injury. Significant burn injury alters the body's metabolic neuroendocrine hormonal control resulting in a hypermetabolic state developing. The hypermetabolic response is the single greatest response to burn injury (Love & Nguyen, 1999). Although metabolic derangement is common in trauma injuries, generally the metabolic rate in burn victims can increase to as much as 2 to 3 times normal (Ramzy, Barret, & Herndon, 1999). The extent of burn injury is directly related to the degree of metabolic response experienced. For example, in burn injuries involving 20% or more TBSA, metabolic demands increase by more than 30% of normal (Flynn, 2004). Similarly, when more than 50% TBSA is involved, metabolic demands increase by 100%.

Metabolic response to burn is manifested as a biphasic pattern of response to acute burn injury, known as an "ebb" phase followed by a "flow" phase (Flynn, 2004; Love & Nguyen, 1999). The ebb phase is evidenced by a decrease in metabolic rate, cardiac function, intravascular volume, and hypoperfusion, commonly called "burn shock" (Flynn). The prolonged flow phase follows the ebb phase and is characterized by more hemodynamic stability, yet hypermetabolism ensues, evidenced by nitrogen loss, increased oxygen consumption, elevated body temperature to 38.5°C, and increased urinary output. The most severely burned individuals experience a severely prolonged flow phase, which results in massive lipolysis, protein catabolism, peripheral muscle wasting, and hepatic fat deposition (Flynn; Love & Nguyen).

Hypermetabolic responses to burn injury endure from stabilization postinjury through wound closure and for a variable time period thereafter. Hypermetabolic nutritional response is essential to matching the body's energy expenditures while providing sufficient nitrogen to replace or restore the body's protein stores to promote healing. The increasing metabolic rate postburn injury is directly proportional to the TBSA and ranges from 15% to 100% of normal basal requirements (Sheridan, 2001). Estimating nutritional needs allows an individualized assessment of the changing nutritional requirements as well as provides a nutritional regimen that encourages wound healing, achieves a zero nutritional balance, and minimizes skeletal muscle wasting (Flynn, 2004). Meeting the necessary levels of nutritional support for burn victims meets the objective of protein therapy during and after burn: to allow for appropriate amino acid production to maximize protein synthesis for optimized wound healing and to avert amino acid outflow from the skeletal muscle (Prelack, Dylewski, & Sheridan, 2007).

Stress-induced hyperglycemia is a result of hypermetabolism. Hyperglycemia is exaggerated in the burn victim due to the presence of counter-regulatory hormones, particularly catecholamines, proinflammatory cytokines, and glucocorticoids produced as part of the physiologic stress response (Flynn, 2004). Here, hyperglycemia is defined as a fasting blood sugar level of 200 mg/dL or higher in absence of diabetes diagnosis. Using high carbohydrate enteral nutrition formulations, if any are available, slows this catabolic response, sparing muscle. Optimized glucose oxidation is achieved with intake levels of approximately 5 mg/kg/min (Sicoutris & Holmes, 2006). Hyperglycemia must be controlled to allow efficient and effective wound healing. Continuous insulin infusion set to maintain blood glucose levels at 80 mg/dL to 110 mg/dL contributes directly to reducing mortality (Flynn, 2004; Supple, 1994; VandenBerge et al., 2001).

Two major principles are involved when pharmaceutical approaches are considered in managing hypermetabolism. First, using anabolics to alleviate severe muscle wasting and preserve lean body mass; second, using antiadrenergics to decrease both myocardial workload and oxygen consumption. Anabolics reduce the skeletal muscle breakdown that normally attends severe burn injury. Concomitant delivery of both insulin and r-HGH, a specific anabolic, accelerate healing time (Ramzy, Barret, & Herndon, 1999). Any modalities that have a positive effect on healing and wound closure result in decreased hospital length of stay, sepsis development, and possible morbidity (Gilpin, Barrow, Rutan, Broemeling, & Herndon, 1994; Ramzy, Barret, & Herndon).

Antiadrenergic drugs modulate the hypermetabolic response by decreasing cardiac work and myocardial oxygen consumption. The most commonly employed antiadrenergic showing great success is propranolol. Merely administering 1 mg/kg/d to 2 mg/kg/d reduces left ventricular work and heart rate by 20% cumulatively, while also decreasing peripheral lipolysis, irritability, and tremulousness (Ramzy, Barret, & Herndon, 1999). Thus, propranolol provides a safe and effective means to mitigate the hyperdynamic cardiac response to thermal injury wounds. Using pharmacological approaches such as anabolics and antiadrenergics in conjunction with appropriate nutrition in the severely burn injured results in faster recovery, wound closure and healing, and rehabilitation while reducing muscle wasting, energy expenditures, and septic morbidity.

Stage 3: Acute Phase Resuscitation: Pain Management

Burn victims suffer pain and anxiety. Having an organized approach to the assessment and treatment of pain and anxiety allows for prompt evaluation of the effectiveness of new interventions. Unfortunately, pain management in the thermally injured is frequently frustrating due to the unpredictable psychologic and physiologic responses to the burn (Sicoutris & Holmes, 2006). Polytraumatized burn victims present a special challenge especially if they are on a ventilator, as pain management similar to general anesthesia with paralytics, opiates, and amnestics given by continuous drip is necessitated (Dougherty & Waxman, 1996). Victims with skeletal injuries of the lower extremities and or thorax may be managed with an indwelling epidural catheter. Total pain elimination in burn wound victims is nearly impossible, short of administering general anesthesia (Sicoutris & Holmes).

Good pain management is achieved by good pain assessment. Therefore, dividing burn wound victims into four categories allows an organized approach to treating with a limited formulary of pain and anxiolytic medications and dosages to prolong developing tolerance (Sheridan, 2001). Additionally, categorization allows the efficient management of procedural pain, background pain, and transition issues for individuals using medications that have the potential to encourage tolerance development and require increasing dosages over time for adequate pain and anxiety management. The four categories of victims and their pain and anxiousness levels are: (a) mechanically ventilated acute, (b) spontaneously breathing acute, (c) acute rehabilitation, and (d) reconstructive. As healing progresses, the need for pain management should decrease.

Initially, administering IV opioid-based analgesia is recommended in severe burn injury victims (DeBoer & O'Connor, 2004). Here, IV morphine or fentanyl are used in conjunction with aggressive fluid resuscitation, and IM-administered versions should be avoided, especially if the patient evidences shock. This is because shunting of the blood to the heart, brain, and lungs takes precedence and adequate perfusion of muscle tissue is sacrificed. Respiratory depression is of concern with the use of opiate pain relief, and disaster nurses should be ready to address severe respiratory depression. Although rates and dosages usually exceed the standard adult administration rate ranges of 1 mg/kg IV to 2 mg/kg IV morphine, the goal is adequate pain relief in extreme pain circumstance (DeBoer & O'Connor, 2004). Over time the pain will lessen, and these levels will be reduced accordingly. It is not surprising however to have varying pain management needs extend 1 to 2 years past the period of rehabilitation.

Where severely injured patients evidence anxiety, the benzodiazepine pharmaceuticals provide safe and effective management. Suggested IV forms are diazepam, administered at rates of 0.6 mg/kg over 8 hours; lorazepam, administered at a rate of 0.05 mg/kg/dose every 2 to 4 hours; and midazolam, administered at a rate of 0.50 mg/kg to 0.10 mg/kg every 2 hours (Dougherty & Waxman, 1996). All of these medications have orally available forms that can be used in the later stages of care and rehabilitation.

Frequent pain reassessment is required to allow quick pain medication titrations to address treatment protocols such as dressing changes and wound debridement, as well as provide steps to wean the victim from pain medication over time (Dougherty & Waxman, 1996). Here, identification of premorbid conditions and underlying disease state allows for safe and effective administration of pain medications. Depending on the severity of the initial injury, pain reassessments should be conducted at a minimum every 3 days to determine when pain medication levels can be lowered, maintained, or even increased depending on upcoming treatments scheduled. Although many healthcare providers are reticent to continue pain medications for extended periods of time, pain management should continue throughout the rehabilitation phase to allow burn-injured patients to fully participate in function-restoring therapy and attain a comfortable recovery during reconstructive procedures, extending through final rehabilitation and outpatient maintenance and support (Dougherty & Waxman).

Stage 4: Final Rehabilitative Phase: Outpatient Maintenance and Support

Stage 4, the final rehabilitative phase, occurs during the first year or two after the burn injury. Here the focus is on scar maturation, preventing wound contractures, and restoring physical function, occupation, and independence (Spires, 2007; Supple, 1994). Burn injury is a catastrophic event, resulting in significant impairment to physical functioning and psychological complications requiring comprehensive rehabilitation efforts. The focus of such treatment is creating strategies to avoid complicating scarring, contractures, and other events that can limit functional mobility (Esselman, 2007; Ramzy, Barret, & Herndon, 1999; Silwa, Heinemann, & Semik, 2005; Spires, 2007). The process usually extends from months to years and requires the commitment of the healthcare providers and patient to ensure maximal outcomes. As the disaster nurse will not be dealing with this phase of the stages, the process of rehabilitation will not be addressed further.

Conclusion

As stated initially, whether the burn injury is thermal or nonthermal in nature, occurring to a single victim or many in a disaster, with or without attendant polytrauma, the physiologic response to burn injury is complex. Understanding the complexity and various components is essential to the assessment, care, and treatment of these victims, to ensure optimal outcome, despite the variable victim characteristics and responses caused by the indiscriminate nature of burn injuries.

Excluding the September 11, 2001, tragedy at the World Trade Centers in New York City, the economic and human toll from burn injuries annually is substantial. Fire kills over 3,900 individuals annually (Spires, 2007). Annually in the United States, approximately 500,000 people are treated for burn injuries with 40,000 requiring hospitalization (Esselman, 2007). Additionally, at least 750 people die annually due to nonthermal burn injuries resulting from motor vehicle accidents, chemical and electrical exposures, and airplane crashes.

Although great strides have been attained in burn wound management since the 1980s, the statistics concerning burn-related mortality are still staggering. In the 1980s, burn wound mortality occurred at 65% TBSA involvement. Today, mortality is basically limited to injuries encompassing 80% TBSA or more. However, because small burn injuries rarely result in death today, these statistics are based on a population of individuals with large wound injuries, defined as encompassing 50% TBSA or more only. Thankfully, in pediatric statistics, where significant burn wound injury is defined as greater than 60% TBSA involvement, there were no mortalities reported between 1991–1997 where 60% or less TBSA was involved (Esselman, 2007).

Should burn injury occur in the mass casualty setting, knowledge and application of the concepts and theories involved in burn injury discussed in this chapter allow the disaster nurse to engage in a cohesive team environment with other EMS present to appropriately triage and stabilize victims on site until appropriate transport to burn centers or ERs can occur. In the next chapter, mass casualty approaches to burn injury are presented, further adding to the disaster nurse's skills and knowledge related to caring for the burn disaster victim.

References

American College of Surgeons, Committee on Trauma. (2004). *Advanced trauma life support for doctors* (7th ed.). Chicago: Author.

Bang, R. L., Gang, R. J., Sanyal, S. C., Modkaddas, E., & Ebrahim, M. K. (1998). Burn septicaemia: An analysis of 79 patients. *Burns, 24,* 354–361.

Beaver, B. M. (1990). Care of the multiple trauma victim. The first hour. *Nursing Clinics of North America, 25,* 11–21.

Brown, T. L. H., & Muller, M. (2004). Damage limitation in burn surgery. *Injury, 35,* 697–707.

Czaja, A. J., McAlhany, J. C., & Pruitt, B. A., Jr. (1974). Acute gastroduodenal disease after thermal injury: An endoscopic evaluation of incidence and natural history. *New England Journal of Medicine, 291,* 925–929.

DeBoer, S., & O'Connor, A. (2004). Prehospital and emergency department burn care. *Critical Care Nursing Clinics of North America, 16,* 61–73.

Demling, R. H., & LaLonde, C. (1989). *Maintaining hemodynamic stability.* In R. H. Demling & C. LaLonde (Eds.), *Burn trauma* (pp. 84–98). New York: Theime Medical Publishers.

Dougherty, W., & Waxman, K. (1996). Complex and challenging problems in trauma surgery: The complexities of managing severe burns with associated trauma. *Surgical Clinics of North America, 76*(4): 923–958.

Esselman, P. (2007). Burn rehabilitation: An overview. *Archives of Physical Medicine and Rehabilitation, 88*(2), S3–S6.

Flynn, M. B. (2004). Nutritional support for the burn injured patient. *Critical Care Nursing Clinics of North America, 16,* 139–144.

Gang, R., Sanyal, S., LalBang, R., Modkaddas, E., & Lari, A. (2000). Staphylococcal septicaemia in burns. *Burns, 26,* 359–366.

Garner, W., & Magee, W. (2005). Acute burn injury. *Clinics in Plastic Surgery, 32,* 187–193.

Gilpin, D. A., Barrow, R. E., Rutan, R. L., Broemeling, L., & Herndon, D. N. (1994). Recombinant human growth hormone accelerates wound healing in children with large cutaneous burns. *Annals of Surgery, 220,* 19–24.

Gomez, R., & Cancio, L. (2007). Management of burn wounds in the Emergency Department. *Emergency Medicine Clinics of North America, 25,* 135–146.

Goodwin, C. W. (1990). Multiple organ failure: Clinical overview of the syndrome. *Journal of Trauma, 30,* S163–S165.

Klein, M., Heimbach, D., & Gibran, N. (2002). Trauma and thermal injury: Management of the burn wound: Introduction. *ACS Surgery Online 2002.* Retrieved March 5, 2008, from http://www.medscape.com/viewarticle/535520_print

Love, R., & Nguyen, T. (1999). Critical care of the burn patient. *Seminars in Anesthesia, Perioperative Medicine and Pain, 18*(1), 87–98.

McAlhany, J. C., Jr., Czaja, A. J., Villarreal, Y., & Pruitt, B. A., Jr. (1974). The gastric mucosal barrier in thermally injured patients: Correlation with gastroduodenal endoscopy. *Surgical Forum, 25,* 414–416.

Merck Manual Professional Edition. (2008). *Burns, injuries, poisoning.* Retrieved January 31, 2008, from http://www.merck.com/mmpe/sec21/ch315/ch315a.html

Morgan, E. D., Bledsoe, S. C, & Barker, J. (2000). Ambulatory management of burns. *American Family Physician, 62,* 2015–2032.

Ninneman, J. L. (1987). Immunological defenses against infection: Alterations following thermal injury. *Journal of Burn Care Rehabilitation, 8,* 475–482.

O'Sullivan, S. T., & O'Connor, T. P. F. (1997). Immunosuppression following thermal injury: The pathogenesis of immunodysfunction. *British Journal of Plastic Surgery, 50,* 615–623.

Prelack, K., Dylewski, M., & Sheridan, R. (2007). Practical guidelines for nutritional management of burn injury and recovery. *Burns, 33,* 14–24.

Ramzy, P., Barret, J., & Herndon, D. (1999). Environmental emergencies: Thermal injuries. *Critical Care Clinics, 15*(2), 333–352.

Rosenkranz, K., & Sheridan, R. (2002). Management of the burned trauma patient: Balancing conflicting priorities. *Burns, 28,* 665–669.

Rossiter, N., Chapman, P., & Haywood, I. (1996). How big is a hand? *Burns, 22,* 230–231.

Sheridan, R. (2001). Current problems in surgery: Comprehensive treatment of burns. *Current Problems in Surgery, 38,* 641–756.

Sicoutris, C., & Holmes, J. (2006). Fire and smoke injuries. *Critical Care Nursing Clinics of North America, 18,* 403–417.

Silwa, J. A., Heinemann, A., & Semik, P. (2005). Inpatient rehabilitation following burn injury: Patient demographics and functional outcomes. *Archives of Physical Medicine and Rehabilitation, 86,* 1920–1923.

Spires, M. C. (2007). Rehabilitation methods for the burn injured individual. *Physical Medicine Rehabilitation Clinics of North America, 18,* 925–948.

Supple, K. G. (1994). Physiologic response to burn injury. *Critical Care Nursing Clinics of North America, 16,* 119–126.

VandenBerge, G., Wouters, P., Weekers, F., Verwaest, C., Bruyninckx, F., Schetz, M., et al. (2001). Intensive insulin therapy in critically ill patients. *New England Journal of Medicine, 345*(19), 1359–1367.

Walker & Morgan, LLC. (2007). *Degrees of burns: First, second, and third degree burns.* Retrieved June 9, 2008, from http://www.walkermorgan.com/html/degree-burns.html

Weaver, L. K., Howe, S., Hopkins, R., & Chan, K. J. (2000). Carboxyhemoglobin half-life in carbon monoxide poisoned patients treated with 100% at atmospheric pressure. *Chest, 117,* 801–808.

Weber, J., & McManus, A. (2004). Infection control in burn patients. *Burns, 30,* A16–A24.

White, D. J., Maass, D. L., Sanders, B., & Horton, J. W. (2002). Cardiomyocyte intracellular calcium and cardiac dysfunction after burn trauma. *Critical Care Medicine, 30,* 14.

chapter 14

Burns in the Mass Casualty Disaster Environment

Deborah A. DeLuca and Deborah S. Adelman

GOAL

The goal of this chapter is to explore the concepts of burn wound identification, burn victim stabilization, and treatment of the burn victim with emphasis on triage and treatment of injuries resulting from explosions or blasts.

OBJECTIVES

At the completion of this chapter, the reader will:

1. Explain what makes burn injuries in the mass casualty incident unique.
2. Summarize the different levels of mass burn casualty management.
3. Discuss concerns specific to triage of the mass casualty burn victim.
4. Review principles of management of burn injuries in mass casualty disasters.
5. Describe the U.S. National Response Plan.

Key Terms

- Mass casualty incident
- Burn disasters
- Mass burn casualty disaster management
- U.S. National Response Plan
- Coordinated burn disaster/mass casualty burn events
- Command, control, and communication
- Triage
- Personnel management
- Rehabilitation
- Burn specialty team

OBJECTIVES *(continued)*

6. Review past disasters and drills relating to mass casualty burn events.
7. Evaluate errors made in the past in caring for mass casualty burn victims.
8. Prepare a plan for management of mass casualty burn victims.

Introduction

This chapter focuses on applying the principles of burn wound injuries and strategies developed in Chapters 12 and 13 to the mass casualty disaster environment generally and, particularly, to the type of burn wounds attending explosion and radiation events in this era of heightened global terrorism concerns. This chapter is divided into two major sections: first, all concepts involved in mass casualty disaster management and burn wound identification, stabilization, and treatment; and, second, concepts involved in understanding all parameters involved in the triage, diagnosis, and management of explosions and blast injuries common with terrorism-based mass disaster events. A brief discussion of natural disaster and natural hazard events producing burn injuries is also presented, with the understanding that the burn concepts developed in this and previous chapters apply equally to the natural disaster scenario.

Mass Casualty Incidents and Burn Disasters

Knowledge and understanding of the various parameters involved in burn wound injury assessment and management are directly related to the morbidity and mortality statistics attending burn wound injury. The stakes are raised significantly when the number of victims that need to be assessed and stabilized increases substantially, such as in a mass casualty disaster incident. This chapter is devoted to exploring some key issues related to improving mortality statistics attending mass casualty burn disasters.

During the last three decades, substantial increases in burn wound injury survival and functional outcomes characterize modern burn wound care (Pham & Gibran, 2007). Successful burn treatment coming forward into this century is based on a multidisciplinary model incorporating surgical wound closure, critical care management, and rehabilitation. This success is directly attributed to the development of specialized burn centers, characterized by highly trained healthcare providers working within a collaborative specialized infrastructure and using care algorithms that address and serve the unique characteristics of burn victims (Pham & Gibran).

There are several elements of commonality that exist across specialized burn centers (Barillo, 2005; Pham & Gibran, 2007). For example, burn centers must deliver all aspects of burn wound care, from initial emergent care through rehabilitation. Regionalization of burn care has increased during the last two decades, with low-volume centers closing, resulting in referral of the seriously injured to regional burn centers for definitive care (Pham & Gibran). The American Burn Association (ABA) actively contributes to the regionalization process by creating and publishing burn center referral criteria (American College of Surgeons [ACS], 1999). In conjunction with the American College of Surgeons, the ABA established a burn center verification program; of the currently existing 139 burn centers in the United States, 43 have been certified through this program (Pham & Gibran). Such commitment to excellence, quality, and improving mortality statistics among the burn victim population suggests that regional certified burn centers will remain as epicenters in the foreseeable future.

Such burn centers come with a price, however. Specialized burn care demands the availability of highly trained healthcare providers, from surgeons, to nurses, psychologists, pharmacists, therapists, and physiatrists, to form the necessary multidisciplinary care team. Scope of practice and training must include both adult and pediatric care, including surgical critical care. Most physicians seek additional certification through burn fellowships, although only five to seven such certified physicians complete the certification annually, leaving many fellowship positions unfilled. A similar plight attends other burn team specialists; proficiency requires months of on-the-job training and many positions remain unfilled for months or years (Pham & Gibran, 2007). These issues raise serious concerns when one considers the need for rapid mobilization of resources and personnel during a mass burn casualty incident.

The Vietnam War provided the first glimpse into the problems attending large scale transport of field burn casualties (Klein, Nathens, Emerson, Heimbach, & Gibran, 2007; Pham & Gibran, 2007). At that time, burn field casualties were flown to the Brooke Army Medical Center in San Antonio, Texas (Pham & Gibran) and respirators were not readily available, causing several complications. Subsequently, burn victim transport today is more sophisticated, especially regarding the availability of respirators that contribute to better patient outcomes (Klein et al.).

Prehospital care and successful transport entails well-synchronized communication and coordination between highly trained personnel at the site of injury and the referring and receiving facilities, along with appropriate assessment and stabilization of the burn victim prior to and throughout transport (Dougherty & Waxman, 1996; Klein et al., 2007; Pham & Gibran, 2007; Rosenkranz & Sheridan, 2002; Sheridan, 2001). In the United States currently, coordinating transport from the burn site to regionalized burn center(s) is no small task, with these burn centers' regions encompassing over a quarter of the nation's total land mass (Pham & Gibran). Fortunately, outcomes are the same for burn victims who are directly admitted to local burn centers compared to those who are long-distance transfers (Klein et al.).

However, regionalized burn centers create challenges as well as address needs, especially in view of possible mass burn casualty incidents. Two important challenges are patient triage and coordinated transport over great distances (Pham & Gibran, 2007). For example, if a referring physician or EMS personnel mistakenly underestimates or overestimates total body surface area (TBSA) involvement, inappropriate initial care, increased morbidity and mortality, and unnecessary use of air transport resources often result, to the detriment of the patient at a minimum (Pham & Gibran; Saffle, Edelman, & Morris, 1999). The problem becomes even more troubling in view of mass burn casualty triage, stabilization, and management.

The Uniqueness of Mass Burn Casualty Management

Fear aside, burn disasters, called mass burn casualty incidents, are uncommon events. The definition of a mass burn casualty incident is "the number of patients and severity of their injuries exceed the capability of the institution" (ACS, 1999, p. 55). This definition implies that as few as five burn victims from a small house fire could overwhelm a burn center where burn nurses frequently work double shifts to cover all of the hospital intensive care units, overflow patients occupy burn center beds due to lack of space elsewhere, and step-down facilities house patients who belong in intensive care. Imagine the problems compounding rapidly in the face of hundreds or thousands of burn casualties resulting from a terrorist attack or large-scale structural fire. It can be seen from this that appropriate burn disaster planning in advance of an incident occurring is necessary on the national, regional, and local levels (Barillo, 2005, 2006; Cancio & Pruitt, 2005).

Terrorist incidents and plane crash experiences demonstrate that burn patients constitute a very small percentage of the tens or hundreds of injured. However, the resources consumed in burn incidents are significant. Consider the following: In the 2 weeks following the terrorist attacks on the World Trade Center (WTC) and Pentagon buildings in the United States in 2001, the massively injured victims quickly died, the "walking wounded" were treated and released, and fractures were reduced, plated, and the victims released from the hospital (Barillo, 2005; Pham & Gibran, 2007). However, burn patients surviving the initial attacks remained hospitalized for several more months, with attentive burn care teams addressing all concerns, while often working overtime (Barillo, 2005).

The terrorist attacks on the World Trade Center buildings and the Pentagon in 2001 served as a wake-up call to the nation regarding the need for quick access to specialized burn centers (Pham & Gibran, 2007; Yurt et al., 2005). Unfortunately, due to the two towers collapsing, the number of actual burn wound or any kind of casualties was relatively small (Pham & Gibran). Had the towers not collapsed, however, the number of burn wound casualties would have been much greater.

Responses of local hospitals in the aftermath of the World Trade Center attack are well documented (Cancio & Pruitt, 2005; Cushman, Pachter & Beaton, 2003; Pryor,

2003; Yurt et al., 2005). Additionally, Yurt and colleagues discussed experiences with casualties from the WTC disaster at the New York Presbyterian Hospital-Weill Cornell Medical Center burn center (Barillo, 2006; Yurt et al.). In the WTC attacks, only 39 surviving casualties sustained significant burn injuries; however, only 28% of these victims were actually triaged to burn centers. Yurt et al. qualified these statistics, quoting, "triage was only possible in the earliest minutes prior to the collapse of the WTC and . . . after that, escape and survival became the mission of the survivors" (Yurt et al., p. 117). Subsequently, only 21 patients were directly triaged to the New York Presbyterian burn center, and 66% of the remaining burn casualties were retriaged and assigned to other regional burn centers. These statistics highlight that improved triage, referral assessment, and transport methods on all levels—local, regional, and national—need to be in place prior to the next mass casualty event (Pham & Gibran, 2007; Yurt et al.).

Another mass casualty event highlighting the need for better disaster management and burn casualty coordination followed the WTC disaster just 17 months later. In February 2003, the nation's fourth deadliest fire occurred in Rhode Island, at the Station Nightclub (Cancio & Pruitt, 2005; Harrington, Biffl, & Cioffi, 2005). Significant time was lost in this event, even though a triage station was set directly across the street from the club soon after the fire. Highlights of the debriefing focus on deficient medical command and control, referral decisions being made by individual ambulance crews, and poor communication between the on-site EMS personnel, the burn center, and among regional hospitals. Thus, an obvious lack of real-time situational awareness of hospital capabilities and patient movement throughout the region existed (Harrington, Biffl, & Cioffi). This event prompted the American College of Surgeons Committee on Trauma to develop a statewide trauma system, complete with central command and communication structures (Cancio & Pruitt; Harrington, Biffl, & Cioffi).

Clearly, principles for appropriate management of burn disasters are identifiable. Basically, these principles are no different from those applicable to other mass casualty events, with the clarifying modifications specifically addressing the unique features of thermal injury and the attendant disaster. Assuming that most fire disasters are chaotic, the events and actions attending the fire disaster are hardly random and certain behaviors by victims, their friends and relatives, and emergency response personnel are predictable (Cancio & Pruitt, 2005). Therefore, effective and efficient response must include efforts to understand, acclimatize, and respond to the ensuing chaos, thereby establishing prompt, reasonable command, and control of all casualty care (Cancio & Pruitt; Harrington, Biffl, & Cioffi, 2007). The primary principles that must be addressed in any mass casualty burn event are disaster planning; command, control, and communication; triage; transport; treatment strategies; personnel needs; equipment and supplies; transfer; rehabilitation and long-term follow-up; and after-action review. Each of these principles is discussed next.

Mass Burn Casualty Management: Disaster Planning

Mass burn casualty disaster management requires establishment of disaster plans for the hospital, community, region, and nation, which anticipate how to handle the massive numbers of burn wound victims attendant to a mass casualty burn event. More importantly, understanding how the local disaster management plan fits within the region, state, and nation's mass casualty disaster management plans, known as the U.S. National Response Plan (USNRP), is essential, due to the USNRP's complexity (Cancio & Pruitt, 2005).

Mass Burn Casualty Management: Command, Control, and Communication

An incident command system (ICS) is essential to coordinate an effective burn disaster response. The ICS, discussed in several previous chapters, serves as a redundant communication format between first-line responders, receiving regional burn centers, and hospitals and triage. Communication capabilities established between the burn center and the regional disaster response system serve to coordinate responses early in the fire disaster timeline. Additionally, activating the ICS as soon as possible during the disaster response ensures efficient flow from triage through referral and transport, ensuring the rational distribution of burn victims to available beds (Cancio & Pruitt, 2005).

Mass Burn Casualty Management: Triage Concerns

As eloquently stated, "for the surgeon facing 30 victims of urban terrorism, the 3–4 badly injured but salvageable patients are the hidden crux of the entire effort" (Hirshberg, 2004, p. 323). In a mass burn casualty disaster, triaging casualties at the scene involves activating state and local response systems, as well as actual assessment and stabilization of the burn victim(s) at the scene (Cancio & Pruitt, 2005; Pham & Gibran, 2007). On the state level, burn specialty teams are specialized disaster medical assistance teams consisting of burn-experienced personnel who provide assistance as needed in the initial care of burn victims (Pham & Gibran). Federally, there are four regional burn specialty teams (Cancio & Pruitt) currently available for federal deployment, formed after the WTC attack and Station Nightclub fire, to support local resources during the initial ensuing minutes and hours postincident.

Locally, triage postburn incidents require quick evaluation of each victim's injury severity, using TBSA estimations as discussed in the previous chapter: age and the presence or absence of inhalation injury or severe mechanical trauma. Assessment is made by seeking those victims with nonsurvivable burns, defined as the lethal area, LA50, for a given age group, or approximately 80% TBSA involvement for young adults. The LA50 assessment estimates that for every individual having 80% TBSA burn wound involvement, 50% are expected to survive, known as the expectant group (Cancio & Pruitt, 2005). Applying this theory to the mass burn casualty environment, triaging victims into expectant groups begins an evidence-based approach to trauma management and similar assessments are performed at the individual burn center and regional burn center levels. Secondary triage assessments are made for inhalation injury and severe mechanical trauma; this calculation adds 10% to the TBSA involvement assessment, thereby reducing the LA50 by 10% to 40% (Cancio & Pruitt; Mackie & Koning, 1990). Similarly, on the opposite end of the triage spectrum, individuals with minimal wounds involving less than 10% TBSA are triaged into the minimal care group. Experience shows that over time, 80% of victims will have non-life-threatening burns of 20% TBSA or less, thereby allowing delay of services to these individuals without significant effect on morbidity and mortality (Cancio & Pruitt).

Concern in triage focuses on who performs the triage assessments. The most qualified individual is normally an experienced burn surgeon (Mackie & Koning, 1990). In mass casualty environments, where inexperienced providers make most of the initial assessments, the likelihood of overestimating TBSA involvement is considerable (Cancio & Pruitt, 2005). Overestimating TBSA involvement usually results in one of two likely outcomes: triaging patients with large but survivable burns to the incorrect expectant group or increasing mortality rates of critically injured victims by inundating overwhelmed hospital facilities or burn centers with noncritical care patients (Frykberg, 2002). Neither outcome is favorable for the victims or the support teams.

These likely results highlight the fact that triage should be conducted outside of the hospital environment, initially at the scene of disaster, in an appropriately tiered manner to avoid overwhelming the system. Tiered triage involves making assessments at three separate levels: (a) Level 1 triage, where victims are separated by designation as acute or nonacute; (b) Level 2 triage, where the acute victims identified in Level 1 are further subdivided and grouped as delayed, immediate, minimal, expectant, or dead; and (c) Level 3 triage, where victims are sorted on referral priority and need to evacuate. When no experienced burn surgeon is available on site to assess and triage victims, victims are triaged into the three aforementioned levels upon arrival at the hospital, *prior to* entering the emergency department (ED). Once triage occurs, those victims identified as nonemergent with minimal injuries are immediately referred to an appropriate outpatient facility in a timely manner and are hence kept away from the ED, avoiding overwhelming the system (Cancio & Pruitt, 2005).

Triage is a dynamic process. Continued assessment of victims is necessary throughout the process every few hours and may result in changes to triage categories for some individuals (Cancio & Pruitt, 2005). Triage does not end when victims arrive at the designated care facility; rather secondary triage ensues, enabling appropriate and timely transfer of victims to available burn unit beds.

Mass Burn Casualty Management: Transfer

Here, the triage process on site focuses on securing appropriate transport for victims. Too often, uncoordinated evacuation of victims occurs, resulting in overwhelming the receiving facility and depriving patients of appropriate and expeditious medical care (Cancio & Pruitt, 2005). However, uncoordinated evacuation will likely occur nonetheless, at rates equivalent to the size and scope of the disaster in question.

Mass Burn Casualty Management: Treatment Strategy and Approaches

As stated in Chapter 13, once a victim arrives at the designated treatment facility, care becomes labor intensive for just that one victim. Extended to the mass casualty burn environment, careful thought is necessary to manage the possibly large number of victims arriving and needing emergent care and to allocate the limited number of burn wound experienced personnel effectively (Cancio & Pruitt, 2005). Since the Advanced Trauma Life Support (ATLS) algorithm is followed to stabilize the victim (discussed in Chapter 13), instituting teams focusing on specific care functions seems to make sense. However, in the current environment of evidence-based practice, this methodology does not appear to be clearly tested and reported upon in currently available literature.

Because of this lack of evidence-based practice, one strategy that appears to be reasonable and supported is assigning a single caregiver, usually a critical care nurse, to the victim (Cancio & Pruitt, 2005; Yurt et al., 2005). The critical care nurse accompanies the victim throughout the initial phases of care, thereby taking full responsibility for all critical interventions and information exchange (Yurt et al., 2005). Incorporating the standardized and simplified clinical practice guidelines for burn management, both before the burn incident and throughout, effectively utilizes skill sets available within the care team and facilitates integration of nonburn personnel during the ensuing crisis period (Cancio & Pruitt; Yurt et al., 2005).

Mass Burn Casualty Management: Personnel Management and Coordination

When mass casualty burn disasters occur, healthcare providers often descend upon the scene in hopes of assisting the survivors. This raises concerns about the balance between appropriate on-site triage and counterproductive efforts, as well as increased danger to all responding from inexperienced and untrained healthcare professionals. As one prudent observer noted during the immediate period subsequent to the WTC events, "Cowboy initiatives begin. Doctors attempt to commandeer transport to go to the site carrying potentially scarce supplies, such as morphine" (Lipkin, 2002, p. 704).

Although the desire to help those in need is admirable, such cavalier action actually places providers at risk and unnecessarily harms victims (Cancio & Pruitt, 2005). "Physicians and nurses . . . scattered in fear when rumors of an adjacent building's imminent collapse circulated" (Cushman, Pachter, & Beaton, 2003, p. 152). Inevitably, volunteers will come to a disaster site to offer assistance, thereby presenting several opportunities for coordination of the volunteers' and disaster medical support personnel's activities. Here, providing psychological debriefing for healthcare providers and coordinating rest schedules, work hours, and meal plans become the focus (Cancio & Pruitt; Cushman, Pachter, & Beaton).

Mass Burn Casualty Management: Supplies and Equipment

Many times during burn disasters, equipment and supplies specific to the care and stabilization of multiple burn victims are in short supply. Appropriate planning by local, regional, state, and federal disaster response teams involves maintaining a list of supplies and equipment needed to support any mass casualty disaster, complete with price lists, catalogs, and ordering information to greatly accelerate obtaining supplies during an emergency (Cancio & Pruitt, 2005; Harrington, Biffl, & Cioffi, 2005). Where burn disaster is concerned specifically, additional information for equipment particular to the prehospital emergency care assessments and stabilization of victims, as discussed in Chapter 13, should be included to cover the first 72 hours postinjury, for on-site stabilization of the victim, surgical care, laboratory support, and rehabilitation as appropriate (Cancio & Pruitt).

Mass Burn Casualty Management: Transfer and Transport Concerns

As discussed in Chapters 12 and 13, appreciation of the capabilities and limitations of the hospital and its personnel, the local and regional support teams, and the nation to appropriately care for burn victims of a mass burn casualty disasters must be recognized. The ABA, in conjunction with the ACS, recognizes that victims with severe thermal injuries require care in nationally recognized burn centers, and both have published guidelines for referral (ACS, 1999; Cancio & Pruitt, 2005; Gomez & Cancio, 2007; Mertens, Jenkins, & Warden, 1997; Rockwell & Erlich, 1990).

Transporting burn victims over short distances is usually undertaken by EMS personnel who do not usually have extensive burn wound stabilization experience. When long-distance transport is needed from a disaster site, the burn flight teams (BFTs) based at the U.S. Army Institute of Surgical Research (USAISR, the U.S. Army Burn Center) are used to coordinate and effectuate aeromedical evacuation of burn victims (Cancio & Pruitt, 2005). Team members include a burn surgeon, a critical care registered nurse, a licensed practical nurse, a respiratory therapist, and an operations sergeant, usually a senior LPN. All personnel included come from burn intensive care units and complete the U.S. Air Force Critical Care Air Transport (CCAT) course.

The Vietnam War again provides historical evidentiary support for using aeromedical evacuation for burn victims, despite risks attendant to transporting unstable burn victims by air (Cancio & Pruitt, 2005; Klein et al., 2007; Pham & Gibran,

2007). During that time, the U.S. Army burn flight teams accomplished 103 aeromedical missions, successfully transporting 824 burn victims from Japan to the U.S. Army Burn Center in San Antonio, Texas (Klein et al.). Only one in-flight death occurred during those air transfers of severely burned, critically ill victims, suggesting the value of aeromedical evacuation from mass casualty disaster settings, provided that appropriate triage occurs first (Cancio & Pruitt; Klein et al.).

Transporting critically injured burn victims from a mass casualty setting occurs only after hemodynamic stability is achieved, yet before the risk for infection developing intervenes. Ideally, air transport occurs between days 1 and 4 postinjury. Statistically, this time period is supported: between 1980 and 1985, the USAISR transported 1196 burn victims, including 542 out-of-state transfers and 59 out-of-country transfers across a cumulative total distance of 850,000 air miles, without a single in-air mortality or major complication (Cancio & Pruitt, 2005). The mean burn size of these air transported victims was 35.9% TBSA, with 52.3% presenting with inhalation injury as well.

Stabilizing the burn-injured victims preflight is required and involves placing an intravenous cannula, nasogastric tube, and Foley catheter (Cancio & Pruitt, 2005; Treat, Sirinek, Levine, & Pruitt, 1980). If needed, endotracheal intubation, escharotomy, fluid volume assessment for burn shock, thoracostomy, and burn wound dressings application should occur preflight as well. Sufficient supplies and equipment are transported with the victim to effect any in-flight changes, including equipment for airway intubation, maintenance, and ventilation (Cancio & Pruitt). Additionally, long-range aeromedical evacuation of intubated victims is facilitated by a pneumatic, time-cycled, pressure-limited transport ventilator and Kevlar–aluminum composite oxygen cylinder (Barillo, Dickerson, Cioffi, Monzingo, & Pruitt, 1997; Cancio & Pruitt). Advanced preparation for unforeseen complications in-flight lessens the risk of mortality to the burn victim.

Mass Burn Casualty Management: Rehabilitation and Long-Term Care

Mass burn casualty disaster response includes the physical, occupational, and psychological rehabilitation of the survivors and is incorporated into the relief operations from onset (Cancio & Pruitt, 2005). This does not overshadow initial lifesaving resuscitation and surgery during the first days and hours postburn injury; however, long-term rehabilitation is necessary for the severely injured and intensifies over time after the initial resuscitation period.

Mass Burn Casualty Management: After-Action Review

Self-critical assessment of the burn disaster team's effectiveness in managing the mass casualty burn event embodies the final consideration in mass casualty burn management generally (Cancio & Pruitt, 2005; Cushman, Pachter, & Beaton, 2003). Assessment focuses on needed changes in the mass casualty burn disaster plan, equipment and supply levels, and staffing.

A Comment on the U.S. National Response Plan

As mentioned above, United States disaster response, based on the National Response Plan (NRP), is multitiered, recognizing the federal government's structure and the limitations placed on federal involvement in local activities; the plan also focuses on containing military involvement (Cancio & Pruitt, 2005; U.S. Department of Health & Human Services, n.d.). Normally, the U.S. government will not intervene in mass casualty disasters, preferring to take a back seat to medical response available. The normal progression of response includes, from most likely to least likely to respond: local, regional/county, and state response, followed by National Disaster Medical System (NDMS) and military support to civil authorities. (See Chapters 1 and 2 for more on this topic.)

Integrating these levels of response is hugely challenging. In the post 9/11 period, the U.S. government attempted to respond to the challenges presented at the WTC and Pentagon sites by forming the Department of Homeland Security (DHS) (Cancio & Pruitt, 2005). Homeland Security Presidential Directive (HSPD) 5, Management of Domestic Incidents, mandated the U.S. government to "establish a single, comprehensive approach to domestic incident management . . . to ensure that all levels of government across the Nation have the capability to work efficiently and effectively together" (Cancio & Pruitt, p. 12). This means that the DHS secretary is wholly responsible for domestic incident management, which means that local and state officials handle the bulk of the response, with the federal government assisting when state capabilities are overwhelmed or federal interests are involved, as described in Chapter 1.

An offshoot of the HSP directive created in 1984 is the NDMS, a federally coordinated system augmenting the nation's medical response capability (U.S. Department of Health & Human Services, n.d.). The NDMS is responsible for coordinating and managing the federal medical response to major emergencies and federally declared disasters, including natural disasters (e.g., Hurricane Katrina), major transportation accidents (e.g., airline carrier crashes investigated by the National Transportation Safety Board [NTSB]), and technological disasters and terrorism attacks involving weapons of mass destruction (WMDs) (Cancio & Pruitt, 2005; U.S. Department of Health & Human Services). The NDMS resides within the Federal Emergency Management Agency (FEMA) and works with the Department of Defense (DOD) and Department of Veterans' Affairs (VA) (Cancio & Pruitt).

Activating the NDMS occurs in one of three ways: (a) the government of a state may request presidential declaration of a disaster or emergency, (b) a state health officer requests NDMS activation through the Department of Health and Human Services (now the CMS), or (c) NDMS activation is requested by the Assistant Secretary of Defense for Health Affairs when patient levels exceed DOD and VA levels (Cancio & Pruitt, 2005). The functions of the NDMS are three-fold: (a) medical response to the disaster site, (b) patient movement from disaster area to unaffected areas of the nation, and (c) definitive medical care at participating hospitals in unaffected areas (Cancio & Pruitt; U.S. Department of Health & Human Services, n.d.)

When a mass casualty burn disaster occurs, the NDMS activates regional disaster medical assistance teams (DMATs), thereby augmenting local existing capabilities for medical response to the disaster (Cancio & Pruitt, 2005). Each DMAT is sponsored by a major medical center or similar institution and includes burn specialty teams (BSTs) for specific response to burn disasters. The BST includes 15 especially burn-experienced personnel:

1. Surgeon team leader
2. Six registered nurses
3. One anesthesia provider
4. One respiratory therapist
5. One administrative officer
6. Five additional support personnel

All of these specialists are selected based on the mission's projected requirements (Cancio & Pruitt). There are only four BSTs nationwide. They are located in Boston, Massachusetts; Gainesville, Florida; Galveston, Texas; and St. Paul, Minnesota. Two more BSTs are planned.

Each BST is affiliated with a local DMAT, ensuring asset sharing (Cancio & Pruitt, 2005). In reality, the DMAT/BST relationship provides the community with resources for state and local requirements, but can be federalized as needed to support national needs (Cancio & Pruitt; U.S. Department of Health & Human Services, n.d.). For example, during the WTC disaster on September 11, 2001, DMATs from Maine, New Jersey, Rhode Island, New York, and the BST from Massachusetts were federalized and deployed to New York City (Sholl & Riley, 2001).

One important contribution of the NDMS that was first mobilized in response to the WTC attack is the Strategic National Stockpile (SNS) program, formerly called the National Pharmaceutical Stockpile. Activating the SNS provides needed pharmaceutical supplies to disaster teams, such as intravenous fluids and medications, airway supplies, dressings, and emergency medications. The SNS is administered in conjunction with the Centers for Disease Control and Prevention (CDC) under the Department of Health and Human Services (Cancio & Pruitt, 2005).

Integrating the nation's burn care capabilities with the NDMS is still challenging (Cancio & Pruitt, 2005). Two primary problems exist: First, because not all burn centers are members of the NDMS, and many are not even located in one of the NDMS metropolitan areas, the burn centers do not receive burn casualties under the NDMS (Wachte, Cowan, & Reardon, 1989). Second, many hospitals that report burn bed availability to the NDMS do not care for burn-injured patients ordinarily. Because of the idea that burn centers should be used for burn casualties, the NDMS recognized a classification scheme for hospitals to receive burn victims: Level 1 burn centers would be verified by the ABA, and Level 2 and Level 3 burn centers would be other hospitals that would occasionally receive and care for burn patients (Cancio & Pruitt; Wachte, Cowan, & Reardon).

Establishing a national burn center bed-reporting system came about as one result of the Gulf War in 1990 to 1991. The principle behind this system was simple: Burn centers should care for burn victims, and full-scale war could exceed the U.S. Army Burn Center's (in San Antonio, Texas) capacity. The current Iraq conflict, which began in March 2003, reinforced this system's implementation. Seventy burn centers in the United States report their daily burn bed availability by electronic mail to the USAISR. This information is coordinated and transferred to the NDMS, the U.S. Air Force, and the American Burn Association, as well as to the appointed liaison officer in the U.S. military hospital at Landstuhl, Germany (Cancio & Pruitt, 2005). This system in theory permits regulation of burn casualties from Landstuhl, Germany, to burn centers with open beds near aeromedical evacuation locations within the United States, if large numbers of burn casualties require burn center care (Barillo, Jordan, et al., 2005; Cancio & Pruitt). Unfortunately, this system has been activated only briefly; the last time in 2004 in response to a fire disaster in Paraguay. Again, recognizing the need and desirability of maintaining such a system on a permanent basis, system testing is being revisited (Cancio & Pruitt).

One last important component of the NDMS is the U.S. Army Special Medical Augmentation Response Teams (SMARTs) created in 1998. SMARTs are designed to provide short-duration medical assistance to local, state, federal, and DOD agencies during disaster response; civil–military cooperative actions; humanitarian missions; WMD incidences; or chemical, biological, radiological, nuclear, or explosive (CBRNE) incidents. Currently, 37 Army SMARTs exist, each consisting of 2 to 12 personnel who specialize in any of the following fields: emergency medicine; medical management of nuclear, biological, or chemical incidents; medical command and control; communications, telemedicine, pastoral care, and stress management; preventive medicine and burns; veterinary medicine; aeromedical isolation transport; and health systems assessments and assistance (Cancio & Pruitt, 2005).

Focusing on mass casualty burn disaster management, there are two specific SMARTs existing at the U.S. Army Burn Center at the U.S. Army Institute of Surgical Research, Brooke Army Medical Center, Fort Sam Houston, Texas. These SMARTs are identical to the burn flight teams established in 1951, discussed previously. These teams specialize in burn triage and resuscitation, managing inhalation injury and respiratory failure, trauma management, evacuation, and aeromedical transfers of burn victims. Additionally, these specialized burn SMART teams provide additional mechanical ventilation expertise regardless of the reason for lung failure, such as mustard gas or nerve agents (Cancio & Pruitt, 2005). Therefore, burn SMARTs are used predominantly for long-range aeromedical evacuation of combat burn casualties and assistance to foreign governments during and following mass burn casualty events (Cancio & Pruitt, 2005).

Clearly, understanding the integration of burn disaster response and management from local to federal levels provides a means by which communities can adequately prepare for mass burn casualty disasters of any type or mechanism. For communities to respond appropriately to mass burn casualty events, communities must have viable disaster plans in place as well as be able to exercise the plan under strenuous and realistic conditions (Cancio & Pruitt, 2005). Commitment by all involved organizations and attendant personnel is the key to effective preparation and response to mass burn casualty disasters. Admittedly, the concept of burn disaster management is evolving from a singly prepared, planned disaster response to embracing all-hazards approaches.

Practical Examples of Coordinated Burn Disaster or Mass Casualty Burn Events

Practicing for disaster events enables burn response teams to appropriately triage mass burn casualty events—writing disaster plans and placing them in binders on shelves alone does not. Generally, primary triage assigns treatment and transportation priorities to multiple casualties, provided adequate preparation of care teams occurs first (Greenfield & Winfree, 2005; Welling et al., in press). Routinely practicing with simulated exercises does not adequately replicate the actual turn of events when mass casualty burn injuries suddenly occur. In the next section, two burn casualty management events are explained to provide examples and proof of their effectiveness. Both concern a medical disaster response with large volumes of burn casualties, the success of which depends on appropriate preparation and planning, prior history, lessons learned, and postevent assessment.

The first incident managed by the U.S. Army Burn Center resulted from an aircraft crash on March 23, 1994, at Pope Air Force Base, Fayetteville, North Carolina, known as the "Disaster on Green Ramp." This event was so named because approximately 500 paratroopers were located on a staging area called the "green ramp" preparing for a training exercise. The crash, which occurred 50 yards from the ramp, created a fireball of burning aviation fuel and flying debris that engulfed the troops. Ten soldiers died immediately; another 130 soldiers were injured. Fifty-one casualties were treated at Fort Bragg, North Carolina; 25 were admitted to burn intensive care units, and 30 were admitted to acute care wards. Six were transferred to local hospitals, and seven were transported to the Jaycee Burn Center in Chapel Hill, North Carolina (Greenfield & Winfree, 2005).

Just one day later, 20 severely injured burn patients from the Green Ramp disaster, each having from 6% to 88% TBSA involvement, were moved to the U.S. Army Institute of Surgical Research (USAISR) in San Antonio, Texas. Of these 20 burn victims, 13 were mechanically ventilated. The next day, another 23 burn victims from Green Ramp were transported to USAISR, bringing the total count to 43 burn patients. Depletion of trained personnel occurred quickly. The first

20 victims sent to USAISR were accompanied by ISR flight team members, specifically by four registered nurses, four licensed practical nurses, three surgeons, and four respiratory therapists, all who flew to Fort Bragg to stabilize the victims and move them to San Antonio (Greenfield & Winfree, 2005). Having all 15 members attending this one set of patients rapidly depleted available personnel as the flight teams worked continuously for 24 hours.

As described later, the first few hours postevent proceeded as a well-choreographed dance without panic or confusion. Transport proceeded smoothly as well, due to the prior training personnel received. Subsequent admission of burn victims was orderly due to coordinated teamwork and regularly rehearsed mass casualty exercises and prior mass casualty experience. However, when the burn center reached 53 total victims, skills and personnel were stretched to capacity, many working 60-hour weeks. Although 33% of the staff had prior experience in mass casualty events, 32% at USAISR had no prior experience, and only 32% had some limited prior experience (Greenfield & Winfree, 2005).

Institutional memory provided the only recollection of after-action assessments completed after previous disasters. The Green Ramp disaster highlighted concerns for appropriate disaster management. As time progressed, communication between team members, family, friends, victims, and military dignitaries degraded. Inconsistencies in reporting and coordinating activities caused confusion. Problems identified in the post-Green Ramp assessment led to the development and implementation of a centralized communication center in the public affairs office; additional recommendations and lessons learned were written into a formal after-action report and incorporated into the USAISR's emergency preparedness plan (Greenfield & Winfree, 2005).

In January 2003, the nation was alerted to a possible war in the Middle East. Historical data quickly gathered indicated that burn wound injuries alone could account for as many as 10–20% of casualties suffered and that 20% of those casualty injuries would be life threatening. The USAISR was designated as the facility for the projected burn wound care should it occur. Expansion to 40 beds was immediately undertaken, with further expansion to 60-bed capacity possible on short notice. The Green Ramp disaster and its lessons provided the USAISR with the requisite knowledge to appropriately plan for any burn contingency and was successfully used to prepare for the possible conflict in the Middle East (Greenfield & Winfree, 2005). The planning became a multidisciplinary effort.

Although burn wound management is also interdisciplinary, it is nursing personnel who spend the most time at the burn victim's bedside. Consequently, having nurses available to augment existing staff is the single most delimiting factor to how many burn victims can be appropriately treated. Therefore, during the preparations for the possible armed conflict, concern quickly developed regarding appropriate preparation of first responders for initial on-site management of burn wound casualties. Personnel staffing databases created during the Green Ramp disaster were activated and expanded to facilitate hiring skilled personnel. Additionally, personnel were encouraged to register with local agencies to confirm credentialing and engage in intensive burn wound training (Greenfield & Winfree, 2005).

These two events demonstrate that the quality of burn wound care available in the hours immediately following mass burn casualty disasters directly affects long-term outcomes (Greenfield & Winfree, 2005). One should not forget that initial burn wound care after the mass casualty event occurs is not provided in a controlled environment but on site, outside of the burn center environment. This means that adhering to the American Burn Association's advanced burn life support course and combat burn life support course algorithms of care could enhance training in stabilization, triage, and aeromedical evacuation of victims sustaining severe or minor burn and attendant polytrauma injuries (Barillo, Jordan, et al., 2005; Greenfield & Winfree, 2005).

The point of these examples is not about how the USAISR handled the two mass burn casualty events but about how effective response to medical disasters involving mass casualties depends upon appropriate planning, preparation, institutional history, and postevent assessment (Greenfield & Winfree, 2005). Consider, if triage is directly related to postburn injury outcomes as postulated, then positioning appropriate medical response in advance of ensuing events ensures successful handling of the mass casualty burn event immediately following the incident. The value of well-conceived disaster planning and training cannot be understated or underestimated. Exemplifying the key role appropriate mass casualty burn disaster planning has, consider the following additional examples of success and failure.

In 1980, during the MGM Grand Hotel fire in Las Vegas, Nevada, 3,000 people were triaged within 3.5 hours of the incident (Cancio & Pruitt, 2005; Barillo, Jordan, et al., 2005). Approximately 726 patients were referred to local hospitals; 1,700 more were classified as minimally injured or displaced and were relocated to a remote refugee area away from the incident site by school bus. One single on-site triage point was established but was quickly overwhelmed. To address this problem, quick action occurred: two additional triage sites were set on the hotel grounds and a common central command post was established to coordinate efforts between the three locations on campus (Barillo, Jordan, et al.). This advanced preparation for a mass casualty burn event certainly provided maximal patient outcomes, at least from the point of triage on site through transport to care facilities.

Now contrast the MGM Grand Hotel fire successes with the world's worst liquid petroleum gas (LPG) disaster in San Juanico, Mexico, in 1984 (Cancio & Pruitt, 2005; Barillo, Jordan, et al., 2005). Here there was no apparent predisaster planning methodology in place. Following the explosion, there was no organized evacuation plan, and chaos characterized both the site and triage efforts. In this burn-based disaster, 625 individuals were hospitalized with burn injuries (Barillo, Jordan, et al.). Of these 625 victims, 350 were admitted to just 2 hospitals, completely overwhelming the respective hospitals' infrastructures, as evidenced by the 140 individuals who died in the first 5 days postinjury. Patient rescue was hampered by refugees who choked the roads surrounding the site, who were given no direction on where to go, how to get there, or how to remain safe and out of the way of harm and rescue efforts. The only disaster preparedness plan available was through the Mexican army's earthquake disaster plan, which clearly provided little benefit (Cancio & Pruitt; Barillo, Jordan, et al.).

Summary on Mass Burn Casualty Disaster Management

These four examples of successes and failures in mass casualty burn incidents management must provide at least one lesson learned or the same mistakes will continue to be repeated, and more and more burn victims will suffer poor outcomes postincident. Some of these incidents are several years old, and others are more recent. What mass casualty lesson(s) learned can come from an almost 25-year spread of incidents? The question is best answered by the following question: What would each burn team know postincident that they only wished they knew preincident? The best single answer upon which all else is based is this: knowing if there was a burn disaster response plan that is adequately integrated at least with other emergency response systems on the local and state levels (Barillo, 2005). A burn disaster plan created in a vacuum is no plan; this is why developing an integrated preevent plan and training for it through drills and tabletop exercises is so important.

As stated previously, fortunately, the mass burn casualty event is not a common one; rather, the next likely burn disaster will be more small scale, involving perhaps 5 to 10 victims locally who experience a thermal or nonthermal incident. The burn center will become the central player in the long-term care and successful outcome of the burn injured victims.

Conclusion

Whether a mass casualty burn event or localized small-scale thermal or nonthermal event occurs becomes irrelevant in a sense. Clearly, burn centers need adequate disaster plans properly drawn and integrated in anticipation of the possible large-scale burn disaster. As suggested, the burn center's disaster response plan should be integrated from the local level to the state level of disaster planning at a minimum, in conjunction with the local prehospital system, the state emergency management system, the hospital emergency department, and trauma services (Barillo, 2005). Advanced preparation and a well-developed plan prevents the chaos that multiple, ill-conceived trauma, burn, prehospital, and emergency department disaster plans cause in the presence of multiple burn victims, when every healthcare provider is following a different protocol and resources are stretched beyond normal limits.

Once the basic concepts, principles, and processes involved in general mass casualty burn incident management are understood, the next step involves applying these concepts, principles, and processes of mass casualty burn incident management to specific types of incidents and wounds encountered: blast burn injuries, chemical burn injuries, and radiation burn injuries. Each of these burn incidents and wound triage required are discussed in the next chapter.

References

American College of Surgeons, Committee on Trauma. (1999). Guidelines for the operations of burn units. Resources for optimal care of the injured patient. *American College of Surgeons, 55,* 55–62.

Barillo, D. J. (2005). Burn disasters and mass casualty incidents. *Journal of Burn Care Rehabilitation, 26,* 107–108.

Barillo, D. J. (2006). Burn centers and disaster response. *Journal of Burn Care Rehabilitation, 27*(5), 558–559.

Barillo, D. J., Cancio, L. C., Hutton, B. G., Mittlesteadt, P. J., Gueller, G. E., & Holcomb, J. B. (2005). Combat burn life support: A military burn education program. *Journal of Burn Care Rehabilitation, 26*(2), 162–165.

Barillo, D. J., Dickerson, E. E., Cioffi, W. G., Monzingo, D. W., & Pruitt, B. A., Jr. (1997). Pressure-controlled ventilation for the long-range aeromedical transport of patients with burns. *Journal of Burn Care Rehabilitation, 18,* 200–205.

Barillo, D. J., Jordan, M. H., Jocz, R., Nye, D., Cancio, L. C., & Holcomb, J. B. (2005). Tracking the daily availability of burn beds for national emergencies. *Journal of Burn Care Rehabilitation, 26,* 174–182.

Cancio, L. C., & Pruitt, B. (2005). Management of mass casualty burn disasters. *International Journal of Disaster Medicine,* 1–16.

Cushman, J. G., Pachter, H. L, & Beaton, H. L. (2003). Two New York City hospitals' surgical response to the September 11, 2001, terrorist attack in New York City. *Journal of Trauma, 54,* 147–154.

Dougherty, W., & Waxman, K. (1996). Complex and challenging problems in trauma surgery: The complexities of managing severe burns with associated trauma. *Surgical Clinics of North America, 76*(4), 923–958.

Frykberg, E. R. (2002). Medical management of disasters and mass casualties from terrorist bombings: How can we cope? *Journal of Trauma, 53,* 201–212.

Gomez, R., & Cancio, L. C. (2007). Management of burn wounds in the emergency department. *Emergency Medicine Clinics of North America, 25,* 135–146.

Greenfield, E., & Winfree, J. (2005). Nursing's role in the planning, preparation and response to burn disaster or mass casualty events. *Journal of Burn Care Rehabilitation, 26*(2), 166–169.

Harrington, D. T., Biffl, W. L., & Cioffi, W. G. (2005). The station nightclub fire. *Journal of Burn Care Rehabilitation, 26*(2), 141–143.

Hirshberg, A. (2004). Multiple casualty incidents: Lessons from the front line. *Annals of Surgery, 239,* 322–324.

Klein, M. B., Nathens, A. B., Emerson, D., Heimbach, D. M., & Gibran, N. S. (2007). Analysis of the long-distance transport of burn patients to a regional burn center. *Journal of Burn Care and Research, 28*(1), 49–55.

Lipkin, M. (2002). Medical ground zero: An early experience of the World Trade Center disaster. *Annals of Internal Medicine, 136,* 704–707.

Mackie, D. P., & Koning, H. M. (1990). Fate of mass burn casualties: Implications for disaster planning. *Burns, 16,* 203–206.

Mertens, D. M., Jenkins, M. E., & Warden, G. D. (1997). Outpatient burn management. *Nursing Clinics of North America, 32,* 343–346.

Pham, T. N., & Gibran, N. S. (2007). Thermal and electrical injuries. *Surgical Clinics of North America, 87,* 185–206.

Pryor, J. P. (2003). The 2001 World Trade Center disaster—summary and evaluation of experiences. *International Journal of Disaster Medicine, 1,* 56–58.

Rockwell, W. B., & Erlich, H. P. (1990). Should burn blister fluid be evacuated? *Journal of Burn Care Rehabilitation, 11,* 93–95.

Rosenkranz, K., & Sheridan, R. (2002). Management of the burned trauma patient: Balancing conflicting priorities. *Burns, 28,* 665–669.

Saffle, J. R., Edelman, L., & Morris, S. E. (1999). Regional air transport of burn patients: A case for telemedicine? *Journal of Telemedical Telecare, 5*(Suppl 1), S52–S54.

Sheridan, R. (2001). Current problems in surgery: Comprehensive treatment of burns. *Current Problems in Surgery, 38,* 641–756.

Sholl, M., & Riley, J. M. (2001). Ground zero: Metro Boston Area DMAT's notes from the field. *Journal of Emergency Nursing, 27,* 556–558.

Treat, R. C., Sirinek, K. R., Levine, B. A., & Pruitt, B. A., Jr. (1980). Air evacuation of thermally injured patients: Principles of treatment and results. *Journal of Trauma, 20,* 275–279.

U.S. Department of Health and Human Services. (n.d.). *National Disaster Medical System.* Retrieved March 20, 2008, from http://www.hhs.gov/aspr/opeo/ndms/index.html

Wachte, T. L., Cowan, M. L., & Reardon, J. D. (1989). Developing a regional and national burn disaster response. *Journal of Burn Care Rehabilitation, 10,* 561–567.

Welling, L., vanHarten, S. M., Henny, C. P., Mackie, D. P., Ubbink, D. T., Kreis, R. W., et al. (in press). Selected topics: Disaster medicine: Reliability of the primary triage process after the Volendam fire disaster. *Journal of Emergency Medicine.*

Yurt, R. W., Bessey, P. Q., Bauer, G. J., Dembicki, R., Laznick, H., Aldenz, N., et al. (2005). A regional burn center's response to a disaster: September 11, 2001, and the days beyond. *Journal of Burn Care Rehabilitation, 26*(2), 117–124.

chapter 15

Upscaling Burn Management: The Mass Burn Casualty Incident Application: CBRN

Deborah A. DeLuca and Deborah S. Adelman

GOAL

The goal of this chapter is to explore the complexities involved in the management of mass burn casualty incidents including the types of burns that the nurse may need to care for.

OBJECTIVES

At the completion of this chapter, the reader will:

1. Discuss how blast burns result in mass casualty incidents.
2. Evaluate the types of victim injuries that result from different types of explosions.
3. Describe the pathophysiology of blast burn injuries.
4. Establish appropriate care for victims of explosive disasters.
5. Describe appropriate disaster nursing care of the radiation burn victim.

Key Terms

- Mass casualty incident
- Blast burns
- Explosions, explosive devices, and weapons of mass destruction
- Blast pressure
- Blast injury levels
- Blast lung
- Special needs of the blast burn victim
- Primary, secondary, tertiary, and quaternary blast injury
- Radiation
- Acute radiation syndrome
- Localized radiation exposure

Introduction

When a mass casualty burn-based trauma incident occurs, having an integrated trauma system is necessary for efficient and effective management of all individuals affected minimally or maximally. Having such a system allows the proper triage, resuscitation, stabilization, and evacuation of the injured, ensuring the best possible medical outcomes for the victims and safe, confident execution of processes and procedures by the first responders and healthcare providers. Specialized care is needed for particular types of burn trauma and, in the field, protecting disaster nurses and responders from the burn source is important. This chapter will address the various types of burns that may ensue from a disaster.

Understanding Blast Burn Mass Casualty Incidents

Understanding blast burn injuries requires understanding the pathophysiology, mechanism of injury, and management recommendations as an additive component to all of the burn wound care processes, from on-site triage through rehabilitation, as presented in Chapters 12, 13, and 14. Incorporating understanding of the concept of terrorism, presented in several previous chapters, sets the stage for the review.

Before engaging in the discussion of mass casualty incidents, particularly blast-based injuries and events management, it is important to briefly differentiate natural disaster mass casualty incidents, as natural disasters can cause similar effects and stressors upon persons, property, infrastructure, and healthcare systems. The difference between natural disaster mass casualty incident management and terrorism-based mass casualty incident management is predictability (United Nations Educational, Scientific, and Cultural Organizations [UNESCO], n.d.). The next section discusses how scientific knowledge concerning the intensity distribution of natural hazards spatiotemporally and the technological developments available to confront those results in a substantial decrement of the consequences of natural hazards, through warning, prevention, and preparedness activities.

Natural hazards beget natural disasters. Natural hazards are naturally occurring physical phenomena occurring slowly or rapidly, originating geologically, hydrologically, or atmospherically, and having effects on a global, regional, national, or local scale. Examples of such events include earthquakes, extreme heat, floods, hurricanes, avalanche, mudslide, landslide, tornados, tsunami, volcano, winter weather, wildfire, and drought (CDC, 2003a; UNESCO, n.d.).

Based on this definition, natural disasters are derived from natural hazards, creating a serious breakdown in the sustainability and disruption of social progress (UNESCO, n.d.). Therefore, losses from natural disasters are dependent on resilience, the ability of the population to resist or support the effects of a natural disaster. Following logically, disasters happen when the population is vulnerable. Hence, it becomes possible to conclude that disasters do not occur when humans are not involved; an example is the effect of a severe earthquake in an uninhabited area. The definition of natural disaster and the assumptions purported herein are supported in the literature; much debate surrounds the inevitability of a natural disaster without human involvement (CDC, 2003a; UNESCO). Interestingly, a key theme developing in the discussions on both natural disaster management and mass casualty incident management is that of preparedness (see Chapter 14).

Overview of Explosions and Mass Casualties

Global reality today includes terrorists using explosive agents in either urban settings or crowded facilities (American Medical Association [AMA], 2005). Blast explosions make a point; they are emphatic, blatant, generally unpredictable, and garner immediate public attention and recognition. Their point is to disrupt normal political and social functioning of a locality and to induce fear. They are unlike natural disasters, which, although devastating, do not have the same impact since they are usually predictable and can be addressed in advance.

Although several types of devices are used by global terrorists such as biological agents, radiation, and chemicals, explosive devices (e.g., bombing attacks) seem to be the favored weapon employed in recent years (Alfici, 2006; Sutphen, 2005). Blast devices are easily accessed, easily created, inexpensive, and highly effective at devastating people, property, and government infrastructures such as buildings, utilities, and transportation systems, including roadways (AMA, 2005). Explosions are not easily forgotten. Medically, explosions result in acute injury, death, dismemberment, psychological stress, entrapment of victims in collapsed structures, emergency medical and surgical care, and forensic disposition of the site, the living victims, the bodies, and body parts.

From the mass trauma perspective, explosive blasts create life-threatening injuries affecting multiple organs in multiple victims simultaneously. The nature and extent of injuries sustained is directly related to the amount and type of explosive materials used, the environmental conditions at the time of the explosion, the delivery device (such as metal or plastic), the distance between the device and the victims, and intervening or complicating hazards or protective barriers present at and immediately surrounding the detonation location (AMA, 2005; Pennardt, Lavonas, & Danzl, 2007). Interestingly, few survivors will actually suffer from life-threatening injuries, assuming appropriate and timely treatment is available (Alfici, 2006).

Immediately postdetonation, explosions create a chaotic environment characterized by shock, confusion, hysteria, panic, and unique, emergent medical challenges. Triage and prehospital assessing and stabilizing victims, as discussed in Chapter 14, take precedence. Hospitals and healthcare providers must be ready to treat hundreds or thousands of burn victims presenting simultaneously with or without polytrauma injuries. Complicating factors include very willing but untrained volunteers, infrastructure losses resulting in difficulty transporting victims, limited supplies and equipment that can arrive at the site of devastation quickly, and possibly even damage to the hospital and other care facilities, limiting where victims can be brought for further assessment, stabilization, and treatment (AMA, 2005).

The United States was introduced to terrorist bombings and their devastating effects starting in the early 1990s, although bombings have been reported since 1886, when a bomb exploded in the Haymarket Square in Chicago, Illinois, during a labor rally and killing 12 people (Sutphen, 2005). Subsequently, the nation was exposed to the concept of suicide bombings in World War II when Japanese pilots attacked Pearl Harbor. Although the number of terrorism-sponsored bombing events continued increasing in frequency and severity throughout Europe, the Middle East, and Asia, the United States was only recently reoriented to them in February, 1993, when the first World Trade Center attack occurred, killing six people and injuring over 1,000 more. In 1996, the Alfred P. Murrah Federal Building in Oklahoma City, Oklahoma, was bombed, resulting in 8,000 injuries and 168 deaths (National Counter Terrorism Center [NCTC], 2008; Sutphen).

More recently, two events are noteworthy that highlight the problems blast incidents cause (Sutphen, 2005). First, on March 11, 2004, a mass terrorist bombing caused substantial damage to life and property in Madrid, Spain. In this event, 10 bombs were hidden in backpacks and detonated on commuter trains, wounding 1,900 people and killing 191. Second, on July 7, 2005, Abu Hafs Al-Masri brigades with a secret organization of Al-Qaeda perpetrated a suicide bombing attack on London's transit system. Although the number of injuries sustained is unpublished, 27 fatalities occurred. Previously, clinicians considered caring for explosions and bombings victims a more remote possibility unless the provider was engaged in the military or overseas aid group (Sutphen). However, these and other recent events indicate this is a no longer practical position.

As stated, terrorist bombings are the most common cause of mass burn casualties with or without attendant polytrauma. For example, statistically, for the period extending from January 1, 1968, through March 25, 2008, the United States NCTC reported 35,688 bombing incidents globally, resulting in 127,854 recorded injuries and 55,758 deaths (NCTC, 2008). These statistics highlight not only the pervasiveness of such mass burn casualty wounds resulting from terrorism-based blast incidents but the sudden and massive burden placed upon emergency, trauma, and critical care systems by these unplanned and often unforeseen incidents. Therefore, understanding mass casualty blast incidents management requires reviewing blast injuries generally, including types of devices employed, the pathophysiology of blast burn wounds, and general mass burn casualty management strategies.

Explosions and Explosive Devices

The rapid chemical conversion of a solid or liquid into a gas with attendant energy release defines an explosion, which is further categorized as either high order (HE) or low order (LE) (CDC, 2003b; Sutphen, 2005). High-order explosives detonate quickly, usually in less than 1/1000th second, generating heat, loud noise, and high-pressure gases. The trademark of a high-order explosive is a defining supersonic overpressurization shockwave (wave front) expanding from the point of detonation outward in a pressure pulse called the blast wave or positive wave (Sutphen). The blast wave moves outward in all directions, exerting a pressure of up to 700 tons. Subsequent shockwaves create a brisance or shattering effect. Displaced air compresses and creates a vacuum, moving backward to the point of detonation, called the negative wave. Examples of high-order explosives include TNT, C-4, Semtex, nitroglycerin, dynamite, and ammonium nitrate fuel oil (ANFO) (CDC, 2003b; Pennardt, Lavonas, & Danzl, 2007; Sutphen). High-order explosives are often deadly and minimally cause severe primary blast injuries (Pennardt, Lavonas, & Danzl, 2007).

Low-order explosives are characterized by a subsonic explosion without the overpressurization wave (CDC, 2003b; Pennardt, Lavonas, & Danzl, 2007; Sutphen, 2005). The trademark of the low-order explosive is a relatively slow energy release with a deflagration burn. Low-order explosions can be deadly but they rarely cause devastating organ and nervous system injuries identified with high-order explosions (Pennardt, Lavonas, & Danzl). Examples of low-order explosives are gun powder fireworks and pyrotechnics, pipe bombs, black powder, most pure petroleum-based bombs such as Molotov cocktails, and aircraft improvised as guided missiles (CDC, 2003b; Pennardt, Lavonas, & Danzl; Sutphen).

Generally, explosives have several effects important for understanding the type of injuries that often occur: a blast pressure wave, blast wind, fragmentation effect, incendiary thermal effect, secondary blast pressure, and ground and water shocks (underground explosions only) (Sutphen, 2005). The blast pressure wave, or primary wave, is described as a function of pressure over time, which occurs due to the intense overpressurization impulse created by the detonated high-order explosive device (CDC, 2003b; Sutphen). The term *blast wave* actually refers to the overpressure component (CDC, 2003b). Graphically, the point of detonation is the arrival time, and the peak overpressure is achieved at this point. The vacuum or negative pressure wave lasts until pressures return to normal postdetonation (Sutphen). Blast wind occurs from the motion of air molecules responding to pressure differentials generated by the blast and is characterized by a superheated, forced air flow (CDC, 2003b). These winds can be as strong as those of a hurricane but are not sustained (Sutphen).

Projectiles attending the blast define the fragmentation effect. These projectiles include particles either from the explosive container, actual projectiles placed within the container, or environmental objects located at and surrounding the point of detonation. Fragments often travel at speeds up to 2,700 feet per second. The incendiary thermal effect refers to temperature over time created by the explosive device. High-order explosives have a higher temperature for a shorter period of time, evidenced by a fireball at the time of detonation (Sutphen, 2005). Comparatively, low-order explosives have a longer thermal effect that usually causes secondary fires.

Secondary blast pressure effects result from the blast wave's reflection off solid surfaces (Severance, 2002; Sutphen, 2005). This results in a prolonged and magnified effect, and is particularly striking in enclosed spaces, where greater energy transfer to the human body occurs than if the secondary blast pressure effect occurred in a more open or larger space, reducing the deflection effect. Finally, ground and water shocks are shockwaves created by underground or underwater explosions (Sutphen). Ground or water actually propagates the wave more forcefully and over greater distances than the same wave occurring in air. Therefore, where high-order and low-order explosive devices are concerned, the resultant injuries vary according to the type, size, and proximity of the device to humans.

Bombs, Improvised Explosive Devices (IEDs), and Weapons of Mass Destruction (WMDs)

Again, injuries sustained in blast incidents vary as much as the weaponry employed. Explosive and incendiary, or fire, bombs are characterized by their source (CDC, 2003b). Generally, bombs are weapons composed of a container filled with explosive material whose explosion is triggered by a clock or other timing device (Sutphen, 2005). Bombs are further classified as either manufactured or improvised, and each causes very different types of injuries. Manufactured bombs are standardized, mass-produced weapons that are quality tested for performance before being issued to the military. They are legal when used by the military in authorized actions (CDC, 2003b). Military-manufactured bombs are exclusively high-order explosive devices.

Improvised explosive devices (IEDs) are often produced in small quantities, are custom made, and employ several different designs and explosive contents (CDC, 2003b; Sutphen, 2005). Generally, improvised devices are regularly existing devices that are modified and used outside of their normally intended use (e.g., plane converted into a guided missile). Most IEDs are composed of either high-order explosives or low-order explosives or may combine both (CDC, 2003b). These bombs are further categorized as either conventional IEDs or dispersive IEDs (Sutphen). Conventional IEDs are those containing chemical explosives. Dispersive IEDs are usually filled with chemicals and other projectiles, such as nails, screws, nuts, or steel pellets, all of which are designed to disperse forcefully, creating secondary injuries and damage.

A special category of IED is the weapon of mass destruction (WMD). The FBI guidelines on counterterrorism define WMD according to the United States Code, 18 U.S.C. 2332 et seq., 18 U.S.C. 2332(a)

> as any weapon designed or intended to: (a) cause death or serious bodily injury through the release, dissemination or impact of toxic/poisonous chemicals or their precursors; (b) release radiation or radioactivity at a level dangerous to human life; (c) any weapon involving a disease organism; and (d) an explosive (greater than 4 ounces), incendiary, poison gas, bomb, grenade, or rocket (United States Federal Bureau of Investigation [FBI], 2001).

A special category of WMD is nuclear bombs, which rely on either nuclear fission or fusion to wreak havoc (Sutphen, 2005). They are always high-order explosive devices and although not used to date in terrorist attacks globally, are particularly concerning. Each type of blast and explosive weaponry used produces unique and varied burn and nonburn mass casualty injuries.

Pathophysiology of Blast Burn Injuries

Blast and explosive devices cause blast injuries, which are generally categorized by physiological and anatomical changes to the body caused either by direct or reflected overpressurization force impacting the body's surface (CDC, 2003b). Explosions and blasts create specific, complex injury patterns with the potential to cause life-threatening multidimensional injuries and multisystem organ failures. The type and pattern of injury sustained is directly related to the type and composition of the device employed, proximity of the victim to the explosive device, the space where the incident occurs (i.e., whether open or closed), and the surrounding barriers or hazards present in the environment at the time of detonation. There are four types of blast injuries: primary, secondary, tertiary, and quaternary (CDC, 2003b, 2008; Severance, 2002; Sutphen, 2005).

Primary Blast Injuries

Primary blast injuries result directly from high-order explosions, in which the overpressurization wave emanating concentrically from the epicenter directly impacts the body's surface (CDC, 2003b, 2008; Severance, 2002; Sutphen, 2005). The actual primary injury generally occurs where tissue interfaces with gas, as in gas-filled organs such as lungs, abdomen, and gastrointestinal tract; liquid, as in lungs, abdomen, eyes, or ears; or at tissue boundary-tethering points (CDC, 2003b, 2008; Severance). Primary blast injury is initially clinically indicated in victims with ruptured tympanic membranes, which rupture at pressures greater than 15 PSI, indicating that the victim experienced possibly deadly pressures. Primary blast injuries account for the majority of on-site fatalities (Severance). If victims survive primary blast injuries on site, they usually expire soon thereafter, which is an important consideration point for triage strategy.

Secondary Blast Injuries

Secondary blast injures result from the fragmentation effect and may be caused by either high-order or low-order explosive devices (Severance, 2002; Sutphen, 2005). Injuries occur when air displacement immediately following the initial detonation creates wind following the blast wave (Severance). This wind accelerates bomb fragments and flying debris, causing penetrating, ballistic, and blunt force injuries not unlike shotgun or bullet wounds. All body parts can be injured, with ocular penetration common (CDC, 2008; Severance; Sutphen). Secondary blast injuries range from minimal to life threatening, depending on the object(s) involved and distance of the victim(s) from the blast. Penetrating thoracic trauma and lacerations of the heart and major blood vessels are a common cause of mortality in secondary blast injury (Pennardt, Lavonas, & Danzl, 2007). However, the majority of blast wound survivors will evidence secondary blast injuries (Severance, 2002).

Tertiary Blast Injuries

Tertiary blast injuries result from the rapid acceleration and deceleration of bodies subjected to blast forces and are attributed to high-order explosions (CDC, 2008; Severance, 2002; Sutphen, 2005). Here, powerful explosions wield forces sufficient to hurl large objects and human bodies located close to the blast through the air (Severance). Extremity amputation(s) occur when acceleration and deceleration forces are either directed at particular body parts or when particular parts of the body strike an existing solid structure in response to those forces. All body parts can be devastated by these forces, and, other than amputation injury, open and closed brain injury and fracture also occur (CDC, 2008; Severance; Sutphen). Crushing injuries are also common. Unless the explosion is focused in some way or of extremely high energy, such as through a hatch or door, a victim suffering a tertiary blast injury is usually very close to the explosion's epicenter (Pennardt, Lavonas, & Danzl, 2007). Clinically, blast amputations usually occur at lethal blast forces, although some victims will survive on site only to die soon thereafter, a key point in triage prioritization strategies (Severance; Sutphen).

Quaternary Blast Injuries

The quaternary blast injury category captures all other sustained explosion-related injuries or illnesses not attributed to primary, secondary, or tertiary mechanisms (CDC, 2003b, 2008; Severance, 2002; Sutphen, 2005). The most common injuries seen in this category include crushing injury from collapsing walls, nuclear radiation contamination, biological or chemical contamination from agents included in terrorist dirty bombs or industrial explosions, and burns (flash, partial thickness, and full thickness) (CDC, 2003b; Severance, 2002). Temperatures of 3000°C are often experienced from the explosive gases (Sutphen). Asphyxia, open and closed brain injuries, and crush injuries are also common (CDC, 2008; Sutphen). Lesser injuries include developing or exacerbating already existing underlying chronic conditions, such as asthma; chronic obstructive pulmonary disease; smoke inhalation; respiratory illnesses attributed to dust, toxic exposures, and fumes; hyperglycemia; and hypertension (CDC, 2003b; Sutphen). Most victims suffering quaternary blast injuries survive. However, victims close to the detonation often suffer third-degree burns that become fatal (Sutphen).

Table 15-1 shows the categories of blast injuries and the corresponding anticipated injuries expected in each category. Note that there is some overlap between

TABLE 15-1 CATEGORIES OF BLAST INJURIES AND CORRESPONDING ANTICIPATED INJURIES

Category	Characteristics	Affected Body Part	Injuries Anticipated
Primary	Due to HE only, from impact of overpressurization wave contact with body surface	Gas-filled organs are most susceptible: eye, lungs, GI tract, and middle ear	Blast lung (pulmonary barotrauma); tympanic membrane rupture, middle ear damage; abdominal hemorrhage and perforation; eye rupture; concussion-traumatic brain injury without physical signs of head injury
Secondary	HE and LE; due to flying debris and bomb fragments	All body parts are vulnerable	Penetrating ballistic fragment or blunt trauma injuries; ocular penetration (can be occult)
Tertiary	Due to HE; victims are thrown by blast wind into solid structures	All body parts are vulnerable	Fracture; traumatic amputation; closed and open brain injuries; crushing injuries
Quaternary	Due to HE and LE; all explosion-related injuries, illnesses, or diseases not due to primary, secondary, or tertiary mechanisms	All body parts are vulnerable	Burns due to high gas heat: flash, partial thickness and full thickness; crushing injuries; closed and open brain injury; developing, complicating, or exacerbating existent conditions (asthma, COPD); other breathing issues from dust, toxic fumes, or smoke; angina; hyperglycemia and hypertension

Source: Adapted from CDC, 2003b; Kluger, Pele, Daniel-Aharonson, & Mayo, A., 2004; Sutphen, 2005.

LE descriptive mechanisms and the HE secondary, tertiary, and quaternary mechanisms; primary mechanisms are associated only with HE blasts.

Once the mechanisms and categories of injuries are identified, it becomes possible to highlight specific expectations anticipated with blast incidents of any type. Bombing casualties generally have higher injury severity scores (16% to 30% versus 10% for other trauma); increased immediate mortality rates (29% for closed space bombings); greater in-hospital mortality rates (6.2% versus 3% for other trauma); higher need for surgical intervention, particularly orthopedic; longer hospital stays; greater need for intensive care support; and generally younger age victims (Sutphen, 2005). This data supports the premise that bombing victims have higher hospital utilization rates than victims of other casualty events. This leads to the need for effective and efficient management of triage efforts on site so that those victims with good possibilities of survival receive immediate medical attention, while those with less serious injuries receive delayed care, leaving those with the poorest survival prognosis receiving minimal care (Severance, 2002; Sutphen). Patients should then be further divided into urgent and nonurgent care categories, upon which care is rendered, in terms of either initial phase resuscitation efforts from on site through referral and arrival at care centers, and a definitive phase, when the volumes of victims arriving lessens and optimized care is deliverable (Sutphen).

One area requiring further delineation is eye injury, which occurs in as many as 10% of all blast survivors. Injuries are usually caused by high-velocity projectiles, occur with little observed discomfort initially, and the victims usually present days, weeks, or months postinjury for care, with symptoms such as irritation, eye pain, foreign body sensations in the eye, altered vision, contusions, or periorbital swelling. Findings on examination often reveal hyphema, globe perforation, subconjunctival hemorrhage, lid lacerations, foreign body intrusion, and decreased vision. Further ophthalmic screening is required.

Table 15-2 presents categorized and summarized anticipated injuries from blast casualty events requiring appropriate and effective triage strategies on site and greater, long-term resource utilization rates. This table represents the primary body systems affected by blast casualty events and the most common injuries or conditions anticipated in each system.

Medical Management of Mass Casualty Burn Incidents

Medical and surgical prioritization of blast victims is well discussed in the literature. The larger issue is whether management is required for a relatively low number of victims from a small blast incident or if a mass casualty burn victim situation occurs (Severance, 2002). Handling small numbers of victims in a burn incident has been thoroughly discussed in Chapters 13 and 14. The differences and concerns between these and large numbers becomes evident when looking at various physiologic parameters of instability associated with a mass casualty burn incident with

TABLE 15-2 BLAST-RELATED INJURIES SUMMARY

Affected System	Common Anticipated Injury or Condition
Auditory	Tympanic membrane rupture; cochlear damage; ossicular disruption and foreign body presence
Circulatory	Cardiac contusion; myocardial infarction from air embolism; vasovagal hypotension; shock; peripheral vascular injury; air embolism-induced injury
Central nervous system	Concussion; open and closed traumatic brain injury; spinal cord injury; stroke; air embolism-induced injury
GI system	Hemorrhage; ruptured liver and/or spleen; sepsis; bowel perforation; air embolism-induced mesenteric ischemia
Eye, orbit, and face	Foreign bodies; air embolism; fracture; perforated globe
Extremities	Traumatic amputation; fractures; crushing injuries; burns (flash, partial thickness, and full thickness); compartment syndrome; lacerations; air embolism-induced injuries; acute arterial occlusions
Renal	Laceration; contusion; acute renal failure due to rhabdomyolysis; hypovolemia and hypotension
Respiratory	Hemothorax; pneumothorax; pulmonary contusion and hemorrhage; air embolism-induced atrioventricular fistulas; airway epithelial damage; aspiration pneumonitis; sepsis and primary blast lung injury (BLI)

Source: Adapted from CDC, 2003b.

several hundred or several thousand burn victims, such as from a terrorist bombing. In theory, although a terrorist bombing is not dissimilar from other mass trauma casualty situations, the mechanism of injury in blasts and explosions is totally different and more complex: There is a blast component, a penetrating wound component, a blunt force trauma component, and a flash burn component (Alfici, 2006; Severance). This suggests an entirely different management and treatment focus, which is the focus of this section. Managing the event is addressed first; victim treatment strategies are addressed second.

First: Managing the Mass Casualty Burn Event

Explosions from intentional bombings and other blasts are one of the few dramatic and instantaneous events that produce massive numbers of casualties in a matter of moments, most of which will require immediate medical attention at some level

(Severance, 2002). Looking at the total number of casualties caused by a blast event, realize that at least half of all initial casualties will seek medical care over the first 1-hour period (CDC, 2003b, 2008). Even more disturbing is the fact that this same population of individuals will arrive at the care facilities *before* the most severely injured; this situation is termed *upside-down triage*. This means there is a very high likelihood that the number of casualties, both remaining on site and presenting at emergency facilities, will exceed the capacity of the local system to respond (Pennardt, Lavonas, & Danzl, 2007).

The goal for managing initial mass casualty burn victims is to provide expeditious and intensive care to the most severely injured and to control victims not severely injured from descending in massive numbers upon local hospitals and clinics. This goal is satisfied by designating medical personnel to a triage area off site, under the control of the local incident commander on site. These off-site, medically staffed and equipped triage location(s) allow(s) for expeditious treatment of minor injuries away from hospital centers, leaving the hospital centers available to care for the critically injured first. Back on site, the critically injured victims, or *red tags,* are assessed, referred, and transported first, followed by the intermediately injured victims, or *yellow tags,* followed by the minimally injured victims, or *green tags,* who could be sent to care facilities away from the hospital setting, such as to area hospitals' outpatient clinics and other community outpatient care centers. In the best case, the green tags who are most minimally injured can be released from care entirely, since their wounds are so minor that no additional treatment is required. This triage plan alleviates the hospital systems from becoming overwhelmed in the initial hours postincident (Severance, 2002).

Second: Caring for the Mass Casualty Burn Incident Victims

Following the triage concept explained in the prior section, approaches to treating each group of casualties in the moments to hours following the blast incident is the next concern. Treatment approaches used for unstable victims are addressed first, followed by treatment approaches used for more stable victims.

Addressing Unstable Victims of Mass Casualty Burn Incidents

As stated above, bombings result in multiple trauma victims both on site and arriving at hospitals shortly after the incident. Effective triage becomes crucial to determine which victims have the best chance for survival, which can receive delayed care due to nonemergent injuries, and which should receive minimal care due to a poor prognosis for survival.

The *ABCs* of the advanced trauma life support (ATLS) algorithm is used to initially assess and stabilize mass casualty burn victims. Airway protection and attention to ventilatory support is paramount, followed by hemodynamic assessment (Sutphen, 2005). Once victims are stabilized, obtain as much information as possible about the distance between the victim and the explosion; and determine whether the victim was located in an open, confined, or closed space at the time of the explosion, and whether the victim wore body armor. It is important to answer these questions to determine the nature and severity of injuries that may not be immediately evident or have not yet been addressed (Alfici, 2006; Pennardt, Lavonas, & Danzl, 2007; Sutphen).

Physiologically unstable victims are prioritized for treatment according to the most common treatable cause of each victim's inherent instability (Alfici, 2006). This means treating the injuries most likely to cause mortality or severe debilitation first, followed by each successively concerning injury until the victim achieves physiologic stability. This may involve not treating actual burn wounds until much later in the process (Alfici, 2006; Pennardt, Lavonas, & Danzl, 2007; Severance, 2002; Sutphen, 2005). Additionally, if some unstable victims present with blast lung injuries and other equally unstable victims do not, the blast lung injury victims are prioritized for care before the nonblast lung injury population (Alfici).

Preliminary triage assessments and treatments conducted on unstable victims, in order, are: (a) examining the lungs, tympanic membranes, and abdomen of all victims exposed to significant explosion, directing particular attention to primary blast lung injury identification; (b) giving hemodynamically unstable patients evidencing significant trauma fresh packed red blood cells, fresh frozen plasma and platelets in a 1:1 ratio; (c) observing pulmonary insufficiency or contusion with radiography, if available, including definitive airway management and ventilatory support as needed; (d) evaluating intestinal hematoma, which usually presents as persistent abdominal pain or vomiting; (e) identifying white phosphorus burns, which require unique treatment; and (f) treating penetrating and or shrapnel wounds (secondary blast injury), blunt trauma (secondary/tertiary blast injury), and burns according to standard treatment protocols (Alfici, 2006; Pennardt, Lavonas, & Danzl, 2007; Sutphen, 2005).

White phosphorus (WP, P4) burns are technically categorized as chemical burns, but since they are a common mass trauma blast event injury, they are often discussed as a traditional burn wound rather than as a chemical burn wound (Irizarry & Williams, 2007). WP causes painful second- and third-degree chemical burns, characterized by a necrotic area with a yellowish color and characteristic garliclike odor. Rapid dermal penetration due to its inherently high-lipid solubility results in heart, liver, and kidney damage and delayed wound healing. Systemic toxicity is evidenced by progressive anuria, decreased creatine clearance, and increased phosphorus blood levels. Developing decreased serum calcium levels and increased serum phosphorus levels, called a reversed calcium-phosphorus ratio, evidenced as prolonged QT segments, ST segment depression, and T wave changes on the ECG, results in bradycardia (Irizarry & Williams; Pennardt, Lavonas, & Danzl, 2007).

Treating WP burns requires substantial caution due to its inherent incendiary nature, increasing the likelihood of further combustion occurring from the particles on the victim. WP reacts with water found on the skin to form phosphoric acid. WP has an inherent characteristic of spontaneous combustion when located on skin, where it can rapidly absorb water (Pennardt, Lavonas, & Danzl, 2007). Therefore, the first priority should be to completely wash any areas on the victim where WP particles are evident. Washing with water or saline neutralizes the combustibility of the particles. Removing any visible WP particles and placing them in water should be part of the lavage process. Additionally, placing saline-soaked gauze on all areas where WP exposure occurred further reduces the risk of incendiarism.

The second step in treating WP burns involves rinsing burned areas with a 1% copper sulfate ($CuSO_4$) solution. Copper sulfate and WP combine to form a blue-black cupric phosphide (Cu_3P_2). The Cu_3P_2 particles are easy to identify and are significantly less likely to combust than the WP particles. Removing the particles carefully and placing them in water further impedes combustion. Once the $CuSO_4$ rinse is completed, saline rinses are necessary to remove the $CuSO_4$ from the burned areas. $CuSO_4$ is easily absorbed systemically and can cause renal failure and intravascular hemolysis. Upon completing the emergent treatment protocol, WP victims should be admitted and placed on cardiac monitoring to watch for ECG changes, particularly life-threatening arrhythmias, as WP injury can cause hypokalemia and hypophosphatemia (Pennardt, Lavonas, & Danzl, 2007). Intravenous calcium may be necessary to reverse hypokalemic effects.

Treating Primary Blast Lung Injury

Primary blast lung injury (BLI) presents complex triage, diagnostic, and management challenges and is a direct consequence of high-order explosive detonations that cause an overpressurization wave to form (CDC, 2003b, 2005, 2006). Of all primary blast injuries, primary blast lung injury has the highest morbidity and mortality rates both at the scene and among survivors (CDC, 2005; Pennardt, Lavonas, & Danzl, 2007). Pulmonary damage sustained includes pulmonary tearing, hemorrhage, edema, and contusion with a resultant ventilation-perfusion mismatch (CDC, 2005). Pulmonary injury occurs when the high-pressure blast wave contacts the body and then travels through the border between alveoli, air, and blood vessels, causing ruptured alveolar septae (Sutphen, 2005). This causes air accumulation in the blood vessels and blood accumulation in the septae. Peribronchial and perivascular disruptions result, alveolar hemorrhages occur, and air embolisms develop.

BLI is characterized by difficult respiration with attendant hypoxia, which could manifest without obvious external injury to the chest (CDC, 2005; Sutphen, 2005). Signs of blast lung injury are usually present by the time of initial evaluation, although symptoms can present as late as 24 to 48 hours postexplosion (CDC, 2003b, 2006, 2008; Sutphen). BLI is clinically diagnosed by presence of the triad bradycardia, apnea, and hypotension (CDC, 2003b). Pulmonary injury ranges from scattered petechiae to confluent hemorrhages. Victims often present with cough, chest pain, tachycardia, hypoxia, decreased breath sounds, cyanosis, wheezing, apnea, and hemodynamic instability (CDC, 2006). One particular characteristic indicating possible BLI is the presence of a butterfly pattern on the chest identified through X-ray of the thoracic cavity (CDC, 2003b, 2008). Determining what further diagnostic testing is required is usually based on details concerning the nature of the explosion, proximity, and trapping of the victim in the area of the explosion and type of event (chemical or biologic involvement) (CDC, 2005, 2006). A generalized blast lung injury management algorithm is presented in Figure 15-1. It should be noted that this algorithm is an initial protocol that can be used for deci-

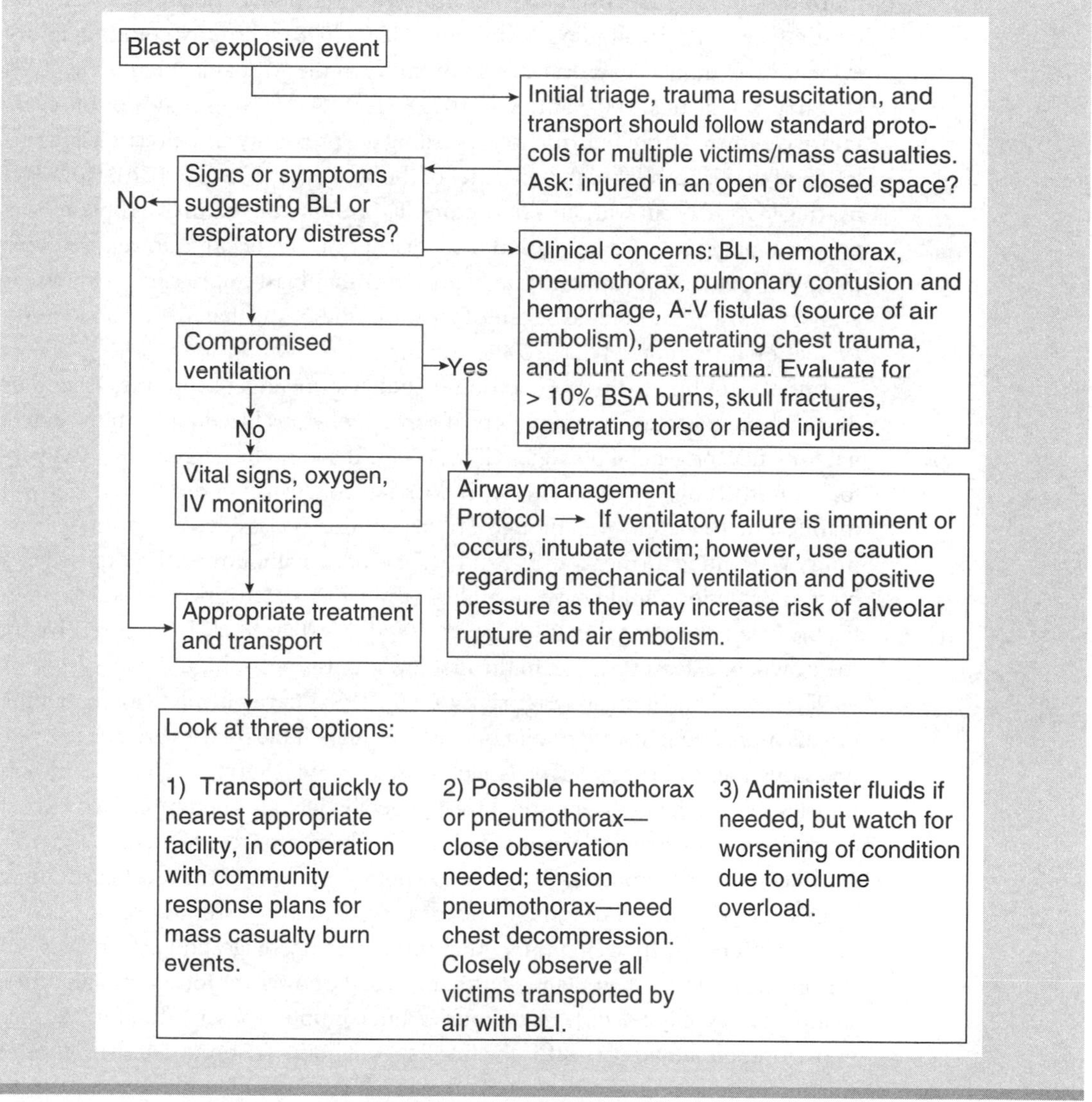

Figure 15-1 Blast Lung Injury Management Algorithm
Source: Adapted from CDC, 2003b, 2005, 2006, 2008.

sion making in primary emergent resuscitation of unstable victims evidencing possible blast lung injury. It is not intended to be a definitive guideline for total care.

Addressing Other Emergent Conditions of Mass Casualty Burn Incidents

There are three other major organ systems requiring careful assessment and resuscitation for unstable victims of mass casualty burn/blast events: ear, abdomen, and brain. These organ systems are briefly discussed.

Primary blast injuries of the auditory system statistically indicate significant morbidity, but are often overlooked by healthcare personnel who are occupied with treating the more visually obvious injuries (CDC, 2008). The most common injury evident on examination is destruction or injury of the tympanic membrane (TM) (Irizarry & Williams, 2007; Sutphen, 2005). Here, the relevant indicator of severe injury is gathered from information regarding the proximity and directional orientation of the victim's ear to the epicenter of the blast event (CDC, 2003b). However, hearing loss can occur without TM rupture. TM rupture can occur at as little as 5 psi pressure, but cochlear damage and ossic disruption can occur at lower pressures (Sutphen, 2005). TM rupture usually predicts other blast injuries may be present even if not visible and should be one of the initial indicators that further blast injury evaluation is warranted (CDC, 2008; Sutphen).

Initial signs on victim presentation include complaints of tinnitus, vestibular dysfunction indicated by complaints of vertigo, obvious bleeding from the external ear canal, or general otoalgia (CDC, 2008). It should be noted that if TM perforation is the only obvious injury, it does not necessarily indicate that BLI will manifest in the victim, even though TM perforation is classified as a primary blast injury warranting further concern and evaluation. Finally, any victim exposed to a blast or explosion should have an otologic assessment performed as soon as practicable by an otolaryngologist (Sutphen, 2005). Most auditory injuries resolve on their own, or at least stabilize, in the first few months postinjury.

The second major organ system is the GI tract. GI injuries involve gas-containing organs more frequently than solid organs, although, if the injuries are due to overpressures, then solid organ involvement is also probable (Sutphen, 2005). Common injuries seen in the gastrointestinal tract generally include abdominal lacerations; contusions to the liver, spleen, and kidney; and hemorrhage. Frequently, abdominal injuries are not immediately evident. Hollow injuries are the most concerning in this category, which can often present up to 14 days postinjury (CDC, 2008). Hollow injuries include circumferential rings of hemorrhage, and petechiae is not uncommon (CDC, 2003b, 2008). Perforations of the bowel are not common injuries, manifesting as only 1% to 1.2% of injuries, but continued observation for evidence of perforation should persist for the first 24 to 48 hours postinjury. If the victim(s) were involved in a significant blast event, several thorough abdominal examinations during inpatient care period(s) should be performed (Sutphen). Here, ileum perforation is concerning and usually requires surgical resection.

Surgical intervention may also be necessary when victims present with diminished bowel sounds, bright red blood per rectum, rebound tenderness, unexplained hypovolemia, and/or guarding (Sutphen, 2005). Other concerning symptoms suggesting surgical intervention include vomiting, nausea with or without vomiting, tenesmus, diarrhea, and testicular or rectal pain (CDC, 2008; Sutphen). Although clinical diagnosis may be adequate, when victims are unconscious or intubated, diagnostic peritoneal lavage may be useful to find perforations or hidden projectiles. Abdominal CT scans, if possible, often reveal extraluminal gas accumulations, solid organ injury or disruption, bowel wall hematomas, large fluid collections around the site of hematoma(s), and hemoperitoneum (Sutphen, 2005). All of these conditions often require surgical repair in the acute treatment phase.

The last of the emergent systems to be presented is the neurological system. "Dead on the scene" events often characterize neurologic injury where blasts are concerned. Subdural and subarachnoid hemorrhages are often found postmortem in blast fatalities, and severe head trauma is the primary cause of mortality in blast victims. Overpressure waves generally seem to be the primary cause of head trauma in blast events. The overpressure theory suggests that the wave, upon contact with the human skull, is transferred to the central nervous system, thereby causing diffuse axonal injury (Sutphen, 2005). From a cellular perspective, it is believed that the overpressure concussive wave creates an inflammatory response, resulting in the release of interleukin 8, which results in mobilization of polymorphonuclear leukocytes into systemic circulation (Pennardt, Lavonas, & Danzl, 2007). Proinflammatory cytokine release occurs, causing expression of the CD11b receptor complex on the polymorphonuclear leukocyte surface, causing adhesion at the injury site, causing brain injury. This phenomenon is sometimes complicated by blast injury to the lungs, which causes inducible nitric oxygen synthase levels to increase in the brain, also causing brain injury. The end result in either case is often mild to severe traumatic brain injury and may cause skull fracture or coup-counter-coup injuries.

Some victims may be able to express complaints including headache, poor concentration, lethargy, depression, insomnia, or fatigue (CDC, 2003b; Sutphen, 2005). In this situation, complaints may evidence either true mild head injury or symptoms attending posttraumatic stress disorder (see Chapter 8) (CDC, 2003b). Therefore, determining the proximity of the victim to the epicenter is helpful in determining if head trauma was sustained, especially since concussion may also be present.

An effective tool for assessing head trauma is the Glasgow Coma Scale (GCS), which ranks head injury according to three general categories: (a) mild, GC score 13–15; (b) moderate, GC score 9–12; and (c) severe, GC score $\leq$ 8 (CDC, 2003a). The GCS is used to assess the depth and duration of coma and consciousness. Table 15-3 presents the Glasgow Coma Scale with care recommendations, along with the points allocated for each sign and symptom evaluated for degree of head trauma present. Care of victims experiencing head trauma due to blast injuries is dependent on proper assessment and allocation of point scores using the GCS (Sutphen, 2005).

Addressing Stable Victims of Mass Casualty Burn Incidents

As stated initially in this section, stable mass casualty blast burn victims usually present at the healthcare facility in advance of the more severely wounded victims. Nonetheless, assessing and treating these victims relies on a separate set of guidelines. Stable victims of a mass casualty burn incident suffer from a range of injuries that are not normally immediately life threatening, ranging from acute psychological stress reactions; serious injuries that are not immediately life threatening but could lead to disability; to minor lacerations, minor penetrating wounds, and minor

TABLE 15-3 GLASGOW COMA SCALE (GCS) FOR VICTIMS OF BLAST TRAUMA WITH HEAD INJURY INVOLVEMENT AND CARE RECOMMENDATIONS BASED ON DEGREE OF SEVERITY

Severity Assessment Scores and Category of Severity

GCS scores are based on totaling points allocated for each of the responses tested in the categories of eye, verbal, and motor responses. The total point scores are interpreted as follows:

Mild brain injury:	13 pts to 15 pts
Moderate brain injury:	9 pts to 12 pts
Severe brain injury:	≤ 8 pts

GCS Testing Cues Used to Assign Points

Point allocations are totaled after each of the responses below are tested in the blast injured victim. Care recommendations are based on the total score assigned.

Eye Responses	Verbal Responses	Motor Responses
Opens on own, blinking at baseline: 4 pts	Alert and oriented: 5 pts	Obeys commands: 6 pts
To verbal command: 3 pts	Confused, disoriented but answers questions: 4 pts	Purposeful to pain: 5 pts
To pain: 2 pts	Inappropriate words: 3 pts	Moves away from pain: 4 pts
Does not open: 1 pt	Moans, unintelligible words: 2 pts	Flexion movements, decorticate posturing: 3 pts
	Does not talk: 1 pt	Extension movements, decerebrate posturing: 2 pts
		No response: 1 pts

(continued)

TABLE 15-3 GLASGOW COMA SCALE (GCS) FOR VICTIMS OF BLAST TRAUMA WITH HEAD INJURY INVOLVEMENT AND CARE RECOMMENDATIONS BASED ON DEGREE OF SEVERITY (Continued)

Recommended Care Guidelines Based on GCS Scores and Head Injury Classification

Care recommendations are made based on the total score assigned after assessment and categorization of the injury as mild, moderate, or severe as follows:

Category	Care Guidelines
Neurologic signs, impaired consciousness or GCS 13–14 points	Refer for urgent CT scan of the head; if abnormal, surgical consult needed. Indications of epidural injury(ies) or subdural injury(ies) or contusion indicate surgery needed
GCS Scores 9–12 points	CT scan of head and C1, C2, C7, T1, and AP lateral X-ray of cervical spine to rule out cervical spine injury(ies)
GCS Scores ≤ 8 points	Neurological management in ICU needed. Intubation, ventilation, maintaining oxygen levels, body temperature, continuous arterial pressure monitoring, pain control, sedation, cervical spine control, and neuromuscular paralysis may be warranted Manage nutrition, seizures, and blood sugar Prevent thromboembolic events

Source: Adapted from CDC, 2003b; Sutphen, 2005.

burn wounds (Alfici, 2006). As discussed in Chapter 14, the primary and secondary surveys are assessment protocols employed with this victim population. The problem here, however, is that initial laboratory studies and radiological examinations will not be available during the first hours postevent. However, part of the primary and secondary survey process is taking a good history and physical examination, looking for signs of injuries that can become life threatening very quickly, particularly a condition called blast lung injury (BLI), which usually develops during the first 24 to 48 hours postblast (Alfici).

Other diagnostics gathered in this stable victim population include respiratory rate, oxygen saturation, chest X-rays, otic examination, and ocular examination (Alfici, 2006). When penetrating injuries are suspected, CT scans when available become important to identify any nonobservable foreign bodies present, including the path the foreign object traveled to reach its end position. Repeated evaluations as needed, based on the severity of the wounds, should be conducted until such time that it is determined that the victim either can be released for further outpatient-based follow-up, admitted for more intensive care, or referred to a specialized burn unit or other clinical setting for additional care (Alfici; Sutphen, 2005).

Regarding optimal duration of observation, the following guidelines are often used. Decisions are based on attendant associated injuries and proximity to blast (CDC, 2008). If no apparent significant injury is evident, if normal vital signs with unremarkable lung and abdominal assessments are made, and if the victim was exposed to an open-space explosive event, the victim usually can be released after 4 hours of observation, with clear instructions regarding return for further evaluation if the victim experiences abdominal pain, vomiting, shortness of breath, or other symptoms not initially present during the initial observation period (Pennardt, Lavonas, & Danzl, 2007).

Second, when closed-space or in-water explosions are experienced with or without TM rupture, there is an automatic higher risk for delayed complications. Before considering release, radiologic study of the chest and other selected organs should be performed, if possible. If no injury is evident, victims should still be admitted for further observation due to the possible development of severe delayed complications. Only totally asymptomatic victims may be released subsequent to a 4-hour observation period. Finally, any victims presenting with suspected air embolism, radiation or WP burns, abnormal vital signs, significant burns, radiographic or clinical signs of pneumothorax or pulmonary contusion, vomiting, abdominal pain, evidence of renal contusion, hypoxia, or with penetrating injuries to the head, abdomen, or thorax must be admitted and observed over several days to weeks, and further stabilization and treatment will be necessary (Pennardt, Lavonas, & Danzl, 2007). Any female in the second or third trimester of pregnancy should be admitted for further monitoring (see Chapter 5) (CDC, 2008).

Radiation Exposure and Burns in the Mass Casualty Event

This section is predicated on the assumption that medical professionals are generally unfamiliar with treating victims of radiation-based events. Threats about existing WMDs, possible terrorist-available WMDs, possible terrorist attacks using nuclear or radiation-based weaponry, and radiation dispersion devices (RDD) all force awareness about the need to recognize the possibility of a mass casualty radiation event occurring and to be prepared for the possible mass casualty radiation-based event. Therefore, the focus of this section is two-fold: discussing the medical treatment approaches to mass radiological casualties and managing the mass casualty radiation or nuclear incident. To begin assessing how medical interventions and management of mass casualties exposed to radiation can be triaged, stabilized, and treated, it is necessary to first understand what the risk is and what it involves.

Etiology of Radiation Events

It is worthy to note that several of the concepts developed in this section apply equally to radiation exposures, regardless of their source: controlled, such as medically warranted exposures; energy production or military-controlled events; or uncontrolled events, such as terrorist attacks. However, the focus of this section is on the unforeseen, unplanned radiation exposure that causes large-scale damage or destruction to individuals or property.

People are regularly exposed to radiation. In the United States, the average annual exposure is estimated at 3.6 milliSieverts (mSv), of which 20% originates from a synthetic source (man-made) and 80% from a natural source (environmental, atmospheric) (Pae & Dill, 2006). It is known that high doses of radiation are carcinogenic; very high-dose, short-exposure effects are immediate and usually lethal; and not much is known about low-dose, long-exposure effects. In the past 50 years, most radiation events resulted in nonlethal consequences. The worst case scenario that can occur is a terrorist-originated nuclear detonation. These events are termed *criticality events,* and even the smallest such event could result in damage equivalent to or greater than the WTC attacks of September 11, 2001 (Koenig et al., 2005). Understanding the dynamics involved in managing and treating victims of such criticality events is necessary since to date there are no experiences upon which post hoc review can lend knowledge and assistance in preparedness plans creation. The purpose of this text is not to be a primer on radiation. Consultation of an appropriate text is advised to provide a deeper understanding of radiation and the different types of exposures that the disaster nurse may see in victims. Care for the patient exposed to radiation is, thus, the next topic.

Principles of Acute Radiation Injury

Acute radiation syndrome (ARS) occurs after whole-body exposure to large doses of ionizing radiation, and involves one of two exposure types: either whole body or localized (Pae & Dill, 2006). In either case, radiation injury occurs when energy is deposited in body tissue and disrupts DNA and other cellular structures (Koenig et al., 2005). Acute exposures are more likely to result in cell death or malignant transformations than protracted exposures. ARS does not occur normally at doses less than 1 Gy and is uniformly fatal at doses greater than 10 Gy (Pae & Dill).

In whole-body radiation exposure, a single acute exposure of penetrating gamma radiation can cause various manifestations of ARS (Koenig et al, 2005). What symptoms appear is dependent on the radiation dosage, type, and individual sensitivity (Neal & Moores, 2002). Since the exact details may not be known concerning the radiation exposure, especially in accidental exposure situations, dose estimates may not be entirely reliable (Pae & Dill, 2006). Therefore, clinical presentations, laboratory measures, and symptomology identified in the early period are often used to determine dosage exposure and prognosis indirectly.

ARS progresses through four stages: prodrome, clinical latency, manifest illness, and recovery or death. The prodrome phase begins with rapid onset of nausea, malaise, and vomiting soon after radiation exposure, and the dose of exposure determines the duration, severity, and onset moments. Common symptoms include nausea, anorexia, fatigue, diarrhea, vomiting, dehydration, and abdominal cramping. At doses greater than 10 Gy, prodrome will begin within 5 to 15 minutes post-exposure; at lower dosages near 2 Gy to 3 Gy, prodrome can be delayed for 12 hours or more. Additionally, severe and rapid onset of prodrome indicates poor prognosis and high-exposure dosage. Immediate onset of diarrhea, fever, and hypotension indicates supralethal exposure (Pae & Dill, 2006). Progression through the subsequent phases depends directly on dosage of exposure.

The latent phase follows and is relatively symptom free (Pae & Dill, 2006). Presence and timing of nausea and vomiting serves as an excellent triage tool to detect those casualties requiring urgent medical attention (Koenig et al., 2005). Serial CBC screens identify casualties with relatively significant radiation doses, because a significant decrease in lymphocyte levels in the first 6 to 48 hours post-exposure indicates that prolonged and intensive medical care is likely required. Manifest illness follows the latent period and either recovery or death occurs (Pae & Dill, 2006). Organ system subsyndromes classic to ARS to watch in the manifest illness phase include the cerebrovascular, gastrointestinal, and hematopoietic (Neal & Moores, 2002; Pae & Dill). Exposure doses of 30 Gy or more (3000 rad) causes cerebrovascular syndrome with central nervous system involvement, which occurs primarily due to the development of hypotension and cerebral edema, and is uniformly fatal (Koenig et al., 2005; Pae & Dill). Attendant signs include nausea, vomiting, hypotension, prostration, ataxia, and convulsions. Death will occur in several days from neurologic and cardiovascular system collapses; from a triage perspective only, palliative care is needed (Pae & Dill). Death occurs within hours post-incident, at radiation exposures of 100 Gy or more.

In cerebrovascular syndrome, coma ensues in hours when exposures occur only between the 20 Gy and 40 Gy levels (Neal & Moores, 2002). Here, the latent phase persists only for a matter of hours before the onset of symptoms. Convulsions may or may not occur; if they present, they are indications of increasing intracranial pressure at a minimum. Survival is unlikely (Pae & Dill, 2006). Blast and thermal effects in a nuclear event would serve only to confound the neurovasculature damage, ensuring 100% lethal consequences for any casualty presenting with these symptoms (Neal & Moores). Again, from a triage perspective, these casualties should be moved to the expectant category when mental status changes occur due to the radiation exposure.

Gastrointestinal syndrome manifests in whole-body radiation exposure dosages between 6 Gy and 20 Gy, usually between 5 Gy and 12 Gy, due to death of mucosal stem cells (Koenig et al., 2005; Pae & Dill, 2006). Hemorrhage, diarrhea, and fluid loss commonly manifests in the prodromal stage, due to denudation of functional cells after microvilli radiation damage (Neal & Moores, 2002). As the normal GI tract boundaries are compromised, sepsis ensues from bacterial proliferation. GI prodrome onset is rapid, followed by a 1-week latent period, after which the symptoms return. If there is attendant injury to the microvasculature as well, death will ensue within 1 to 2 weeks (Neal & Moores). Treatment strategies for gastrointestinal syndrome focuses on infection prevention and maintaining electrolyte and fluid balances, but from a triage perspective this care is merely palliative, as death usually ensues in 3 to 10 days on average (Pae & Dill).

Hematopoietic syndrome occurs at much lower exposure levels, of 2 Gy to 5 Gy (Pae & Dill, 2006). In this situation, radiation-induced apoptosis occurs, causing lymphocytes to die. Bone marrow suppression results thereby preventing formation of new leukocytes and platelets, causing an increased risk of infection and anemia to develop from 10 to 60 days postradiation (Neal & Moores, 2002; Pae & Dill). Anemia does not appear without hemorrhage. If neutropenia develops secondary to radiation exposure, the treatment is no different than treating neutropenia due to nonradiation causes (Neal & Moores). From a triage perspective, early supportive care, neutropenia treatment and infection prevention are the primary procedures to follow for these patients; however, despite treating the hematopoietic syndrome, death commonly occurs due to multiple organ failure (Pae & Dill).

Prehospital Triage Approaches and Casualty Management in Mass Casualty Radiation Exposure Incidents

Potential radiation injury diagnosis is missed 15% of the time when a full medical history is relied upon for the assessment (Koenig et al., 2005). Delayed diagnosis is also problematic. Between 1987 and 2000, the time from the beginning of the radiation exposure incident and definitive diagnosis averaged 22 days. This is not to suggest that a thorough medical history and victim description of the event and symptom onset and severity discussion should not occur. However, when critical time may be lost that could otherwise be used to avert a possible fatal outcome, alternative methods should be considered and employed to estimate exposure levels. Laboratory studies when possible are one of the key components involved in managing whole-body ARS. Several different evaluations are available from simple blood and urine sampling, and are presented in the following sections.

Using Time to Emesis (TE) to Estimate Dosage Exposure Levels

Time to emesis (TE) has been proposed as a clinical parameter for indirectly estimating dosage exposures. As dosage increases, TE decreases. Therefore, for TE less than 1 hour postexposure, the estimated whole-body dose is estimated to be greater than 4 Gy. Similarly, for a TE between 1 and 2 hours postexposure, the estimated whole-body dose is approximately greater than 3 Gy; for TE greater than 4 hours, whole-body dose is estimated to be minimal, at 1 Gy (Pae & Dill, 2006).

Using the Serial CBC with Differential in Whole-Body ARS Management

Laboratory studies, particularly an early baseline complete blood count (CBC) with differential, should be obtained whenever possible and repeated every 4 to 6 hours or every 6 to 12 hours, as needed, to monitor neutrophil and leukocyte counts (Koenig et al., 2005; Pae & Dill, 2006). Minimum lymphocyte counts (MLC) are inversely proportional to absorbed dose, with higher MLCs indicating better prognosis and lower MLCs indicating poor prognosis. Here, an MLC of 1000/mm^3 to 1499/mm^3 corresponds to an approximate absorbed dose of 0.5 Gy to 1.9 Gy. Prognosis is usually good for these victims, as this level of absorbed dose is usually nonlethal, despite the presentation of other clinically significant symptoms (Pae & Dill).

Additionally, MLC levels ranging from 500/mm^3 to 999/mm^3 correspond to an absorbed dose of 2.0 Gy to 3.9 Gy, usually accompanied by severe injuries and a fair prognosis. Lower MLC levels, from 100/mm^3 to 499/mm^3 indicate an approximate absorbed dose of 4.0 Gy to 7.9 Gy, predicting severe injury and poor prognosis. Finally, MLC levels indicating a high likelihood of death and absorbed dose of 8 Gy or more are lower than 100/mm^3. Bone marrow stimulation will not help these patients. For any patient with an absorbed dose of greater than 10 Gy, survival is not documented (Pae & Dill, 2006). Obviously, from a triage and care perspective, a simple CBC with differential can provide incredibly helpful information when resources are stretched by mass casualty needs.

Prehospital Triage and ED Approaches to Mass Casualty Victim Management and Treatment

Medical and emergency response personnel should assume that a radiation exposure event will create a chaotic situation among the public and victims; hospitals and clinics need to be prepared to manage large numbers of agitated and potentially contaminated victims. Initial triage focuses on separating and moving the nonphysically injured victims to a designated area away from the on-site and hospital locations, with EDs prepared to receive injured casualties from the incident site (Petersen, Benedek, & Grieger, 2007). Field personnel should ascertain the type of radioactive material involved and extent of exposure (Pae & Dill, 2006). Exposure limits will be controlled and regulated by field supervisors.

Significant clinical experience exists with victims who have received large amounts of external body radiation exposure (Koenig et al., 2005). Generally, no treatment is required unless victims have received external radiation exposures with absorbed doses in excess of 1 Gy (100 rad). When radiologically contaminated victims present with physical trauma and require medical care, treatment is first directed at stabilizing the patient and treating physical injuries, as reviewed previously in Chapter 14 (Pae & Dill, 2006; Petersen, Benedek, & Grieger, 2007). Remember that a victim presenting with radiation exposure and physical trauma has significantly more severe injuries than a victim presenting with either (Petersen, Benedek, &

Grieger). The literature reveals no cases of healthcare workers becoming acutely ill from radiation exposure due to caring for and decontaminating victims involved in radiation accidents.

Decontaminating victims who are sufficiently stable should occur first, with injury treatment following (Pae & Dill, 2006). Decontamination should occur as close to the event site as possible, as simple clothing removal eliminates 90% to 95% of total contamination (see Chapter 11) (Neal & Moores, 2002; Pae & Dill). Open wounds should be covered during clothing removal. Hypochlorite 0.5% can be used to wash the body (Neal & Moores). Any removed clothing and liquids used for lavage should be collected in appropriately marked biohazard containers. If biohazard containers are not available, the fluids and water should be flushed to standard drains, with notification to the local water treatment facility occurring immediately thereafter. Avoid rubbing or irritating wounds as irritation causes accelerated absorption of certain radioactive particles. Once decontamination occurs, severely injured and critically ill victims should be relocated after BLI/ATLS protocols are initiated (Chapter 14); unstable casualties should be transported rapidly to appropriately equipped facilities with decontamination procedures occurring after arrival (Neal & Moores; Pae & Dill).

Upon hospital arrival, critically ill and injured victims should be moved to critical care facilities within the hospital structure, and decontamination should proceed during resuscitation according to the hospital's incident command structure (HICS; Chapter 4) (Petersen, Benedek, & Grieger, 2007; Pae & Dill, 2006). Treatment is focused on stabilizing the patient and treating physical injuries in order from greatest concern to least concern (Petersen, Benedek, & Grieger). The ATLS algorithm should be followed to secure airway, breathing, and circulation. Physiologic studies should include tissue and blood typing and a CBC with differential to look for drops in lymphocyte levels over 24 hours or an absolute neutrophil count (ANC) of less than 100/mm^3, indicating significant exposure (Koenig et al., 2005; Petersen, Benedek, & Grieger). Any wounds are cleaned and extensively debrided prior to the onset of immunosuppression to reduce the risk of latent severe infection developing (Petersen, Benedek, & Grieger). Open wounds are closed primarily in this case, rather than allowing normal closure over time to occur. Any surgical interventions should be performed within the first 24 hours postexposure, and medication should be employed to sedate agitated victims.

Once medical stabilizing is achieved, assessing casualties for radiation injury on the basis of dose, isotope type, and presence of internal contamination takes precedence. Within 24 hours of arrival at the facility, blood should be drawn for a rapid-sort, automated chromosome aberration biodosimetry. Additionally, TE, measured from the time of irradiation, and lymphocyte depletion kinetics estimate radiation dose in mass casualty victims (Koenig et al., 2005). Estimates of radiation dose using a combination of patient history, serial lymphocyte counts (MLC), and TE may be calculated with the Armed Forces Radiobiology Research Institute's free Biological

Assessment Exposures Tool (BAT), available from http://www.afrri.usuhs.mil. Final assessment after initial medical stabilization is for localized radiation exposure.

Localized Radiation Exposure (LRE) Assessment and Care

Localized radiation exposure (LRE) occurs from direct contact with radioactive sources (Koenig et al., 2005; Pae & Dill, 2006). Absorbed doses are usually very high, but victims usually survive the exposure. Systemic manifestations tend to resolve quickly, as distance from the radiation source causes the dose rate to drop proportionally to distance. Therefore, local injury tends to be severe, and systemic symptoms tend to be less severe. Unlike thermal injuries, cutaneous radiation injury (CRI), characterized by delayed desquamation, blistering, and erythema, is common in LRE, occurring 12 to 20 days postevent (Koenig et al.; Petersen, Benedek, & Grieger, 2007).

In LRE, a CBC should be performed on a 24-hour basis if clinical presentation is consistent with CRI (Petersen, Benedek, & Grieger, 2007). Victims presenting with localized irradiation and cutaneous injury are treated according to the same protocols used in thermal burn wound management, as indicated in Chapter 14 (Koenig et al., 2005; Pae & Dill, 2006). Treating localized radiation injuries include pain management, grafting, surgery, and amputation (Koenig et al.). Infection control is also prioritized. When treating victims with suspected CRI, clinicians need to recognize several factors. First, the severity of the cutaneous injury depends on both the depth of radiation penetration into the tissue and exposure dose. Second, whereas chemical and blast casualty events cause immediate obvious damage to the skin layers, radiation exposures rarely do until days or weeks later, and when the damage manifests, the damage will appear and heal in a cyclical fashion. Third, for healthcare providers to adequately address and treat CRI, secondary infection must be prevented and adequate pain management must be made available (Petersen, Benedek, & Grieger, 2007).

There are five stages to CRI, similar to ARS: (a) prodromal, (b) latent, (c) manifest illness, (d) third wave of erythema, and (e) latent effects stage. The prodromal stage occurs within hours of exposure and is characterized by the first wave of erythema, pruritus, and sensations of heat that define the exposed areas. This phase occurs within hours of exposure. The second or latent stage occurs within 1 to 2 days postexposure. At this time, no outward injury is present, but, depending on the body part involved, the general rule is that the larger the exposure dose, the shorter the duration of the latent period. Therefore, skin of the face, neck, and chest will have a shorter latent stage than skin on the soles of the feet and palms of the hands (Petersen, Benedek, & Grieger, 2007).

The third stage, called the manifest illness stage, occurs from days to weeks postexposure. Here, the basal layer is repopulated through surviving clonogenic cell proliferation. The manifest illness stage initiates at the time of main erythema development and is evidenced by sensations of heat and slight edema, accompanied by slightly increased pigmentation. Here, symptoms vary from dry desquamation or ulceration to necrosis, all of which depend directly on the severity of the CRI generally. The fourth stage is the third wave of erythema, which occurs 10 to 16 weeks postexposure. Here the victim experiences late erythema, increasing pain, and edema due to blood vessel destruction or injury. The skin often takes on a blue pallor. Epilation may subside, but will be replaced by dermal necrosis, thinning, and atrophy of the dermis and new ulcer formation (Petersen, Benedek, & Grieger, 2007).

The fifth and final stage is the late effects stage. This stage begins months to years after radiation exposure. Symptoms range widely, from slight dermal atrophy to continual ulcer generation, dermal necrosis, and deformity. Telangiectasia (small blood vessel occlusion with subsequent disturbance to the blood supply), lymphatic network destruction, regional lymphostasis, and increasingly invasive keratosis, fibrosis, subcutaneous sclerosis, and vasculitis may develop as well. Pain and pigment changes present, and skin cancer development is possible in subsequent years (Petersen, Benedek, & Grieger, 2007).

Basically, unless the most severe radiation exposure dose is encountered where poor prognosis for survival is almost guaranteed, most radiation exposure injuries are treatable and survivable. Nearly all radiation exposure casualties have treatable injuries provided that medical care is accessible. Casualties with unsurvivable irradiation injury usually die immediately on site, or they are severely injured by the blast and thermal effects from detonation, such as by overpressurization wave, flash, and flame burns, such that their death results secondary to radiation exposure. Unfortunately, it is possible that significant radiation dose exposures below the level necessary to cause outward symptoms alter the body's immune responses significantly, making infection risk a real medical management concern after initial resuscitation and stabilization procedures are completed. Therefore, understanding pharmacologic approaches used in radiation injuries is important to increasing victim survivability (Armed Forces Radiobiology Research Institute, 2008).

Pharmacologic Treatment of Radiation Exposures

Pharmacologic treatment of mass casualty wounds of any sort is termed *medical countermeasures.* These countermeasures fall into three basic categories: drugs preventing radiation-induced cellular and molecular damage (including amifostine and phosphonol, keratinocyte growth factor, angiotensin-converting enzyme inhibitor captopril, isoflavone genistein, nonandrogenic steroid androstenediol, and α-tocopherol succinate); radiation mitigators that accelerate recovery and repair after radiation injury (including colony-stimulating factors and cytokines, androgenic steroid androstenediol, glutamine, and pentoxifylline); and radionuclide eliminators used to discorporate and block internalized radionuclide absorptions (including potassium iodide, ferric hexacyanoferrate [Prussian blue], and calcium and zinc diethylenetriaminepentaacetate [Ca- and Zn-DTPA]) (Koenig et al., 2005; Pae & Dill, 2006). Generally, pharmacological management occurs early in the postresuscitation phase of care since conventional injuries and illnesses are treated before radiation concerns are addressed, because it is these secondary effects that usually result in less optimal outcomes for survivors of radiation exposure (Pae & Dill). It is not possible to go into a thorough discussion of drugs in this text. The reader is advised to seek out further texts dealing with these pharmaceuticals.

Conclusion

There is no quick approach to handling a mass casualty event due to radiation or blast exposures. However, when the unpredictable event occurs, chaos should give way to logic, recognizing that common diagnostic and treatment algorithms apply and should be instituted. In this regard, acuity, dose, and duration of exposure in radiation disasters and amount and type of explosive materials used, the environmental conditions at the time of the explosion, the delivery device (such as metal or plastic), the distance between the device and the victims, and intervening or complicating hazards or protective barriers present at and immediately surrounding the detonation location in blast disasters provide guidance on how to assess, resuscitate, stabilize, and treat irradiated victims of mass casualty CBRN disasters.

Treatment objectives in caring for victims of radiation disasters are the following:

1. Resuscitate and provide first aid as needed.
2. Stabilize medically and surgically as needed.
3. Treat serious injuries in the order from most life threatening or confounding to least concerning.
4. Minimize and prevent internal contamination.
5. Assess external contamination sources and radiation method used and decontaminate accordingly with appropriate hazardous waste disposal.
6. Treat other minor, observed injuries.
7. Contain contamination to treatment area if decontamination cannot be performed at the incident site prior to transfer.
8. Take adequate precautions to protect healthcare providers from unnecessary contamination exposure.
9. Reassess internal contamination.
10. Treat internal contamination; may be handled concurrently with any of the steps 1–7 as warranted.
11. Assess local radiation exposure injuries and radiation dose.
12. Counsel patients regarding long-term exposure risks and effects.
13. Provide for long-term follow-up assessment of patients suffering whole-body radiation exposure or internal contamination (Koenig et al., 2005).

Following these guidelines should ensure the best outcome possible in the mass radiation exposure casualty event for each of its surviving victims, understanding that in certain exposures, death will be inevitable.

Reviewing bombings and blast-related mass casualty events, and all other mass casualty events in general, the reality is that severe demands are placed upon prehospital and in-hospital systems. The resultant volume of victims requiring care can easily overwhelm the resources of any facility not already possessing a preparedness plan. When radiation exposure is added into the mass burn casualty event equation, which is the most likely event to occur from dirty bomb (RDD) terrorist activities, the challenges become even more daunting; rapid control and processing of contaminated victims becomes critically important to avoid unnecessary contamination of the hospital and healthcare providers.

The WTC destruction in 2001 brought the need for effective and efficient disaster management and preparedness to the forefront. Federal agencies are now established to address mass casualty events in conjunction with local, state, and regional agencies and first response teams, but none of these systems are able to respond sufficiently, expeditiously, or effectively when massive needs occur from an unplanned mass casualty incident. Local community response in cooperation with hospitals and EMS providers must take the lead to coordinate appropriate assessment, resuscitation, stabilization, and referral of the massive number of victims. Additionally, these first-level responders must be able to quickly adapt existing protocols and procedures to meet the various demands presented when radiation exposure and contamination is added into the equation. Therefore, the disaster nurse must take the lead in preparing for the unplanned mass casualty event to ensure optimal outcomes for the largest number of survivors.

References

Alfici, R. (2006). *Military medicine: Management of victims in a mass casualty incident caused by a terrorist bombing: Treatment algorithms for stable, unstable and in extremis victims* [Electronic version]. *Israeli Medical Association Journal*, Retrieved December 2006 from http://www.findarticles.com/p/articles/mi_qa3912/is_200612/ai_n17185624

American Medical Association. (2005). *Mass trauma and explosive events.* Retrieved March 24, 2008, from http://www.ama-assn.org/ama1/pub/upload/mm/415/05_masstrauma.pdf

Armed Forces Radiobiology Research Institute. (2008). Biodosimetry Exposure Assessment Tool [Software application]. Bethesda, MD: Author. Retrieved March 30, 2008, from http://www.afrri.usuhs.mil

Centers for Disease Control and Prevention. (2003a). *Mass casualties: Glasgow Coma Scale.* Retrieved March 27, 2008, from http://www.bt.cdc.gov/masscasualties/pdf/glasgow-coma-scale.pdf

Centers for Disease Control and Prevention. (2003b). *Mass casualties: Explosions and blast injuries: A primer for clinicians.* Retrieved March 24, 2008, from http://www.bt.cdc.gov/masscasualties/pdf/explosions.blast-injuries.pdf

Centers for Disease Control and Prevention. (2005). *Mass casualties: Blast lung injuries: What clinicians need to know.* Retrieved March 24, 2008, from http://www.bt.cdc.gov/masscasualties/pdf/blastlunginjury.pdf

Centers for Disease Control and Prevention. (2006). *Mass casualties: Blast lung injury: An overview for prehospital care providers.* Retrieved March 24, 2008, from http://www.bt.cdc.gov/masscasualties/pdf/blastlunginjury_prehospital.pdf

Centers for Disease Control and Prevention. (2008). *Mass casualties: Blast injuries: Essential facts.* Retrieved March 24, 2008, from http://www.bt.cdc.gov/masscasualties/pdf/blastinjuries.pdf

Irizarry, L., & Williams, G. M. (2007, August 22). CBRNE-incendiary agents, white phosphorus. *Medscape Journal.* Retrieved March 26, 2008, from http://www.emedicine.com/EMERG/topic918.htm

Kluger, Y., Pele, K., Daniel-Aharonson, L., & Mayo, A. (2004). The special injury pattern in terrorist bombings. *Journal of the American College of Surgeons, 199,* 875–879.

Koenig, K. L., Goans, R. E., Hatchett, R. J., Mettler, F. A., Schumacher, T. A., Noji, E. K., et al. (2005). Medical treatment of radiological casualties: Current concepts. *Annals of Emergency Medicine, 45*(6), 643–652.

National CounterTerrorism Center. (2008). *MIPT terrorism knowledge database.* Retrieved March 25, 2008, from http://www.tkb.org/IncidentDateModule.jsp

Neal, C. J., & Moores, L. E. (2002). Weapons of mass destruction: Radiation. *Neurosurgical Focus, 12*(3), E4. Retrieved March 6, 2008, from http://www.medscape.com/viewarticle/431313_print

Pae, J. S., & Dill, C. E. (2006, November 9). CBRNE: Radiation emergencies. *eMedicine Journal.* Retrieved March 11, 2008, from http://www.emedicine.com/emerg/TOPIC934.htm

Pennardt, A., Lavonas, E., & Danzl, D. (2007, December 19). Blast injuries. *Medscape Journal.* Retrieved March 24, 2008, from http://www.emedicine.com/emerg/TOPIC63.htm

Petersen, K. M., Benedek, D. M., & Grieger, T. A. (2007, January 8). Terrorism and disaster—What clinicians need to know: Radiation attack: Medical & psychosocial management. *Medscape Journal.* Retrieved March 11, 2008, from http://www.medscape.com/viewprogram/6507_pnt

Severance, H. W. (2002). Mass-casualty victim "surge" management, Preparing for bombings and blast-related injuries with possibility of hazardous materials exposure. *National Contract Management Journal, 63*(5), 242–246.

Sutphen, S. K. (2005, November 9). Blast injuries: A review. *Medscape Journal.* Retrieved March 16, 2008, from www.medscape.com/viewprogram/4714_pnt

United Nations Educational, Scientific, and Cultural Organizations. (n.d.) *About natural disasters.* Retrieved March 25, 2008, from http://www.unesco.org/science/disaster/about_disaster.shtml

United States Federal Bureau of Investigation. (2001). *CounterTerrorism: FBI policy and guidelines.* Retrieved March 24, 2008, from http://jackson.fbi.gov/cntrterr.htm

chapter 16

Bioterrorism: The Use of Biological Agents

Deborah S. Adelman and Timothy J. Legg

GOAL

The goal of this chapter is to provide an understanding of the different types of biological agents that may be used in a bioterrorism attack.

OBJECTIVES

At the completion of this chapter, the reader will:

1. Discuss the various categories of biological agents that may be used in a bioterrorism attack.
2. Assess patients presenting with exposure to various types of bioterrorism agents.
3. Design nursing interventions based on signs and symptoms of exposure to a biological agent.
4. Understand the proper treatments for each category of biological agent.

Key Terms

- Bioterrorism
- Biological agent
- Category A agents
- Category B agents
- Category C agents

Introduction

Up to this point we have examined a myriad of disasters that can impact a given society. We shall now turn our attention to a particularly frightening type of disaster. Envision an attacker who cannot be seen—an invisible presence that cannot be touched or smelled. An attacker who does not kill or hurt in one swift strike, but who instead forces us to become slowly ill long after the attack has been made; an attacker who makes us suffer while family and friends watch; an attacker who may spread to friends and family; an attacker who, by the time it is detected, may have killed thousands. Herein lies the true terror of biological disasters.

The subject of biological disaster is one that has both fascinated and terrified humans for centuries. Throughout recorded history, violence and devastation from the unseen world of microorganisms has left its mark on humanity. The omnipresent threat of biological disaster has manifested itself in many people's belief systems regarding personal health practices and hygiene: How many of us have heard the famous lament "Don't go outside after you get out of the shower! Your hair is wet and you will get sick"? There is also the specter of epidemics and pandemics, naturally occurring throughout history, much less man-made bioterrorism: the Black Plague, the Spanish Flu, and others.

Biological disaster and its possibility have even managed to appear in our popular movies and films. How many can recall the 1971 film *The Andromeda Strain* in which alien bacteria threatened to destroy humanity (Internet Movie Database [IMDB], 2008a). Although *The Andromeda Strain* is based in science fiction, we also found ourselves fascinated by the 1993 film *And the Band Played On*, which chronicled the unfolding AIDS epidemic (IMDB, 2008b).

Whether an accidental release of microorganisms into the general public by a laboratory error or the intentional release of disease-causing organisms by a terrorist group or "simply" as a natural history event, the danger of biological agents is real. In this chapter, we will explore the common classes of biological agents.

Understanding Biological Agents

Biological agents include microorganisms such as bacteria, viruses, and fungi. The microorganisms, in addition to their associated toxins (i.e., substances secreted by the microorganisms as they grow and proliferate) can affect human health in a multitude of ways, ranging from mild symptoms of allergic reaction to severe illness and death. These organisms are naturally found in nature, in plants, soil, water, and animals. Because of their ability to reproduce rapidly with minimal resources, they pose a serious threat to health (Occupational Safety and Health Administration [OSHA], 2006). Although all of these agents exist in nature, they can be cultivated for a variety of uses. Consider the use of botulism for cosmetic and plastics procedures. Some bacteria are used for medical research. Just as these biological agents are used for the good of humanity, they can also be used in terrorist acts.

Brief History of Biological Agents

There is an immediate propensity to consider biological agents to be a specter of this century. However, biological agents have existed since the beginning of recorded history. In fact, probably since the beginning of humanity itself. Let us consider plague, which has been "responsible for some of the worst catastrophes in the story of humankind, and more than once has changed the course of history" (Dobson, 2007, p. 8). Naturally occurring and spread by rats and fleas, the plague has killed over 75 million people worldwide. Other biological agents have appeared throughout history such as dengue fever, measles, yellow fever, rabies, polio, influenza, leprosy, syphilis, typhus, and cholera. New, naturally occurring diseases and microorganisms are appearing all the time. Some of the latest include Ebola, Marburg, and hanta viruses.

There is also a mistaken idea that the use of biological agents as weapons of terror is a modern day phenomenon. Let us not forget American history: British officers gave blankets and handkerchiefs taken from a smallpox hospital to Indians who threatened the safety of Fort Pitt, Pennsylvania (Fenn, 2001). Biological weapons have been in existence for centuries and have been used for at least the same amount of time by various groups.

Categories of Biological Agents

Biological agents have been categorized into three separate categories of agents. In this section, we will explore each of these categories and see examples of the agents belonging to each category. A brief overview will be provided and extensive tables will support the text.

Category A Agents

Category A agents are those agents which have been given highest priority because they include pathogens that are rarely seen in the United States. They pose a risk to national security for several reasons: (a) these agents can be easily disseminated or transmitted from one person to another, (b) diseases resulting from these agents have high mortality rates and have the potential to have a major public health impact, (c) they have the potential to cause panic and social disruption, and (d) they require special attention for public health preparedness (Centers for Disease Control and Prevention [CDC], n.d.). Category A agents include *Bacillus anthracis* (anthrax; see examples of cutaneous and inhalation anthrax in Figures 16-1 through 16-5), *Clostridium botulinum* toxin (botulism), *Variola major* (smallpox; see Figure 16-6), *Yersinia pestis* (plague; see Figure 16-7), *Francisella tularensis* (tularemia), and several viruses belonging to a group known as the "viral hemorrhagic fevers" (e.g., filoviruses such as Ebola and Marburg as well as arenaviruses such as Lassa fever and Machupo).

Cutaneous Anthrax

The following figures show the progression of symptoms of cutaneous anthrax.

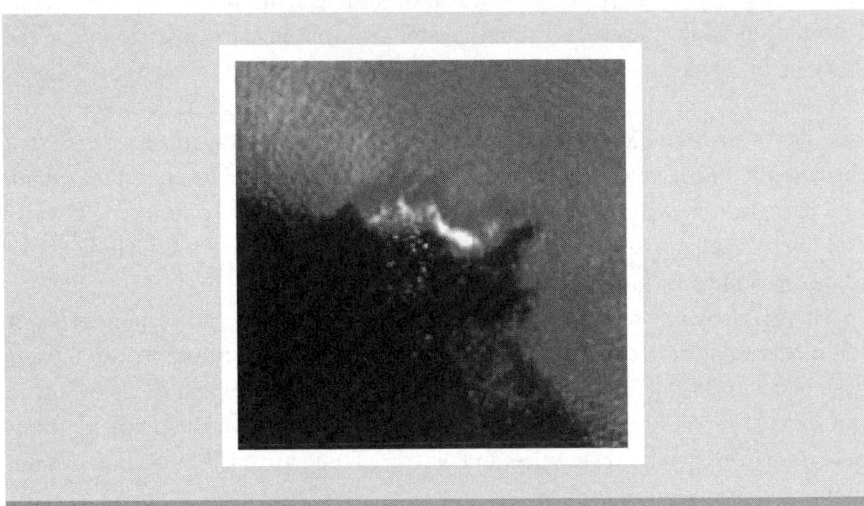

Figure 16-1 Symptoms of cutaneous anthrax: day 2 postexposure.
Source: Courtesy of CDC.

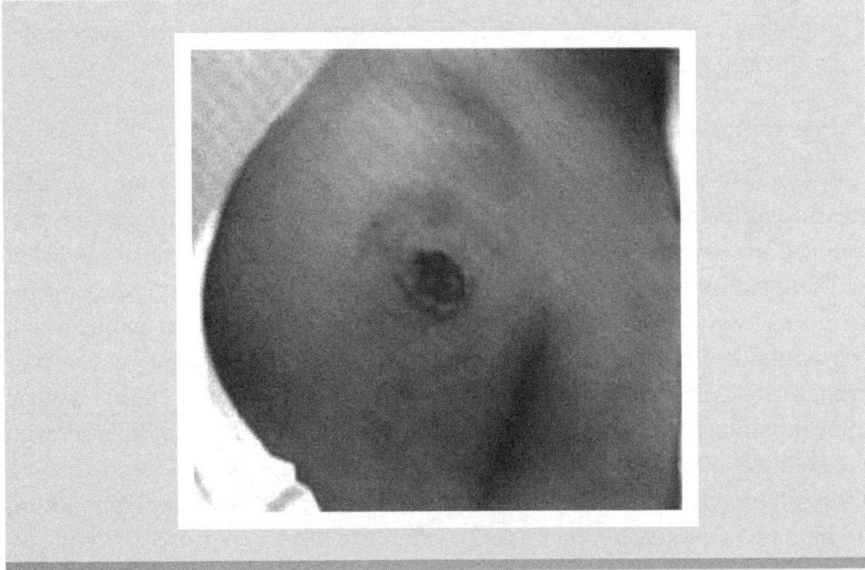

Figure 16-2 Symptoms of cutaneous anthrax: day 4 postexposure.
Source: Courtesy of CDC.

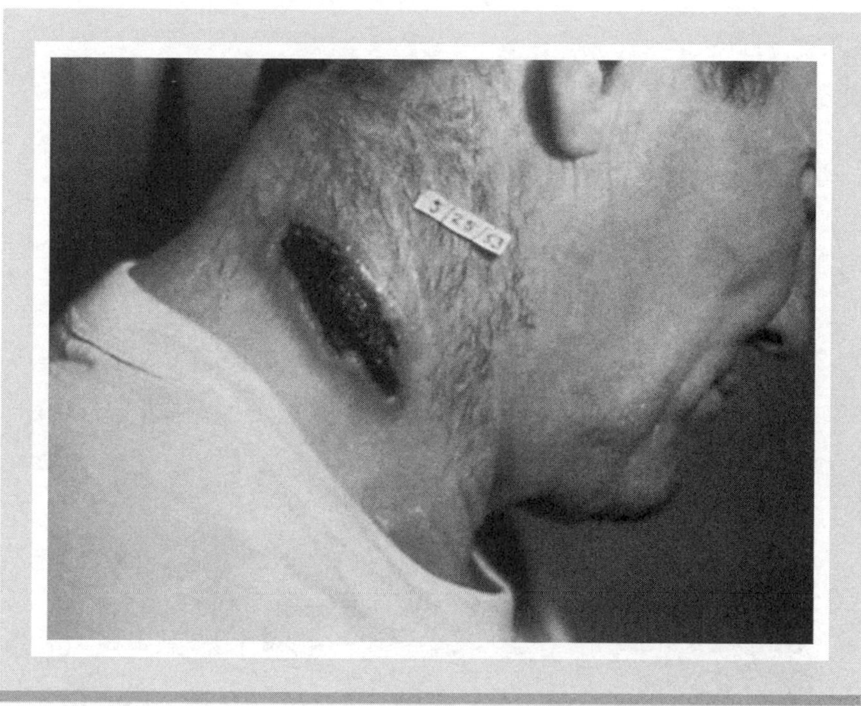

Figure 16-3 Symptoms of cutaneous anthrax: day 6 postexposure.
Source: Courtesy of CDC.

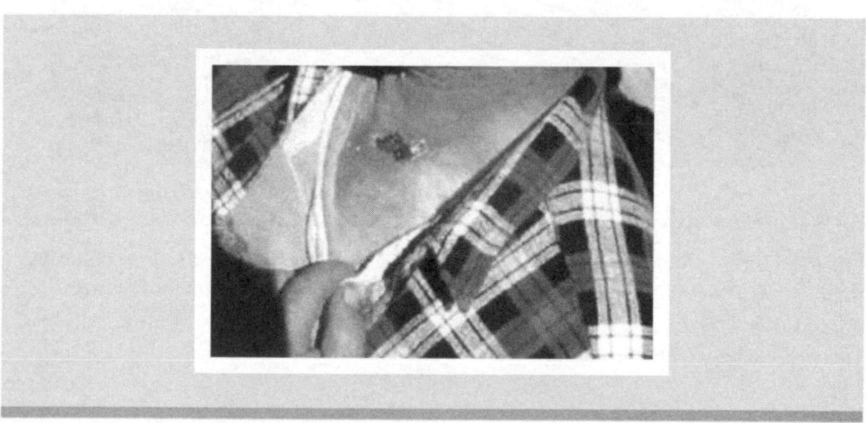

Figure 16-4 Symptoms of cutaneous anthrax: day 10 postexposure.
Source: Courtesy of CDC.

Anthrax Inhalation

Figure 16-5 displays the classic X-ray picture of anthrax inhalation.

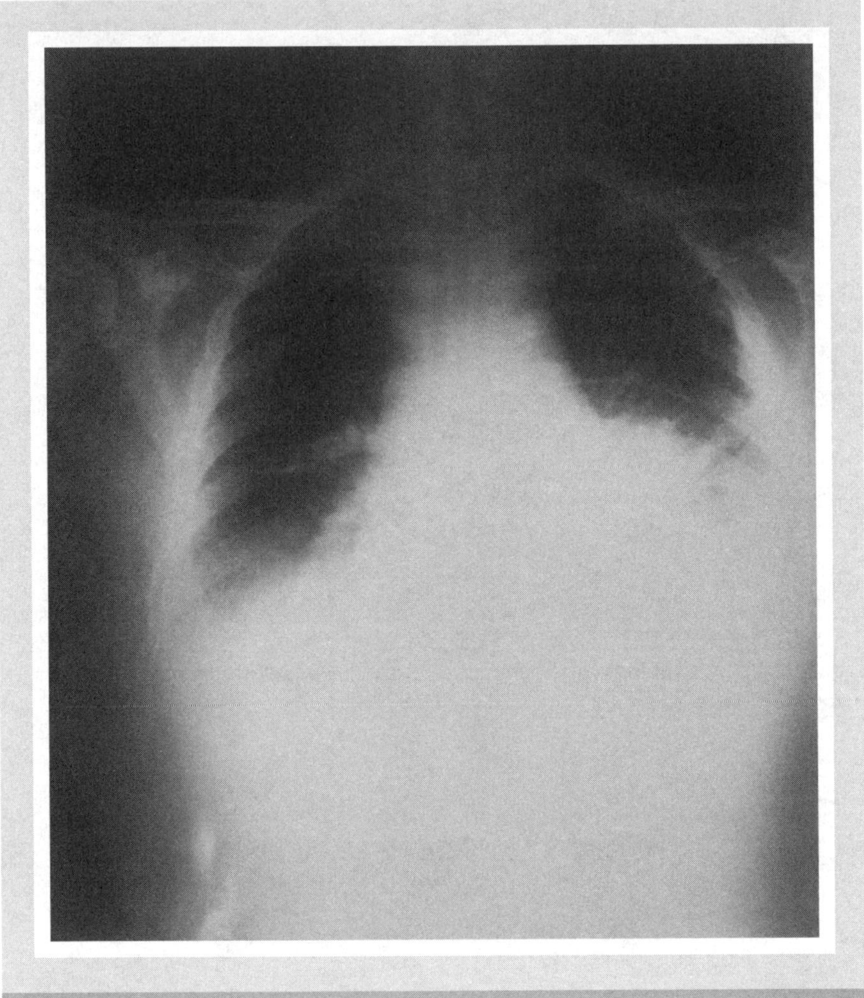

Figure 16-5 The photographic X-ray presents anthrax inhalation. Note enlarged mediastinum and whiteout of bases of lungs, classic X-ray presentation of anthrax inhalation.
Source: Courtesy of Dr. P.S. Brachman/CDC.

Smallpox

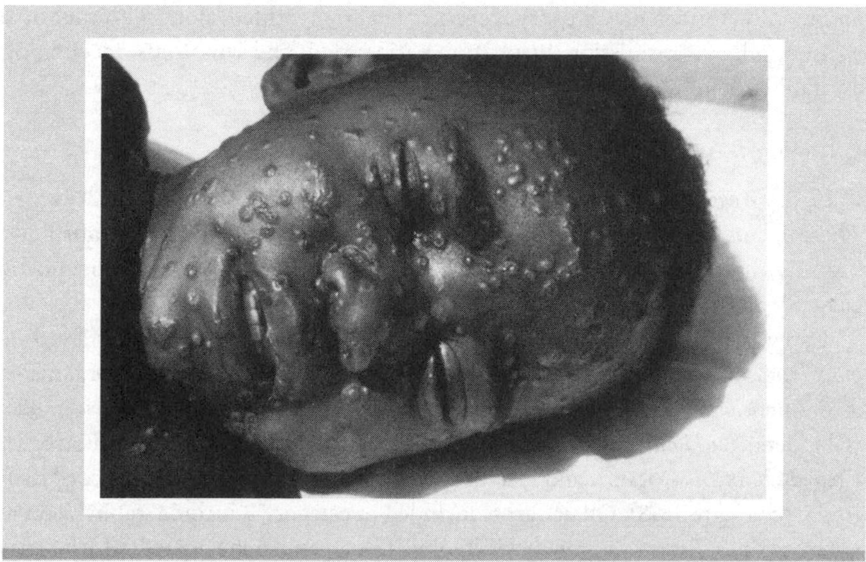

Figure 16-6 A smallpox victim.
Source: Courtesy of CDC.

Plague

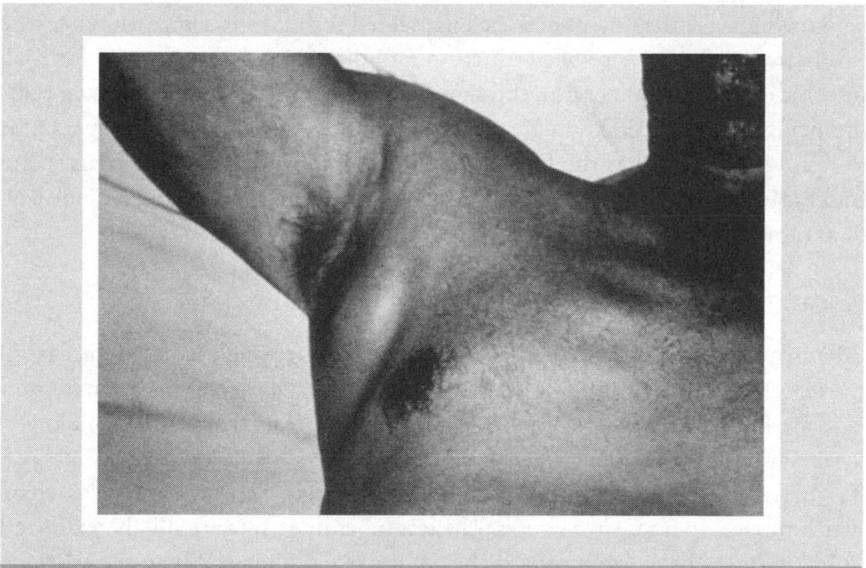

Figure 16-7 Plague buboe at lymph node under arm.
Source: Courtesy of CDC.

In Table 16-1, Category A agents are presented along with causative agent, mode of transmission, incubation period, signs and symptoms, vaccination availability, and medical treatment. Category B agents are also presented, along with causative agent, mode of transmission, incubation period, signs and symptoms, vaccination availability, and medical treatment.

Category B Agents

Category B agents have been given the second highest priority of biological agents. These agents are moderately easy to disseminate and result in moderate morbidity but low mortality rates and would require enhancements to CDC's diagnostic capacity and enhanced disease surveillance (CDC, n.d.).

Category B agents include *Brucella* species (brucellosis), *Clostridium perfringens* (the source of epsilon toxin), food safety threats (caused by such organisms as *Salmonella, Escherichia coli,* and *Shigella;* see Table 16-2), *Burkholderia mallei* (Glanders), *Burkholderia pseudomallei* (melioidosis), *Chlamydia psittaci* (psittacosis), *Coxiella burnetii* (Q fever), and *Ricinus communis* (castor beans—the source of ricin toxin; see Figure 16-8). Other agents included in category B include staphylococcal enterotoxin B, *Rickettsia prowazekii* (typhus fever), and alphaviruses (which cause viral encephalitis), as well as water safety threats from organisms such as *Vibrio cholera* and *Cryptosporidium parvum* (CDC, n.d.)

Category C Agents

These agents have been given the third highest priority and include emerging agents that have the potential to be engineered for mass dissemination because of their availability, ease of production and dissemination, potential for high morbidity and mortality rates, and the overall impact that they can have on public health (CDC, n.d.). Category C agents include zoonotic diseases such as Nepal virus, which has the fruit bat as host, as well as tick-borne viruses and rabies. Figure 16-9 contains photographs of the rabies virus and a patient who had rabies.

Conclusion

Bioterrorism and natural biological epidemics are terrifying events. In the case of bioterrorism, the perpetrator is long gone when signs and symptoms begin to show and are finally diagnosed. With the downfall of the Soviet Union, many biological agents were lost from their public health facility that stored these agents. Smallpox test tubes kept there and at the CDC in Atlanta, Georgia, were the only places left on Earth thought to house live viruses. The test tubes in Atlanta are still there; the test tubes in Russia have disappeared—the nightmare continues: Where and when do we have to worry about these biological agents popping up?

(*text continues on page 319*)

TABLE 16-1 CATEGORY A AND CATEGORY B BIOLOGICAL AGENTS

Name	Causative Agent	Mode of Transmission	Incubation Period	Signs and Symptoms	Vaccination Availability	Medical Treatment
Category A Agents						
Anthrax	*Bacillus anthracis*	Human-to-human contact has not been documented. Transmission is from animal to human through handling or breathing in spores from infected animals. GI anthrax can result from eating undercooked meat from infected animals (CDC, 2003a).	As short as 7 days, up to 42 days for inhalation anthrax (CDC, 2003a).	Cutaneous: small sore that develops into a blister that develops into a skin ulcer with a black area in the center. Sore, blister, and area do not hurt. Gastrointestinal: nausea, loss of appetite, bloody diarrhea, fever, and stomach pain. Inhalation: cold or flulike symptoms (sore throat, mild fever, muscle aches)—later symptoms include cough, chest discomfort, shortness of breath, fatigue, and muscle aches (CDC, 2003a).	Although a vaccine has been developed, it is not available to the general public (CDC, 2003a).	Antibiotics such as ciprofloxacin, levofloxacin, doxycycline, or penicillin can be used to treat anthrax. Treatment is usually a 60-day course of antibiotics. Treatment success depends on how soon the disease is identified and antimicrobial agents are begun (CDC, 2003a).

(continued)

TABLE 16-1 CATEGORY A AND CATEGORY B BIOLOGICAL AGENTS (Continued)

Name	Causative Agent	Mode of Transmission	Incubation Period	Signs and Symptoms	Vaccination Availability	Medical Treatment
Botulism	The disease is caused by the release of a neuroparalytic toxin produced by the bacterium *Clostridium botulinum.*	Transmission is primarily foodborne, and it cannot be transmitted from person to person. Botulism can also result from wound infection (contamination of a wound with *Clostridium botulinum*). May be seen in IV drug users because of puncture wounds from needles (CDC, 2006a).	Symptoms of foodborne botulism occur within 12–36 hours after ingestion of the toxin but have been reported to range from 6 hours to 10 days. Wound botulism is difficult to estimate because actual exposure time cannot be ascertained (CDC, 2006b).	Victims of foodborne botulism may experience symmetric cranial neuropathies such as diplopia, drooping eyelids, dry mouth, altered voice/difficulty speaking, or difficulty swallowing. Symmetric descending flaccid paralysis in a proximal-distal pattern may be seen. Some have reported abdominal pain, nausea, and vomiting. Wound botulism results in the same neurological findings as foodborne botulism with the exception of gastrointestinal symptoms.	There is no botulism vaccine, and antitoxins cannot prevent it. Natural immunity to botulism does not exist. Prevention is essential. Foods should be properly cooked to appropriate temperatures for appropriate length of times. Also, IV drug use should be discouraged (CDC, 2006c).	Botulinum antitoxin is available. This does not reverse paralysis, but merely halts its progression. Before administering, skin testing to evaluate sensitivity should be undertaken. Treatment is otherwise supportive, and the person will recover when new neuromuscular connections regenerate (CDC, 2006d).

				Neurological findings are indistinguishable from foodborne botulism without gastrointestinal symptoms The wound itself may not appear grossly infected but these wounds are usually deep and contain areas that are avascular (CDC, 2006c).		
Plague (Bubonic and Pneumonic)	*Yersenia pestis*	Bubonic plague is the more common type of plague and is caused by a bite from a flea infected with *Y. pestis.* Bubonic plague does not spread from person to person. Pneumonic plague occurs when *Y. pestis* infects the lungs. This type of	A person usually manifests signs and symptoms of bubonic plague within 2–6 days after being infected (CDC, 2001). Pneumonic plague symptoms appear within 1 to 6 days after initial exposure (CDC, 2005a).	The typical sign of the most common form of human plague is a swollen and very tender lymph gland, accompanied by pain. The swollen gland is called a "bubo." Bubonic plague should be suspected when a person develops a swollen gland, fever, chills, headache, extreme	There is no plague vaccine currently available in the United States (CDC, 2001). If persons must live or work in an area where a plague outbreak has occurred, they can render themselves immune for up to 3 weeks by taking prophylactic antibiotics.	Streptomycin is FDA approved for treatment of plague. Problems with availability may result in other antimicrobial choices, for example, the aminoglycosides, tetracyclines, and chloramphenicol. Newer antimicrobial agents such as the fluoro-

(continued)

TABLE 16-1 CATEGORY A AND CATEGORY B BIOLOGICAL AGENTS (Continued)

Name	Causative Agent	Mode of Transmission	Incubation Period	Signs and Symptoms	Vaccination Availability	Medical Treatment
		plague can be transmitted from person to person. This type of plague requires direct and close contact to spread (CDC, 2001).		exhaustion, and has a history of possible exposure to infected rodents, rabbits, or fleas (CDC, 2005b). With pneumonic plague, the first signs of illness are fever, headache, weakness, and rapidly developing pneumonia with shortness of breath, chest pain, cough, and sometimes bloody or watery sputum. The pneumonia progresses for 2 to 4 days and may cause respiratory failure and shock. Without early treatment, patients may die (CDC, 2001).	Tetracyclines or sulfonamides are preferred for plague prophylaxis (CDC, 2005c).	quinolones may also be considered (CDC, 2007a).

Smallpox	*Variola major*	Direct contact with infected body fluids or fomite-to-person contact. There is no animal- or insect-to-human transmission as humans are the only carriers of the *Variola* virus. The last known case of smallpox in the United States was in 1949. However, events of 9/11/01 resulted in the concern that smallpox may be used as an agent of biological warfare (CDC, 2007b).	Incubation period following exposure can range from 7 to 17 days (CDC, 2007b).	From 7 to 17 days following initial exposure, the infected patient may complain of no symptoms and is not contagious. After the incubation period, first symptoms that are nonspecific appear and include fever, fatigue, achiness, and in some cases, emesis. Fever can range from 101°–104°F. This stage may last 2–4 days. Following the nonspecific symptom stage, small red spots manifest on the tongue and inside the mouth. Following this, a skin rash appears beginning on the face and spreading to the arms and	There is a vaccine which can be used against smallpox. In fact, this very vaccine was used to eradicate smallpox from the human population (CDC, 2007d).	There is no cure for smallpox, and the disease must be allowed to run its course. Medical management involves supportive measures such as IV therapy, controlling fever, and antibiotics for secondary bacterial infections (CDC, 2007c).

(continued)

TABLE 16-1 CATEGORY A AND CATEGORY B BIOLOGICAL AGENTS (Continued)

Name	Causative Agent	Mode of Transmission	Incubation Period	Signs and Symptoms	Vaccination Availability	Medical Treatment
				legs, next to hands and feet, and usually spreading to all body parts within 24 hours. This rash turns into raised bumps that eventually become pustules. The pustules then form a crust and then scab over. By the end of the second week, most of the pustules have scabbed over. Scabs then begin to fall off leaving scars that appear as shallow craters (CDC, 2007c).		

Tularemia	*Francisella tularensis*	The bacterium is found in animals and can be transmitted to humans through a bite from an infected tick, deerfly, or other insect. It can also be transmitted through handling infected animal carcasses, eating or drinking food or water that has been contaminated by *F. tularensis*, or through inhalation of the bacteria (CDC, 2003b).	Incubation period ranges from 1 to 14 days (Dennis et al., 2001).	Abrupt onset with fever, headache, chills, and rigors. Patient may complain of generalized body aches (especially in the lower back) and dry or slightly productive cough with complaints of chest tightness. Patient may not have objective signs of pneumonia (purulent sputum, dyspnea, tachypnea, pleuritic pain, etc.). Some patients may complain of nausea, vomiting, and diarrhea. Sweating, chills, progressive weakness, malaise, anorexia, and weight loss are noted with progressing illness (Dennis et al., 2001).	In the United States, live attenuated vaccine has been used to protect laboratory workers who routinely work with the bacteria, but it is not available to the general public (CDC, 2003c).	Parenteral streptomycin is the drug of choice for treatment of tularemia. Gentamicin can also be used IV and is more widely available. Treatment should continue for at least 10 days. Tetracyclines and chloramphenicol may also be used, but primary treatment failure and relapses have been noted with these drugs. Doxycycline and ciprofloxacin may be used in a mass casualty setting. Doxycycline should be continued for 14–21 days, and ciprofloxacin should be continued for at least 10 days (Dennis et al., 2001).

(continued)

TABLE 16-1 CATEGORY A AND CATEGORY B BIOLOGICAL AGENTS (Continued)

Name	Causative Agent	Mode of Transmission	Incubation Period	Signs and Symptoms	Vaccination Availability	Medical Treatment
Category B Agents						
Brucellosis (a.k.a. Undulant fever)	Organisms from the *Brucella* species. Different organisms are associated with different animals, for example *B. abortus* is usually harbored by cattle, whereas *B. melitensi* and *B. ovis* are more common among sheep and goats. *B. canis* is associated with dogs (CDC, 2005d).	There are three primary mechanisms of infection in humans: oral, inhalation, or via wound infection. Consumption of contaminated milk products remains the most prevalent means of transmission. Direct person-to-person contact is rare, but possible. Transmission via breast milk and sexual contact and tissue transplantation have also been reported (CDC, 2007e).	Although no specific information about incubation period was found, it can be inferred that individuals who have been exposed should be monitored for fever for up to 4 weeks. Passive monitoring of broader symptoms should continue for up to 6 months (CDC, 2007e).	Depend upon point in the disease process. In the acute form (less than 8 weeks from onset of illness), flulike symptoms have been reported (including fever, anorexia, headache, and myalgia). In the undulant form (less than 1 year from the onset of illness), symptoms such as undulant fevers (fevers that appear in patterns, i.e., wax and wane), arthritis, epididymoorchitis in males, and neurological symptoms (in about 5% of cases). Depression and chronic fatigue syndrome have also been reported (CDC, 2005d).	There is no vaccine available for humans (CDC, 2007e).	Doxycycline and rifampin in combination for 6 weeks to prevent recurrent infection (CDC, 2007e).

Glanders	*Burkholderia* (formerly known as *Pseudomonas mallei*), a gram-negative bacillus (CDC, 2008b)	Direct contact with infected animals through skin and mucous membranes of the eyes and nose. Pulmonary transmission has also been documented (CDC, 2008a).	Depends upon method of transmission. Localized infection through cutaneous route, within 1 to 5 days. In pulmonary infections, signs and symptoms of pneumonia are noted. Chest X-ray reveals localized infection. Bloodstream infection is severe usually resulting in fatality within 7 to 10 days (CDC, 2008a).	Symptoms depend upon mode of transmission. General symptoms include fever, muscle aches and tightness, headache, excessive tearing of the eyes, photophobia, and diarrhea. Localized signs and symptoms of localized infection include erythema, warmth to touch, and ulceration at the site where bacteria entered the body. Lymph node swelling and infections involving mucous membranes of the eyes, nose, and respiratory tract will result in increased mucous production (at infected sites).	There is no vaccine available for glanders. In countries where glanders is endemic in animals, prevention of the disease in humans involves identification and elimination of the infection in the animal population. Within the health-care setting, transmission can be prevented by using common blood and body fluid precautions (CDC, 2008a).	Because human cases of glanders are rare, there is limited information about antibiotic treatment of the organism in humans. Sulfadiazine has been found to be an effective in experimental animals and in humans. *Burkholderia mallei* is usually sensitive to tetracyclines, ciprofloxacin, streptomycin, novobiocin, gentamicin, imipenem, ceftrazidime, and the sulfonamides. Resistance to chloramphenicol has been reported (CDC, 2008a).

(continued)

TABLE 16-1 CATEGORY A AND CATEGORY B BIOLOGICAL AGENTS (Continued)

Name	Causative Agent	Mode of Transmission	Incubation Period	Signs and Symptoms	Vaccination Availability	Medical Treatment
				Pulmonary infections result in signs/symptoms of pneumonia. Chest X-ray demonstrates localized infection. Chronic infection is possible and manifests as multiple abscesses within the arms and legs or in the liver or spleen (CDC, 2008a).		
Q-fever	*Coxiella burnetii* (CDC, 2006e)	*C. burnetii* can be excreted in milk, urine, and feces of infected animals; however, human transmission via this route is not common. Humans are generally infected through inhalation of the organism via	Incubation period depends on number of organisms that initially infect the host. The greater the number of organisms, the shorter the incubation period. In general, illness manifests itself within 2–3 weeks	Approximately one half of persons infected with *C. burnetii* will demonstrate signs of illness. Those individuals that do may have a sudden onset of symptoms such as fever (up to 104°–105°F), headache, myalgia,	A vaccine for use in humans was developed in Australia, but it is not commercially available in the United States (CDC, 2006g).	Doxycycline is the treatment of choice for acute Q fever (100 mg PO for 15–21 days). Quinolones have also demonstrated utility against Q fever. Therapy should be initiated within 3 days of

	droplets or inhalation of barnyard dust contaminated with the organism. Transmission via tick bites and human-to-human transmission are rare (CDC, 2006e).	after exposure, but approximately half of all persons infected will remain asymptomatic (CDC, 2006e).	chills and/or sweats, nonproductive cough, nausea, vomiting, abdominal pain, and diarrhea. Fever persists for approximately 1 to 2 weeks. Up to 50% of those with symptoms will develop pneumonia. 30 to 50% of patients with a symptomatic infection will develop pneumonia. Other patients may go on to develop abnormal liver tests, hepatitis, myocarditis, encephalitis, osteomyelitis, and miscarriages in pregnant women. Mortality rate is approximately 1–2%. Chronic infection is		symptoms onset. Doxycycline therapy is the recommended antibiotic. Antibiotic treatment is most effective when initiated within the first 3 days of illness (CDC, 2006h).

(continued)

TABLE 16-1 CATEGORY A AND CATEGORY B BIOLOGICAL AGENTS (Continued)

Name	Causative Agent	Mode of Transmission	Incubation Period	Signs and Symptoms	Vaccination Availability	Medical Treatment
				possible, but rare. Fatality rates of 1–2% are reported for acute Q fever (CDC, 2006f).		
Ricin	Castor beans (ricin is part of the waste product of castor oil production).	Transmission is deliberate, that is, one must deliberately make ricin and then transmit it. Accidental exposure is highly unlikely unless the individual were to accidentally consume castor beans (CDC, 2008e).	Symptoms depend upon route of exposure and are dose dependent. Inhalation: symptoms occur within 8 hours following exposure. Ingestion: symptoms occur within 6 hours following exposure (CDC, 2008e).	Inhalation: cough, respiratory distress, fever, nausea and sweating. Cyanosis may also be noted. Eventually, low blood pressure and respiratory failure result. Ingestion: a significant amount must be consumed. Vomiting, diarrhea (turning bloody), dehydration, and low blood pressure	There is no antidote for ricin poisoning (CDC, 2008e).	If exposure is through skin and mucous membranes, get ricin off the body quickly (including eye flushes). If ingested, get out of the body quickly (via activated charcoal if ingestion was recent). Medical supportive care is provided including mechanical

		result. Other symptoms may include hallucinations, seizures, hematuria, and eventual hepatic and/or renal failure. Skin and mucous membrane exposure: contact with powdered products containing ricin are unlikely to be absorbed through the skin. Redness and pain of skin and eyes can occur. Death could result within 36 to 72 hours of exposure, depending upon route of transmission and dose (CDC, 2008e).		ventilation, IV therapy, seizure control, and hemodynamic support.

TABLE 16-2 FOOD SAFETY THREATS

Food Safety Threat	Causative Agent	Mode of Transmission	Incubation Period	Signs and Symptoms	Vaccination Availability	Medical Treatment
Salmonellosis	*Salmonella*	Fecal–oral route through the consumption of contaminated food (CDC, 2008c).	Symptoms usually develop within 12 to 72 hours after ingestion (CDC, 2008c).	Most persons will develop diarrhea, fever, and abdominal cramps persisting for approximately 4 to 7 days. In some patients, *Salmonella* may spread from the intestines to the bloodstream and travel to other body areas. This can result in death, especially in immunocompromised individuals (CDC, 2008c).	There is no vaccine against *Salmonella* (CDC, 2008c).	Infection generally resolves within a week, without treatment. Some patients may require supportive therapy if dehydration develops or if infection spreads to other areas. In these cases, ampicillin, gentamicin, trimethoprim/sulfamethoxazole, or ciprofloxacin can all be used. Some resistance to antimicrobial agents has been noted (CDC, 2008c).

Shigellosis	*Shigella* (CDC, 2008d)	Fecal–oral contact through poor hygienic practices and contaminated food (CDC, 2008d)	Initial symptoms begin within 1 to 2 days after exposure (CDC, 2008d).	Signs and symptoms include diarrhea, fever, and stomach cramps. Diarrhea may turn bloody. Severe infection may be accompanied by high fever, and young children are at risk for seizures (CDC, 2008d).	There is no vaccine (CDC, 2008d).	Most persons will recover without need for medical intervention. In the case of dehydration, IV therapy may be indicated. Antimicrobial therapy can shorten the course of illness; however, ampicillin, trimethoprim/sulfamethaxazole, ceftriaxone or ciprofloxacin can be used, if indicated. Some antimicrobial resistance has been reported, and antibiotics should be used only if deemed necessary. Antidiarrheal agents such as loperamide, and diphenoxylate with atropine should be avoided (CDC, 2008d).

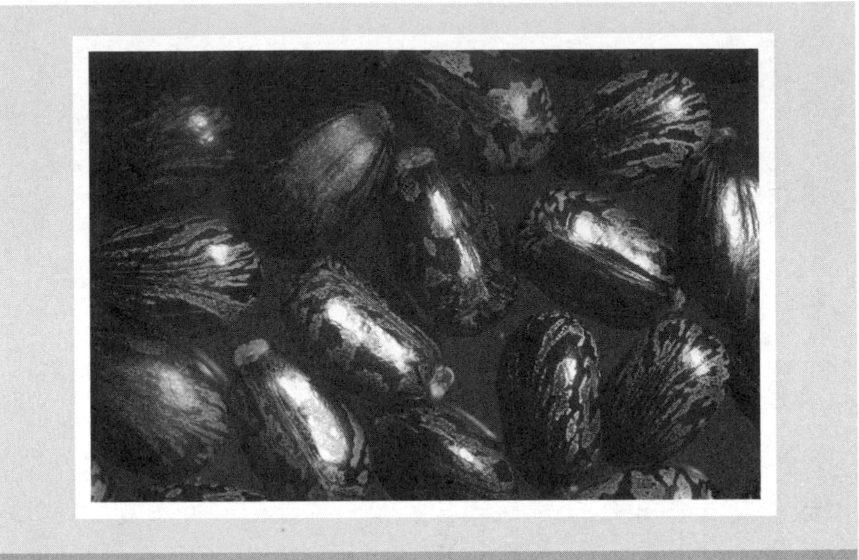

Figure 16-8 Castor beans—the source of ricin.
Source: Courtesy of Brian Prechtel/USDA.

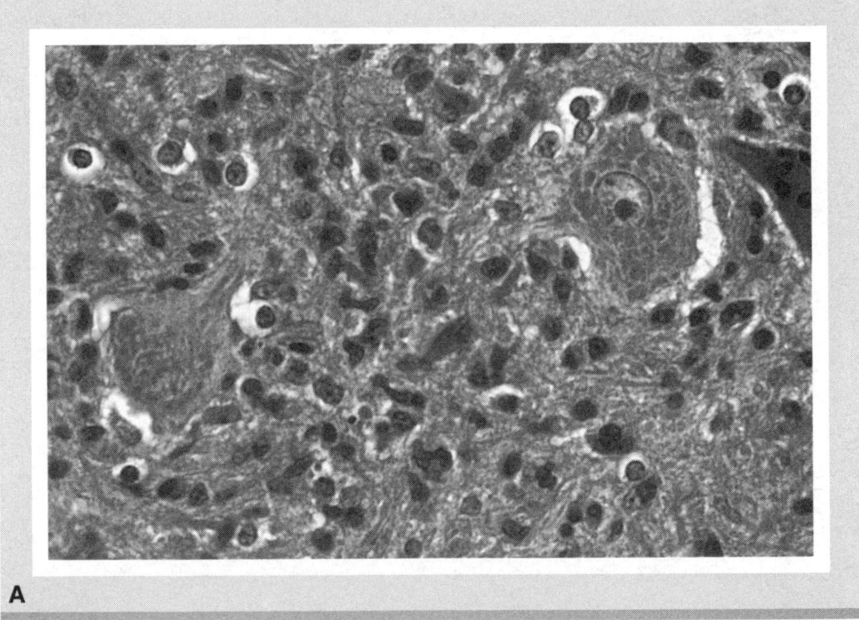

A

Figure 16-9 Rabies virus (a) and a patient with rabies (b).
Source: Courtesy of CDC.

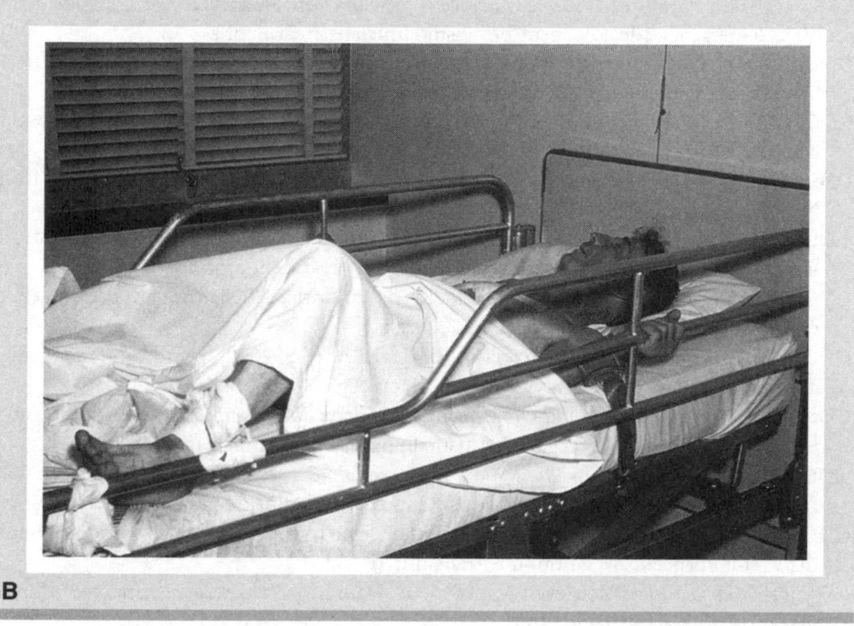

Figure 16-9 (Continued)

References

Centers for Disease Control and Prevention (CDC). (2001). *Facts about pneumonic plague.* Retrieved April 5, 2008, from http://emergency.cdc.gov/agent/plague/factsheet.pdf

CDC. (2003a). *Anthrax: What you need to know.* Retrieved April 5, 2008, from http://emergency.cdc.gov/agent/anthrax/pdf/needtoknow.pdf

CDC. (2003b). *Key facts about tularemia.* Retrieved April 5, 2008, from http://emergency.cdc.gov/agent/tularemia/facts.asp

CDC. (2003c). *Frequently asked questions (FAQ) about tularemia.* Retrieved April 5, 2008, from http://emergency.cdc.gov/agent/tularemia/faq.asp

CDC. (2005a). *Frequently asked questions (FAQ) about plague.* Retrieved April 5, 2008, from http://emergency.cdc.gov/agent/plague/faq.asp

CDC. (2005b). *Plague: Diagnosis.* Retrieved April 5, 2008, from http://www.cdc.gov/ncidod/dvbid/plague/diagnosis.htm

CDC. (2005c). *Plague: Prevention and control.* Retrieved April 5, 2008, from http://www.cdc.gov/ncidod/dvbid/plague/prevent.htm

CDC. (2005d). *Brucellosis.* Retrieved April 6, 2008, from http://www.cdc.gov/ncidod/dbmd/diseaseinfo/brucellosis_t.htm

CDC. (2006a). *Botulism: Background information for clinicians.* Retrieved April 5, 2008, from http://emergency.cdc.gov/agent/Botulism/clinicians/Background.asp

CDC. (2006b). *Botulism: Clinical description.* Retrieved April 5, 2008, from http://emergency.cdc.gov/agent/botulism/clinicians/clindesc.asp

CDC. (2006c). *Botulism: Prevention overview for clinicians.* Retrieved April 5, 2008, from http://emergency.cdc.gov/agent/botulism/clinicians/prevention.asp

CDC. (2006d). *Botulism: Treatment overview for clinicians.* Retrieved April 5, 2008, from http://emergency.cdc.gov/agent/botulism/clinicians/treatment.asp

CDC. (2006e). *Q fever: Epidemiologic overview for clinicians.* Retrieved April 6, 2008, from http://emergency.cdc.gov/agent/qfever/clinicians/epidemiology.asp

CDC. (2006f). *Q fever: Clinical description.* Retrieved April 6, 2008, from http://emergency.cdc.gov/agent/qfever/clinicians/clindesc.asp

CDC. (2006g). *Q fever: Prevention overview for clinicians.* Retrieved April 6, 2008, from http://emergency.cdc.gov/agent/qfever/clinicians/prevention.asp

CDC. (2006h). *Q fever: Treatment overview for clinicians.* Retrieved April 6, 2008, from http://emergency.cdc.gov/agent/qfever/clinicians/treatment.asp

CDC. (2007a). *Plague: Medical management.* Retrieved April 5, 2008, from http://emergency.cdc.gov/agent/plague/trainingmodule/5/06.asp

CDC. (2007b). *Smallpox disease overview.* Retrieved April 5, 2008, from http://emergency.cdc.gov/agent/smallpox/overview/disease-facts.asp

CDC. (2007c). *What you should know about a smallpox outbreak.* Retrieved April 5, 2008, from http://emergency.cdc.gov/agent/smallpox/basics/outbreak.asp

CDC. (2007d). *Frequently asked questions about smallpox vaccine.* Retrieved April 5, 2008, from http://emergency.cdc.gov/agent/smallpox/vaccination/faq.asp

CDC. (2007e). *Brucellosis.* Retrieved April 6, 2008, from http://www.cdc.gov/ncidod/dbmd/diseaseinfo/brucellosis_g.htm#howtransmitted

CDC. (2008a). *Glanders.* Retrieved April 6, 2008, from http://www.cdc.gov/nczved/dfbmd/disease_listing/glanders_gi.html

CDC. (2008b). *Glanders* (Burkholderia mallei). Retrieved April 5, 2008, from http://www.cdc.gov/nczved/dfbmd/disease_listing/glanders_ti.html

CDC. (2008c). *Salmonellosis.* Retrieved April 6, 2008, from http://www.cdc.gov/nczved/dfbmd/disease_listing/salmonellosis_gi.html

CDC. (2008d). *Shigellosis.* Retrieved April 6, 2008, from http://www.cdc.gov/nczved/dfbmd/disease_listing/shigellosis_gi.html

CDC. (2008e). *Facts about ricin.* Retrieved April 6, 2008, from http://emergency.cdc.gov/agent/ricin/facts.asp

CDC. (n.d.). *Bioterrorism agents/diseases by category.* Retrieved April 4, 2008, from http://emergency.cdc.gov/agent/agentlist-category.asp

Dennis, D. T., Inglesby, T. V., Henderson, D. A., Bartlett, J. G., Ascher, M. S., Eitzen, E. E., et al. (2001). Tularemia as a biological weapon: Medical and public health management [Electronic version]. *Journal of the American Medical Association, 285*(21), 2763–2773.

Dobson, M. (2007). *Disease: The extraordinary stories behind history's deadliest killers.* London: Quercus.

Fenn, E. A. (2001). *Pox Americana: The great smallpox epidemic of 1775–82.* New York: Hill and Wang.

Internet Movie Database. (2008a). *The Andromeda Strain.* Retrieved April 5, 2008, from http://www.imdb.com/title/tt0066769

Internet Movie Database. (2008b). *And the Band Played On.* Retrieved April 5, 2008, from http://www.imdb.com/title/tt0106273

Occupational Safety and Health Administration. (2006). *Safety and health topics: Biological agents.* Retrieved April 5, 2008, from http://www.osha.gov/SLTC/biologicalagents/index.html

chapter 17

Issues That Arise in a Disaster

Timothy J. Legg and Deborah S. Adelman

GOAL

The goal of this chapter is to review disaster nursing education, research, and its future, and evaluate international disaster nursing.

OBJECTIVES

At the completion of this chapter, the reader will:

1. Describe the differences between national and international disaster responses.
2. List at least three issues specific to disaster nursing education.
3. Analyze the appropriate level of disaster nursing education in the classroom.
4. Categorize different types of disaster nursing education.
5. Summarize basic competencies in disaster nursing education.
6. Discuss the relevance of evidence-based practice to disaster nursing.

Key Terms

- National disaster nursing
- International disaster nursing
- Level of education
- Nursing professional development
- Joint Commission
- Centers for Medicare and Medicaid Services
- Disaster nursing education in the classroom
- Disaster nursing education in staff development
- Disaster nursing continuing education
- Evidence-based disaster nursing practice

Introduction

Disaster nursing on a national and international scale and the future of nursing research in disaster nursing are topics that have not been adequately explored in the nursing literature as yet. Along with these issues, the issue of education for all registered nurses in a disaster is still being debated in nursing and healthcare circles. This chapter will begin with a discussion of national and international nursing.

National and International Disaster Nursing

When considering responding on a national or international level to a disaster, the disaster nurse has several issues to consider, issues that go beyond the usual local disaster response. Some of these issues were discussed in Chapters 1 and 2, but others still exist.

National Disaster Response

Responding to a national disaster can sometimes be a spur-of-the-moment impulse based on the nature of the disaster. A good example was the outpouring of volunteers who walked into their local Red Cross chapters after September 11, 2001. These people sincerely wanted to assist in any way they could with the national tragedy that occurred that day. Many were saddened and even angry to find out they could not just walk in and be sent to New York without specialized disaster training, even if they were healthcare professionals. Many did not even go to their local Red Cross chapters; they jumped in their cars or volunteer fire trucks and such, driving straight to New York and inundating an already resource-strapped city with over 30,000 more people to feed, shelter, and protect.

Many disaster agencies offer the trained disaster nurse an opportunity to volunteer for national disaster relief work. As mentioned in Chapter 2, such groups as the Illinois Medical Emergency Response Team send volunteer healthcare professionals and supplies to major national disasters when requested by another state as well as responding within Illinois. American Red Cross disaster health nurses who wish to do national work also may be sent to another state when that state's Red Cross lead chapter requests help. The Community Emergency Response Team has been asked to help in national disasters, as well, responding to the 2005 series of hurricanes that struck Florida when almost every other emergency response agency on state and national levels was tapped out.

The key to responding on a national level is simple: Be prepared. Volunteer at a local disaster response agency. Take all the disaster training courses available, even those that are not health care related. Be sure that you have the time needed, as many agencies want a minimum of 2 to 3 weeks committed to such a large-scale response. It is important to check with an employer about these plans, as some do allow release time, some allow paid time off, some disaster agencies may reimburse employers, and some employers may refuse the time away from work.

It is also important to plan for family and pets. Keeping a jump kit, with enough food, water, clothing, and medications for 3 weeks ready is a must. Ensuring that pets are going to be cared for, mail picked up or held, and communications established with family and emergency contacts is also part of planning for that emergency response call. Ask the agency how they plan to help you return to "civilian" life before you go, too. Disaster responders often find that the transition home is a difficult one, and knowing where to turn for help when back in normal life and problems arise is part of the key to successful national disaster volunteer work (see Chapter 8).

When responding as an American Red Cross disaster health nurse, the local chapter will keep copies of nursing licenses and register the volunteers so that there is no issue with working in a state in which one does not have a license (see Chapters 2 and 10). Registering your license with the Emergency System for Advance Registration of Volunteer Health Professionals (ESAR-VHP) is one of many avenues to ensure that a valid nursing license is on record with the federal government so that the disaster nurse can respond on a national level. ESAR-VHP was a direct response by Congress to the inability of New York disaster agencies to identify who was and who was not a licensed healthcare professional in the wake of 9/11. Congress, in 2002, enacted a public law called the Public Health Security and Bioterrorism Preparedness and Response Act (Public Law 107-188). This law allowed states and those concerned with disaster health responses to verify licensing and allow disaster healthcare volunteers to work (American Hospital Association, 2005).

International Disaster Response

Much of what is true for national disaster work is true of international disaster response, though there are extra issues to consider. An up-to-date passport will be needed, as will immunizations for travel to some other countries. Even countries where no immunizations are required may become countries where a disaster changes the nature of travel and response, suddenly requiring immunizations. A jump kit with clothing and medications for a 6-month commitment is necessary to volunteer on an international level in some cases. For example, when the International Committee of the Red Cross sends disaster nurses to a disaster, they call upon Red Cross societies in the area at the national level. These national-level Red Cross societies then find local volunteers who have indicated a willingness to respond on an international level.

At times, other agencies may send disaster volunteers and, if interested, the disaster nurse should contact the agency he or she volunteers for about the process involved in international disaster work. Some considerations before volunteering on an international level are:

1. Do you have the time necessary to volunteer internationally?
2. Do you know the customs and languages of countries you may have to travel to?

3. Do you have the proper immunizations?
4. Do you have a valid passport?
5. Have you considered the possible danger, including death, which may result from volunteering in foreign countries?

These are but a very few of the many considerations one must think about before volunteering for international disaster work.

Disaster Nursing Education

Despite the inclusion of disaster content in the National Council Licensure Examination for Registered Nurses (NCLEX-RN), the topic of disasters receives little attention in entry into practice programs. This is equally true for masters- and doctoral-level nursing education (Weiner, 2006). The result of this curricular omission is a nursing workforce that is disadvantaged in terms of its ability to meet the comprehensive care needs of any given segment of our population that finds itself thrust into a state of vulnerability due to a disaster. It has been further acknowledged that education is integral to disaster preparedness, yet many of the practices that are taught are neither standardized nor evidence-based (Hsu et al., 2006).

When one considers the myriad of disasters that can befall humankind and the volume and complexity of the material that is available on the subject, coupled with the relative lack of healthcare providers trained in disaster response, it becomes more apparent as to why the subject of disasters is not included in nursing programs. Questions that nursing must address include such issues as:

1. Should disaster nursing content be included in the entry into practice program and, if so, what amount of complexity of content should be included?
2. Should disaster nursing content be taught at the master's level and, if so, which types of program should include this information?
3. Should disaster nursing be taught to all registered nurses via a continuing education approach and, if so, what about those states that require no continuing education for registered nurses?
4. Should the knowledge, skills, and abilities needed by registered nurses in disaster situations be the subject of a unique master's or doctoral program?
5. Should education specific to the role of the registered nurse in the disaster situation be the responsibility of the healthcare organizations that employ registered nurses?
6. What curricular content should be included in disaster education?

Let us attempt to answer these questions.

Should Disaster Education Be Included in Nursing Programs?

We need to begin this discussion with the understanding that there are no national mandates for nursing education that require registered nurses to be educated to respond to mass casualty incidents (MCIs) (Stanley, 2005). Does this lack of a specific mandate requiring registered nurses to be educated in MCIs indicate that registered nurses should not be instructed in this area? Tyler (1949) posed several questions to the educational establishment. His first and most compelling question centered on the purposes of the educational establishment within a given society. Tyler noted, "many sociologists and others concerned with the pressing problems of contemporary society see in an analysis of contemporary society the basic information from which objectives may be derived" (p. 5). Whereas Tyler realized that contemporary social problems were not the only source of objectives for a school, he did recognize their importance. Since curricular content is not prescribed by those agencies that accredit nursing programs, it is up to the individual nursing programs and the faculty who decide upon the curricular content to evaluate whether or not their curriculum is responsive to societal needs in terms of the inclusion of disaster nursing content.

Some authors have advocated the mandate of inclusion of MCI content by state boards of nursing as a requirement for registered nurse licensure candidates or as a continuing education program that must be taken by currently licensed registered nurses who seek licensure renewal (Stanley, 2005). Some opponents to this approach argue that this type of mandate undermines the autonomy of faculty in terms of establishing the curriculum in schools of nursing. A similar argument had been used in the past regarding the mandate of state boards of nursing to include gerontological nursing content in schools of nursing (in order to respond to an aging population), to which Fulmer and Nyack (1995) responded by reminding us that the same could be said of pediatrics, obstetrics, and psychiatric nursing, but "to date these areas are not perceived as problematic" (p. 31).

Whereas there is definitely a level of temptation to want to see essential areas of care that would meet the needs of society included in nursing programs through legislation, we feel that this temptation should be avoided. Faculty in nursing programs need to shed the mantra of "We have always done it this way" and should be challenged to take a good look at the social forces surrounding them. As Tyler (1949, p. 1) asked, following his question about the educational purposes of a school, "what educational experiences can be provided that are likely to attain these purposes?" Faculty needs to ask themselves if they are preparing their students for the unique challenges that their students may face once they are released into the professional nursing workforce and begin practicing in a world where terrorism and natural disasters are spreading across the globe.

Disaster Education: Ah, Yes, but at Which Level?

We readily acknowledge that inclusion of disaster education into existing nursing curricula is not easily achieved. We further acknowledge that existing nursing curricula includes some content specific to safety of patients (e.g., fire safety and patient handling techniques during evacuations). Whereas this content constitutes a start, it is also insufficient in terms of what the registered nurse needs to be adequately prepared to respond to a disaster situation and only exists as a result of OSHA regulations.

There are a plethora of questions that educators must consider before attempting to infuse disaster education into any existing nursing curricula. For instance, at which level of nursing education should disaster education be provided? The reflex answer to this question would be at the entry-into-practice level; however, in an already packed curriculum, how much time could be devoted to disaster education for registered nurses? If disaster education were provided to registered nurses during their entry-into-practice program, would sufficient time be able to be devoted to this topic or would the subject receive superficial treatment rendering what was taught insufficient resulting in a waste of time? Baccalaureate degree programs have the luxury of 4 years to include content specific to disasters, but what of the new 2+2 BSN programs, second bachelor degree programs, and associate degree and hospital-based diploma programs? Would the inclusion of content specific to disasters be another topic that would differentiate baccalaureate-level education from associate degree or diploma-level education?

It is interesting to note that, in one small study, students enrolled in a baccalaureate of nursing program demonstrated interest in learning about disasters. In this study, completed by Bond and Beaton (2005), 96% of juniors in a 4-year baccalaureate nursing program were interested in receiving didactic content specific to disaster nursing and, of that number, 83% were "somewhat" or "extremely interested" in clinical applications of disaster nursing content (p. 448). Clearly, these students saw the need for disaster nursing content. It would be interesting to see how other BSN students felt in other parts of the United States and the world.

Disaster Education in Graduate Programs

The next possibility is the inclusion of disaster content at the graduate level. This is another tempting solution. In the case of graduate study, the professional registered nurse makes a conscious choice to seek advanced preparation in a given area of study. It has been noted that several colleges and universities are establishing new programs in topics surrounding emergency and disaster preparedness for a wide range of healthcare professionals in order to meet the needs of those registered nurses and other healthcare professionals who seek advanced study in these areas. However, there are several issues associated with this approach. The first issue that must be addressed is whether or not there is a need for this content to be taught at the graduate level. Is the content specific to disaster nursing of sufficient complexity that it should be taught at the master's or doctoral level?

Another issue to consider is the recognition of an advanced degree in this area. Specifically, what can the graduate "do" with the degree? Whereas there are certainly agencies that would and do hire registered nurses with graduate degrees in emergency and disaster management, how many agencies need registered nurses with this type of graduate preparation? Currently, most graduate programs for registered nurses prepare their graduates for careers as advanced practice registered nurses, including nurse practitioners, clinical nurse specialists, nurse midwives, and nurse anesthetists. Each of these nursing professionals must obtain a graduate degree in order to move into specialty practice. In most of the 50 states, the terms *nurse practitioner, clinical nurse specialist, nurse midwife,* and *nurse anesthetist* have some form of title protection. That is, individual registered nurses cannot arbitrarily identify themselves as a "nurse practitioner" unless they have a license or certification to practice as a nurse practitioner. The same is not true of emergency and disaster nursing, at least at this point in time. There are no entry-level or advanced certifications, no specific scope of practice guidelines, and no title protections for the use of the term. There are not even any established disaster nursing standards to use as benchmarks for developing certification exams, though several nursing organizations are in the process of developing such standards.

Would employers be willing to pay registered nurses with graduate education in emergency and disaster nursing what they were worth? How would that worth be determined? Would the possession of a graduate degree result in those registered nurses who held the degree being considered too "pricey"? That is, would employers seek registered nurses with knowledge, skills, and abilities specific to emergency and disaster situations but with less educational preparation? Would employers consider hiring those registered nurses with "compelling" experience and/or continuing education, in the hopes of paying a lesser salary? Although we certainly believe that advanced education is something that should be undertaken for the sake of advancing nursing as a scientific discipline, professional growth, and personal self-actualization, we would be naïve if we did not acknowledge that many registered nurses do enter into graduate programs with the hope of making more money upon completion. We also know that, upon graduation, advanced practice registered nurses do make more money than nonadvanced practice registered nurses. Can we make this same claim for registered nurses who would have graduate preparation in disaster nursing?

A logical approach to overcome these issues would be the creation of a specialty tract within existing nursing graduate programs. For example, an adult or community health nurse practitioner or clinical nurse specialist program could include a specialty tract that offers coursework and specialization in disaster nursing. This could be considered a value-added approach to a conventional advanced nursing degree. It would prepare the registered nurse to assume an advanced practice nursing role, while at the same time, assuring that registered nurses received education in the response to emergency and disaster situations.

Disaster Education Through Continuing Education Programs

Not every registered nurse will engage in or see value in formal education beyond his or her entry-into-practice program. This is where continuing professional education programming can help bring registered nurses the knowledge they need specific to emergency and disaster situations. Continuing education should not be considered a panacea, however, as not every state requires continuing education for registered nurses for licensure renewal. Depending upon the state, a registered nurse may receive his or her initial professional nursing license and never be required to pick up a book or journal ever again. As long as the appropriate licensure renewal fees are paid, registered nurses in these states can continue to practice nursing without any type of continuing education. For those states that do mandate continuing education for professional nursing licensure renewal and those registered nurses who are not required to obtain continuing education credits but wish to do so, coursework in emergency preparedness and disaster nursing could be offered.

A logical question that arises when discussing continuing education programs in disaster nursing is "Would registered nurses be interested in this topic?" One study found that 88% of registered nurses surveyed were "somewhat or extremely interested" in didactic continuing educational offerings that had disaster nursing content (Bond & Beaton, 2005, p. 448). To meet the needs of those registered nurses, coursework in the various aspects of emergency preparedness and disaster response could be developed and delivered using a multiplicity of approaches, including home/self-study (correspondence), synchronous and asynchronous distance education, and interactive CD-ROM.

Disaster Education Through Nursing Professional Development

Nursing professional development is the newest term endorsed by the American Nurses Credentialing Center (ANCC) to refer to those who engage in the practice of "staff development." The term *professional development* was selected to replace *staff development,* and the ANCC defines the role of the nurse in professional development as follows:

> The nurse in professional development practice provides nonacademic learning activities intended to build on the educational and experiential bases of professional nurses and other personnel who assist in providing nursing care. These learning activities are designed to enhance nursing practice, education, administration, research, or theory development with the goal of improving the health of the public. The purpose of these learning activities includes supporting learner attitudes on the value of lifelong learning; contributing to the development, maintenance, and enhancement of competent nursing practice; promoting professional development; and advancing career goals. Nursing professional development practice is based on the principles of adult education. (ANCC, 2008, ¶ 1)

Nurses who engage in the practice of nursing professional development are usually employed in hospitals, nursing homes, and other healthcare organizations as staff development directors or nurse educators. These individuals have an incredible responsibility in terms of providing continuing educational programs aimed at enhancing the professional competence and skills of nurses and those that provide nursing-related services within their respective organizations. The nursing professional development registered nurse also plays an even more important role in those states where there are no continuing education requirements as the nursing professional development registered nurse often provides the only educational experiences that nurses employed in those states may receive.

The nursing professional development registered nurse develops continuing education programs from a variety of sources. Some programs are based on the need for the assurance of nursing competency (i.e., skills that are considered high risk such as blood transfusions). Some programs are remedial in nature (e.g., a nurse makes a medication error and is referred to the staff development department for remedial education). Other programs conducted by the nursing professional development registered nurse include those programs that are designed to meet the requirements of licensing or regulatory agencies such as the state health department or the Joint Commission.

Nestled within the requirements of licensing and regulatory agencies are some requirements for emergency preparedness and/or disaster training. The Joint Commission requires that all organizations that it accredits have some type of emergency management plan, also referred to as a disaster plan (see Chapters 3 and 4). The goal of this plan is to assure that the organization is capable of providing continued care in the event of an emergency situation regardless of source of emergency or disaster, whether it is an internal or external disaster. The Joint Commission (2008, ¶ 1) specifies in its requirements that

> the emergency management program shall be based on the priorities identified in the Hazardous Vulnerability Analysis (HVA). The Joint Commission discourages the development of separate plans for each contingency because these would be impractical to use and difficult to keep updated. Based on an evaluation of incident probability/frequency specific to the organization, disasters that might be considered in an organization's emergency management plan include, but are not limited to (based on definitions of Red Cross and the Disaster Relief Act of 1974) natural disasters, including the following types:
>
> - Meteorological disasters: cyclones, typhoons, hurricanes, tornadoes, hailstorms, snowstorms, and droughts
> - Topological disasters: landslides, avalanches, mudflows, and floods
> - Disasters that originate underground: earthquakes, volcanic eruptions, and tsunamis (seismic sea waves)
> - Biological disasters: communicable disease epidemics and insect swarms (locusts)
>
> Man-made disasters, including the following types:
>
> - Warfare: conventional warfare (bombardment, blockade and siege) and nonconventional warfare (nuclear, chemical, and biological)
> - Civil disasters: riots, demonstrations, and strikes

- Criminal/terrorist action: bomb threat/incident; nuclear, chemical, or biological attack; hostage incident
- Accidents: transportation (planes, trucks, automobiles, trains, or ships), structural collapse (buildings, dams, bridges, mines, or other structures), explosions, fires, chemical (toxic waste and pollution) and biological (sanitation)
- Equipment in long-term care smoking rooms

The requirements of the Joint Commission are quite comprehensive. Once this plan has been developed by the accredited healthcare organization, the nursing professional development registered nurse must help disseminate the content relevant to the appropriate staff. Training should occur upon time of hire and should logically be provided on at least an annual basis.

Not all healthcare organizations are accredited by the Joint Commission. Skilled nursing facilities are but one example. Skilled nursing facilities operate under licenses from their respective state health departments and must adhere to regulations outlined by the Centers for Medicare and Medicaid Services (CMS) in order to receive reimbursement to care for their client populations (primarily older adults receiving Medicare or Medicaid funding). CMS has its own requirements for disaster planning and emergency preparedness that are a bit more nebulous than the outline provided by the Joint Commission. According to CMS (2007), "the facility must have detailed written plans and procedures to meet all potential emergencies and disasters, such as fire, severe weather, and missing residents" (p. 532) and "the facilities must train all employees in emergency procedures when they begin to work in the facility, periodically review the procedures with existing staff, and carry out unannounced staff drills using those procedures" (p. 533). Clearly these requirements do not spell out what the program of each skilled nursing facility should include as CMS recognizes that every facility should tailor its program to meet the unique needs of the geographic area in which the facility is situated. The nursing professional development registered nurse must become knowledgeable about the individual disaster management and emergency preparedness plans of their organization and convey this information to new staff at the time of hire as well as periodically, usually annually, thereafter.

It goes without saying that nursing professional development registered nurses must, themselves, have some degree of expertise in terms of disaster nursing in order to meet the learning needs of those whom the nursing professional development registered nurse is charged with teaching. What training should the nursing professional development registered nurse have specific to disaster nursing in order to convey knowledge and assess competency of other nurses in this area? Clearly there must be a defined body of knowledge, and the nursing professional development registered nurse must either possess these core competencies or be able to procure the educational services of those individuals who do possess the core competencies. Which takes us to our last and perhaps most compelling question: What competencies are needed to respond to disasters?

Competencies in Disaster Nursing Education

Up to this point we have discussed several concepts related to disaster nursing. We have talked about emergency and disaster preparedness as well as mass casualty incidents, and we have done so as if there were a finite body of knowledge with identified core competencies and a curricular model which upon completion resulted in the ability of individuals to take up and use the title *disaster nurse.* This is not the case, however. Waeckerle (2004, as cited in Slepski, 2005) "stated that there is no single source of authority or approved body of emergency preparedness content or curriculum, and as a result, there has been unfocused training and educational efforts" (p. 421). Multiple groups have either attempted or are currently attempting to develop competencies that will enable nurses to respond to disasters. Some individuals (Bond & Beaton, 2005) sought to identify competencies that were geographically specific. As of the time of this writing, the newest efforts are being made by the American Nurses Association (ANA) in partnership with the Medical College of Georgia (Disaster Preparedness and Response Competencies for Health Professionals Identified, 2008).

Whereas the efforts of individuals and groups are certainly acknowledged and important, one of the best known and most cited groups of educational competencies for registered nurses responding to disasters has been developed by the International Coalition for Mass Casualty Education (INCMCE). With support from the American Association of Colleges of Nursing (AACN) and a committee consisting of approximately 16 nursing organizations and nursing school faculty members, the INCMCE (2003) developed "Educational Competencies for Registered Nurses Responding to Mass Casualty Incidents."

The INCMCE (2003) notes that whereas not all nurses can or should be prepared as first responders, every nurse should be capable of recognizing when a mass casualty incident (MCI) has occurred, how to protect oneself, how to care for persons who have been injured or otherwise involved in the incident, and how to appreciate their own professional limitations. The competencies proposed by the INCMCE are capable of being applied to nurses in a wide range of practice settings and should be interpreted in the context of the role that the nurse occupies in a given practice setting. The competencies include core competencies and core knowledge. Core competencies include critical thinking, assessment (general and specific to the disaster incident), technical skills (i.e., nursing interventions), and communication. Core knowledge is of such areas as health promotion, the healthcare system (including policy), illness and disease management, information and healthcare technology, ethics, and human diversity. Also included in their educational competencies is the concept of professional role development (INCMCE).

Regardless of educational setting, nurse educators should consult these competencies and be aware of development of additional competencies by related organizations specific to disaster nursing. They should work towards further developing these competencies and doing research into disaster nursing theory, as well.

Disaster Nursing Research

Topics for disaster research have been well defined elsewhere. In an exceptional contribution on this subject, Walker, Garmon Bibb, and Elberson (2005) provided nursing researchers with an excellent perspective on the types of research that has been done and has yet to be done specific to disasters, mass casualty events, war, and terrorism. It is not our intent to examine problems that can be explored through research. Instead it is the individual disaster nurse, through his or her own practice, who will generate their own priorities for research in this area. Instead, we would like to focus on the broad area of research and how it relates to disasters in general and nursing knowledge in this area in particular. It is also not our intent to treat the reader to a review of the mechanics of research. Issues surrounding identifying and refining research questions, defining variables, and use of parametric and nonparametric tests to answer various levels of research questions are also beyond the scope of this text.

Instead, we want to discuss disaster nursing research from the vantage point of evidence-based practice (EBP), one of nursing's newest and favorite buzzwords. Evidence-based practice should result from research. It differs from research utilization in that research utilization involves implementation of interventions based on the findings of a single research study. Evidence-based practice has been defined as

> a problem solving approach to practice that involves the conscientious use of current best evidence in making decisions about patient care; EBP incorporates a systematic search for and critical appraisal of the most relevant evidence to answer a clinical question along with one's own clinical expertise and patient values and preferences. (Melnyk & Fineout-Overholt, 2005, p. 587)

In an evidence-based approach to nursing practice, nurses are expected to examine existing evidence (research), rate it based on strength of the evidence, and then disseminate the best practices.

We have noted through our own experience (as well as the results of published studies) that evidence-based practice may not be much more than a "flavor of the week" in terms of nursing buzzwords. The basis of this statement has to do with the willingness of nurses (as well as other healthcare providers and healthcare organizations) to alter practices based on the current evidence. Brandt (2005) noted in an article entitled "The Evidence Is Changing, But Will The Practice," that although findings on episiotomies and fasting are in opposition to current practice, practice relative to these two areas has yet to change. Far too often, nursing is wed to many of its practices based on "tradition" versus evidence. Perhaps evidence-based practice is still too new as a concept. Perhaps nursing will evolve to accept evidence-based practices as it is integrated into nursing programs and new graduates come to the practice with an appreciation of the tentative nature of science. Only the future will tell.

The Future of Disaster Nursing

It is sad to say, but the future of disaster nursing is strong as this area develops into a specialty within nursing. Between natural and man-made disasters, including terrorism, the need for nurses who are willing to volunteer their time or work in this area will continue to grow. What is also sad is that any nurse in any location may find him- or herself called upon to respond to a disaster or find him- or herself actually in a disaster. There is no luxury in thinking "It can't happen here or to me" any longer. All nurses must be prepared when, not if, the need arises.

Conclusion

Regardless of the source of a disaster, the fact remains that disasters emerging from a multiplicity of sources will most likely plague humankind forever. Nurses must be prepared to respond both nationally and internationally to the needs of a global society. Generation of new knowledge from research is only part of the way in which we will prepare nurses to respond to disaster situations. Dissemination of this newly generated knowledge via educational opportunities is essential. Multiple stakeholders need to take an active role in assuring that the nursing workforce of today and tomorrow is adequately prepared to respond to disasters—wherever and whenever they may occur.

References

American Hospital Association. (2005). *Emergency system for advanced registration of volunteer health care personnel—Hospital implementation issues and solutions focus group meeting report.* Retrieved December 31, 2007, from www.hrsa.gov/esarvhp/FocusGroupReport0705/default.htm

American Nurses Credentialing Center. (2008). *Nursing professional development certification: Description of practice.* Retrieved March 29, 2008, from http://www.nursecredentialing.org/cert/eligibility/ProfDev.html

Bond, E. F., & Beaton, R. (2005). Disaster nursing curriculum development based on vulnerability assessment of the Pacific Northwest. *Nursing Clinics of North America, 40,* 441–451.

Brandt, D. (2005). The evidence is changing, but will the practice [Electronic version]. *American Journal of Nursing, 105*(8), 20.

Centers for Medicare & Medicaid Services (CMS). (2007, August 17). *State operations manual, Appendix PP—Guidance to surveyors for long-term care facilities.* Retrieved March 29, 2008, from http://cms.hhs.gov/manuals/Downloads/som107ap_pp_guidelines_ltcf.pdf

Disaster preparedness and response competencies for health professionals identified. (2008). *Journal for Nurse Practitioners, 4*(3), 162.

Fulmer, T., & Nyack, M. T. (1995). Incorporating geriatrics into the licensure and accreditation process. In T. Fulmer & M. Matzo (Eds.), *Strengthening geriatric nursing education.* New York: Springer.

Hsu, E. B., Thomas, T. L., Bass, E. B., Whyne, D., Kelen, G. D., & Green, G. B. (2006). Healthcare worker competencies for disaster training [Electronic version]. *BMC Medical Education, 6*(19). Retrieved March 22, 2008, from http://www.pubmedcentral.nih.gov/articlerender.fcgi?artid=1471784

International Nursing Coalition for Mass Casualty Education. (2003, August). *Educational competencies for registered nurses responding to mass casualty incidents.* Retrieved March 29, 2008, from http://www.cumc.columbia.edu/dept/nursing/chphsr/pdf/masscasua.pdf

Joint Commission. (2008). *What kinds of situations should be included in an organization's emergency management plans?* Retrieved March 29, 2008, from http://www.jointcommission.org/AccreditationPrograms/Hospitals/Standards/FAQs/Management+of+Env+of+Care/Planning+and+Implementation+Activities/Emergency_Management.htm

Melnyk, B. M., & Fineout-Overholt, E. (2005). *Evidence-based practice in nursing & healthcare.* Philadelphia: Lippincott, Williams & Wilkins.

Slepski, L. A. (2005). Emergency preparedness: Concept development for nursing practice. *Nursing Clinics of North America, 40,* 419–430.

Stanley, J. M. (2005). Disaster competency development and integration in nursing education. *Nursing Clinics of North America, 40,* 453–467.

Tyler, R. W. (1949). *Basic principles of curriculum and instruction.* Chicago: University of Chicago Press.

Walker, P. H., Garmon Bibb, S. C., & Elberson, K. L. (2005). Research issues in preparedness for mass casualty events, disaster, war, and terrorism. *Nursing Clinics of North America, 40,* 551–564.

Weiner, E. (2006). Preparing nurses internationally for emergency planning and response. *Online Journal of Issues in Nursing, 11*(3). Retrieved March 22, 2008, from http://nursingworld.org/MainMenuCategories/ANAMarketplace/ANAPeriodicals/OJIN/TableofContents/Volume112006/Number3/PreparingNurses.aspx

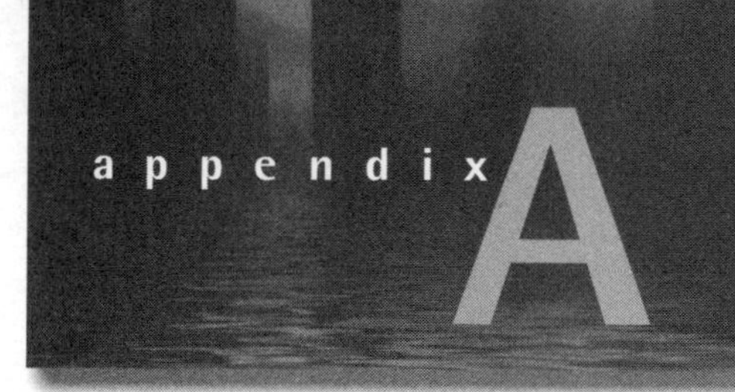

Disaster Terminology Internet Resources

Susan Sonnier

Name of Site	URL
Disaster terminology	http://pdm.medicine.wisc.edu/vocab.htm
Core terminology of disaster reduction	http://www.ehs.unu.edu/moodle/mod/glossary/view.php?id=1&mode=&hook=ALL&sortkey=&sortorder=&fullsearch=0&page=7
International strategy for disaster reduction: Terminology: Basic terms of disaster risk reduction	http://www.unisdr.org/eng/library/lib-terminology-eng%20home.htm
Glossary of public health emergency preparedness terms and acronyms	http://www.doh.wa.gov/phepr/pheprglossary.htm
FEMA: ICS resource center—Glossary of related terms	http://training.fema.gov/EMIWeb/IS/ICSResource/ICSResCntr_Glossary.htm
National Disaster Management Authority: Terminology of disaster risk reduction	http://www.ndma.gov.pk/Publications/Terminology_Disaster%20Risk%20Reduction.doc

appendix B

Measures for Dealing with Hazardous Materials

Susan Sonnier

Type of Agent	Physiological Effects Signs and Symptoms of Exposure	Medical Response
Nerve Agents: • Most potent and deadly • Several routes of exposure possible Agent Names: • Cyclohexyl sarine (GF) • GE • Sarine (GB) • Soman (GD) • Tabun (GA) • VE • VG • V-gas • VM • VX	Break down neurotransmitter acetylcholine in peripheral and central nervous system Symptoms develop quickly: • Salivation • Urination • Sweating • Bradycardia • Hypotension • Convulsions • Respiratory depression • Runny nose • Chest tightness • Death due to respiratory failure	Respiratory failure will require intubation, mechanical ventilation, and suctioning. Prevention of seizures with anticonvulsants Medications to reverse neuromuscular effects and to reestablish neurotransmitter functions
Blistering/Vesicating Agents: • Often used in military conflicts • Mustard and sulfur mustard compounds frequently used	Absorbs through the skin, eyes, and respiratory and gastrointestinal tract Interacts with RNA, DNA, and proteins to interrupt cell functions	Careful cleaning of skin lesions and topical antibiotics Symptomatic treatment of systemic effects

(continued)

Type of Agent	Physiological Effects Signs and Symptoms of Exposure	Medical Response
Agent Names: • Distilled mustard (HD) • Lewisite (L, L-1, L-2, L-3) • Mustard gas (H) • Nitrogen mustard (HN-1,2,3) • Phosgene oxide (CX) • Ethyldichloroarsine (ED) • Methyldichloroarsine (MD) • Mustard/Lewisite (HL) • Phendichloroarsine (PD) • Sequi mustard	Symptoms may not appear immediately and up to 12–24 hours after exposure. Symptoms may be blistered, open skin on exposed areas. Systemic absorption may cause GI, respiratory, cardiac, or hematologic effects.	
Blood Agents: • Usually cyanide based • Rapidly toxic • Can be ingested or inhaled Agent Names: • Arsine • Cyanogen chloride (CK) • Hydrogen chloride • Hydrogen cyanide (AC)	Absorbed into the blood through ingestion, inhalation, or cutaneous absorption of the specific compound Blood levels are normally detectable after exposure. Signs and symptoms of exposure or consumption: • Rapid breathing • Restlessness • Dizziness • Weakness • Headache • Nausea and vomiting • Rapid heart rate • Convulsions • Low blood pressure • Slow heart rate • Loss of consciousness • Lung injury • Respiratory failure leading to death	Treatment should begin before blood levels known since these agents are rapidly toxic. • Removal from area of exposure and possible inhalation • Clothing removal and disposal • Showering with copious water and soap to cleanse skin surfaces • Eye irrigations, remove contact lenses • Use of a cyanide antidote kit: 1. Amyl nitrate–nasally inhaled 2. IV administration of sodium nitrate and sodium thiosulfate
Respiratory Agents: • Primary agents: Chlorine and phosgene	Absorption primarily through respiratory tract. Eye irritation and exposure possible with these gasses.	Optimize respiratory functions: Oxygenation and ventilation by: • High-flow oxygen • Pulse oximetry monitoring

(continued)

Type of Agent	Physiological Effects Signs and Symptoms of Exposure	Medical Response
• Chlorine: Rapid onset of action. • Phosgene: Symptoms may not appear for up to 24 hours. Agent Names: • Chlorine (CL) • Diphosgene (DP) • Cyanide • Nitrogen oxide (NO) • Perfluoroisobutylene (PHIB) • Phosgene (CG) • Red phosphorous (RP) • Sulfur trioxide—clorosulfonic acid (FS) • Teflon and perfluror-isobutylene (PHIB) • Titanium tetrachloride (FM) • Zinc oxide (HC)	Signs and symptoms of inhalation: • Cough • Choking • Gasping • Stridor • Wheezing • Shortness of breath • Pulmonary edema • Respiratory failure	• Intubation and mechanical ventilation • Beta-2 agonists to prevent bronchospasm
Radiation Exposure: Presenting symptoms and organ systems affected are largely dependent on what type of radiation exposure has occurred and what the length of exposure to the agent is. Alpha radiation: Heavy atoms: Uranium, radon, radium, and plutonium Beta radiation: Less dense and nondamaging particles. Only penetrates the skin. Gamma radiation: Photon radiation similar to X-rays. Penetrates the entire body.	Exposure to radiation is commonplace with sunlight and naturally occurring radiation in the environment. Acute radiation syndrome: Heavy doses of radiation in a short period of time can be dangerous or fatal. Signs and symptoms: Vary to amount of exposure and time of exposure. Symptoms may go through a prodromal syndrome to changing symptoms over several weeks that may include: • Nausea, vomiting, diarrhea, anorexia • Erythema, blistering, ulcerated tissue, possible necrotic tissue	Treatment is largely dependent on the time and amount of radiation exposure. Many of the following interventions could be considered in a radiation exposure patient. • Secure ABCs (airway, breathing, circulation) • Physiologic monitoring (blood pressure, blood gases, electrolyte and urine output) as appropriate • Treat major trauma, burns, and respiratory injury if present. • Blood samples for CBC (complete blood count), with attention to

(continued)

Type of Agent	Physiological Effects Signs and Symptoms of Exposure	Medical Response
	• Bone marrow suppression of RBCs and WBCs • Chromosomal abnormalities • Disorientation, seizures, coma, death	lymphocyte count, and HLA (human leukocyte antigen) • Treat contamination as needed. • If exposure occurred within 8 to 12 hours, repeat CBC, with attention to lymphocyte count, 2 or 3 more times (approximately every 2 to 3 hours) to assess lymphocyte depletion. • Reverse isolation techniques for immunosuppression to prevent infections.

Source: Adapted from Centers for Disease Control and Prevention. (n.d.). *Chemical emergencies: Chemical agents A-Z.* Retrieved February 8, 2008, from http://www.bt.cdc.gov/agent/agentlistchem.asp; Karam, A. (2003). Chapter 20: Radiological incidents and emergencies. In T. G. Veenema (Ed.), *Disaster nursing and emergency preparedness for chemical, biological, and radiological terrorism and other hazards.* New York: Springer Publishing; Veenema, T. G., & Wax, P. (2003). Chapter 19: Chemical agents of concern. In T. G. Veenema (Ed.), *Disaster nursing and emergency preparedness for chemical, biological, and radiological terrorism and other hazards.* New York: Springer Publishing.

Index

C